D0908130

Lamaze

Oxford Studies in International History

James J. Sheehan, series advisor

Lamaze

An International History

Paula A. Michaels

OXFORD
UNIVERSITY PRESS

OXFORD
UNIVERSITY PRESS

Oxford University Press is a department of the University of
Oxford. It furthers the University's objective of excellence in research,
scholarship, and education by publishing worldwide.

Oxford   New York
Auckland   Cape Town   Dar es Salaam   Hong Kong   Karachi
Kuala Lumpur   Madrid   Melbourne   Mexico City   Nairobi
New Delhi   Shanghai   Taipei   Toronto

With offices in
Argentina   Austria   Brazil   Chile   Czech Republic   France   Greece
Guatemala   Hungary   Italy   Japan   Poland   Portugal   Singapore
South Korea   Switzerland   Thailand   Turkey   Ukraine   Vietnam

Oxford is a registered trademark of Oxford University Press
in the UK and certain other countries.

Published in the United States of America by
Oxford University Press
198 Madison Avenue, New York, NY 10016

© Oxford University Press 2014

Portions of this book have appeared previously. Parts of chapters three and four were published in
"Comrades in the Labor Room: The Lamaze Method of Childbirth Preparation and France's Cold
War Home Front, 1951–1957," *American Historical Review* 115 (October 2010): 1031–1060 and in
"A Chapter from Lamaze History: Birth Narratives and Authoritative Knowledge in France,
1951–1957," *Journal of Perinatal Education* 19 (Summer 2010): 35–43. Passages in chapters five, six
and seven appeared in "Pain and Blame: Psychological Approaches to Obstetric Pain, 1950–1980,"
in *Knowledge and Pain*, eds. Esther Cohen, Leona Toker, Manuela Consonni, and Otniel Dror,
231–55. At the Interface/Probing the Boundaries 84. Amsterdam: Rodopi, 2012.

"Lamaze" is a trademark of Lamaze International and is registered in the U.S. and other
countries. Lamaze International has not participated in the development of this publication. Its
contents are solely the responsibility of the author and do not necessarily represent the official
views of Lamaze International.

Library of Congress Cataloging-in-Publication Data
Michaels, Paula A., 1966–
Lamaze : an international history / Paula A. Michaels.
pages cm.—(Oxford studies in international history) Includes bibliographical
references and index. ISBN 978–0–19–973864–9 (hardback)   1. Natural childbirth.
2. Natural childbirth—Cross-cultural studies.   3. Lamaze, Fernand, 1890–1957.   I. Title.
RG661.M48 2014
618.4'5—dc23
2013042938

1 3 5 7 9 8 6 4 2
Printed in the United States of America
on acid-free paper

To Dan and Misha,
who fill my life with love and so very much laughter

CONTENTS

ACKNOWLEDGMENTS

Convention dictates that the author thank first the organizations that bankrolled a project, and then acknowledge the contributions of colleagues, friends, and family, but for a book about childbirth it seems appropriate to begin at conception. My son, Misha Coleman, was still in utero when this book was just a flicker of an idea and, were it not for him, I would have never embarked on this journey. He was five years old when I began to work on it in earnest. When he was around seven or eight years old, he delighted in quizzing adults about whether they knew what the word "psychoprophylaxis" meant. By the time this book appears in print he will have turned thirteen. He cannot remember a time when the Lamaze method was not part of our lives, a daily topic of conversation in our home. I am grateful to him as the original spark for this book and as the most delightful sidekick along the path to its fruition.

My other constant companion has been Dan Coleman, who has gone above and beyond the call of duty in support of this work. Dan has been a sounding board for ideas and my first reader for every chapter. He shouldered the lion's share of our domestic duties, freeing me to devote countless hours to research and writing. He joined me on research trips to Boston, Washington, London, and Paris, which allowed me get done what I needed to at archives and libraries during the day, but still come home to him and Misha at night. Dan has been a partner to me in the fullest sense. It was my lucky day when I met him and he's brought me nothing but good luck ever since.

I have had the good fortune to draw on the wisdom and knowledge of two wonderful scholars: Marilène Vuille and Jacqueline Wolf. I appreciate the foundations that they laid and on which I have attempted to build. Our conversations pushed me to think more deeply about the history and social meanings of childbirth, and their enthusiasm for this project encouraged my efforts. They gave generously of their time, reading the draft manuscript and offering careful, detailed feedback. Crossing paths and becoming friends with them is a happy byproduct of this study.

Several other friends and colleagues deserve to be singled out for their special contributions. Roberta Manning first suggested to me that I extend my study beyond the Soviet Union, following Lamaze back to France and then on to the US. Mary Schaeffer Conroy has been an enthusiastic supporter in ways too numerous and varied to recount. I profited from the comments and camaraderie of a writing group comprised of the smart and wonderful Emily Burrill, Gigi Dillon, Anne Drapkin Lyerly, and Sarah Shields.

A dizzying number of people played a part in this work's realization. I benefited from research assistance of various sorts, including people schlepping hundreds of pages of photocopies halfway around the globe for me. I relied on the expertise of colleagues in fields well outside my comfort zone for advice and suggestions. Many people read early drafts of portions of the text. Equally important to this work's completion was the tremendous hospitality that I enjoyed when I was far from home. For their diverse contributions, it is a pleasure to express my appreciation to: Jennifer Amos; Beth Bailey; Rob Craig; Allison Connolly; Marko Dumančić; Deborah Furey; Jocelyne George; Colin Gordon; Betsy Hemenway; Beth Holmgren; Gene Hughes; Guzel Idelbaeva; Linda Kerber; Richard Kerber; Wendy Kline; Marjorie Levine-Clark; Josh Lobert; Marie-France Morel; Kevin Mumford; Scott Ninnemann; Lyubov Obraztsova; Jennifer Parks; Rebecca Jo Plant; Rebecca Pulju; Jacki Rand; Anne Regourd; Ed Roslof; Lara Roslof; Heather Sarkissian; Eric Schaefer; Anne Schnell; Jennifer Sessions; Anne Silver; Debbie Sokoloff; Shel Stromquist; Jessica Werneke; Anton Yasnitsky; El'vira Yershova; and Ben Zajicek. My thanks also for comments and criticisms from my colleagues at meetings of the Association for Slavic, East European and Eurasian Studies, the American Association for the History of Medicine, the European Association for the History of Medicine and Health, La Société d'histoire de la naissance, and the Western Society for French History. I appreciate the feedback I received on presentations at Duke University, Eastern Mediterranean University, Hebrew University, Loyola University of Chicago, and the University of North Carolina at Chapel Hill.

I also wish to thank the staff of the many repositories where I worked. At the helm of Ukraine's state archives, Hennadi Boriak did a wonderful job supporting my efforts. I gratefully acknowledge the assistance I received from the staffs of Ukraine's Central State Archive of Higher Agencies of Authority and Administration and the State Archive of Kharkov Oblast. Affiliation with Kyiv's Taras Shevchenko National University and Kharkiv's National Pharmaceutical University facilitated my work, and I appreciate the help of P. O. Bekh, V. S. Trukh, and T. P Tsapko at these institutions.

Olesya Hulchiy at the O. O. Bohomolets National Medical University and the staff of the university's library were also of great assistance, as were B. V. Mikhailov and members of his department at the Kharkov Medical Academy of Postgraduate Education. In Moscow, I benefited from staff support at the State Archive of the Russian Federation and Central Scientific Medical Library. In Paris, Jean-Pierre Elbaz and Zahoua Goudjil proved patient and generous hosts at the General Confederation of Labor of Metallurgy's Institute of Social History. Staff at the Arthur and Elizabeth Schlesinger Library on the History of Women in America, especially Ellen Shea, provided terrific help, as did the librarians at the National Library of Medicine, most notably Stephen Greenberg. My thanks also go to the University of Iowa Libraries, especially the Interlibrary Loan staff.

Editor Susan Ferber and the anonymous reviewers at Oxford University Press provided helpful suggestions at the final stage of this project. I appreciate the work of the copy editors, designer, and marketing staff at OUP. My thanks also to Karen Kletter for indexing the book.

I benefited from generous financial backing to research and write this book. I thank the University of Iowa for the many ways that it supported this project. The Office of the Vice President for Research's Faculty Scholar Award gave me time away from the classroom, funding to study French, and the opportunity to conduct research in the United States, France, and Great Britain. The UI College of Arts and Sciences and International Programs supported travel to several conferences, where I was able to present my work at an early stage and get feedback from knowledgeable colleagues. My wonderful comrades in the History Department provided thoughtful input and a collegial environment over many years and it was my pleasure and honor to be a member of that distinguished department. I am grateful to Monash University's Department of History for providing a welcoming new home and the last bit of funding needed to take this project over the finish line.

Major support for researching this book was provided by the International Research and Exchanges Board, with funds provided by the National Endowment for the Humanities, the United States Information Agency, and the US Department of State; the National Council for Eurasian and East European Research under authority of a Title VIII grant from the US Department of State; the Schlesinger Library, Radcliffe Institute for Advanced Study, Harvard University; and the Wellcome Trust.

Grants from the American Council of Learned Societies, the John Simon Guggenheim Foundation, the National Endowment for the Humanities, and the National Institutes of Health underwrote additional research and the writing of this book. These funds enabled me to spend two highly productive years in residence at the National Humanities Center. NHC librarians Brooke Andrade, Josiah Drewry, Jean Houston, and Eliza Robertson and copyeditor Karen Carroll made the most direct contributions to this book's completion, but I am grateful to the entire Center staff for providing such a perfectly blissful environment. I appreciate Sarah Payne, Don Solomon, Carol Vorhaus, and others for indulging my steady chatter about psychoprophylaxis over lunches and on post-lunch power walks. I am also grateful to the fellows who participated in the Feminist Reading Group (2008–09) and the Working Group in Gender Studies (2011–12), especially Karen Hagemann and Ellen Ross.

Despite all the financial, intellectual, and emotional resources poured into this project, no funding agencies or individuals other than the author are responsible for the views expressed in the text. Accountability for all errors and omissions is mine alone.

ABBREVIATIONS AND ACRONYMS

ABC   Alternative Birth Center
AF   Archives du féminisme (Archive of Feminism), Angers
ANF   Archives nationales de France (National Archive of
           France), Paris
ASD   l'accouchement sans douleur (painless childbirth)
ASPO   American Society for Psychoprophylaxis in Obstetrics
BACE   Boston Association of Childbirth Educators
CCES   Council of Childbirth Education Specialists
CGT   Confédération Général du Travail (General Confederation
           of Labor)
CNFF   Conseil National de Femmes Françaises (National Council of
           French Women)
CWPEA   Childbirth Without Pain Education Association
DAKhO   Derzhavnyi arkhiv Kharkivskoi oblasti (State Archive of
           Kharkiv Oblast), Kharkiv
FCMC   Family-Centered Maternity Care
GARF   Gosudarstvennyi arkhiv Rossiiskoi Federatsii (State Archive
           of the Russian Federation), Moscow
GP   General practitioner
ICEA   International Childbirth Education Association
IV   Intravenous
KhMAPO   Khar'kovskaia meditsinskaia akademiia poslediplomnogo
           obrazovanii (Kharkiv Medical Academy of Postgraduate
           Education)
LHSL   Augustus C. Long Health Sciences Library Archives and
           Special Collections, Columbia University, New York
LI   Lamaze International
MCA   Maternity Center Association
Minzdrav   Ministerstvo zdravookhraneniia (Ministry of Public Health)
MPP   la méthode psychoprophylactique (psychoprophylactic
           method)

MZ SSSR	Ministerstvo zdravookhraneniia Soiuza Sovetskikh Sotsialisticheskikh Respublik (Ministry of Public Health of the Union of Soviet Socialist Republics)
MZ USSR	Ministerstvo zdravookhraneniia Ukrainskoi Sovetskoi Sotsialisticheskoi Respubliki (Ministry of Public Health of the Ukrainian Soviet Socialist Republic)
NBTF	National Birthday Trust Fund
NCT	National Childbirth Trust
NHS	National Health Service
Ob/gyn	Obstetrician-gynecologist
OMD	Okhrana materinstva i detstva (Protection of Maternity and Childhood)

TRANSLATION OF FOREIGN TERMS

active management of labor	*L'accouchement dirigé*
Department of Maternity Wards and Women's Clinics	*Upravlenie rodil'nykh domov i zhenskikh konsul'tatsii*
district	*raion*
express preparation	*ekspress-podgotovka; skorostnaia podgotovka*
Institute for the Protection of Maternity and Childhood	*Institut okhrany materinstva i detstva*
maternity ward; maternity home	*rodil'nyi dom; roddom*
Obstetrics and Gynecology	*Akusherstvo i ginekologiia*
Obstetrics Commission	*Komissii rodovspomozheniia*
physical therapy	*lechebnaia gimnastika*
region	*oblast'*
Sécurité sociale	France's social welfare and healthcare system, inaugurated in 1946
USSR Central Pharmaceutical Administration	*Tsentral'noe aptechnoe upravlenie SSSR*

Lamaze

Introduction

In the spring of 2000, I was delighted to find myself pregnant. Like many first-time mothers-to-be, I set about researching pregnancy and childbirth with gusto. Hunting for the requisite childbirth education class, I did what no doubt other expectant American women did at the dawn of the twenty-first century. I googled the one word I associated with prenatal preparation, the word often used as a synonym for childbirth education: Lamaze. My search took me to the home page of Lamaze International, the world's largest nonprofit organization dedicated to prenatal education. There I spied a link marked "history." A historian by profession, I reflexively clicked on it. The brief narrative opened with a tantalizing sentence about French obstetrician Fernand Lamaze, pictured in Figure 0.1, traveling to the Soviet Union in 1951 and discovering in use there a method of childbirth known as psychoprophylaxis, which he brought back to France and popularized.

To the extent that I had thought about the Lamaze method at all previously, I had some vague idea that maybe it was of French origin, but I certainly never heard that it began in the USSR. For the run-of-the-mill expectant mother, that might not have been such a shocking revelation, but I am a historian who specializes in the history of Soviet medicine. How did I, of all people, not know that something that was a household word in the United States had Soviet roots? I turned over in my mind the likelihood that the Soviet origins of what we called the Lamaze method had been deliberately obscured. Amid the Cold War, it seemed plausible that proponents cloaked psychoprophylaxis's Communist pedigree, in part by changing the method's name, to make it acceptable to the American public.

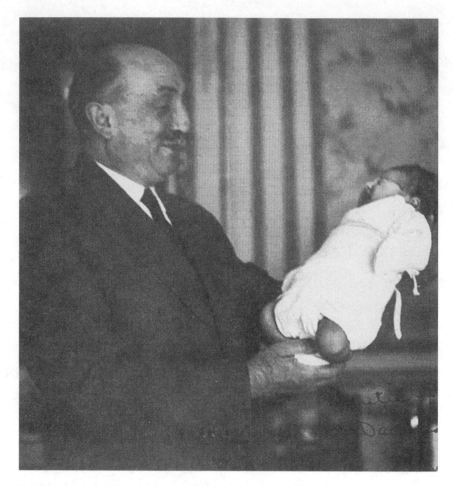

Figure 0.1: Fernand Lamaze holds the newborn baby of actress Deanna Durbin, mid-1950s. Caroline Gutmann, *The Legacy of Doctor Lamaze: The Story of The Man who Changed Childbirth*. Translated by Bruce Benderson. New York: St. Martin's, 2001. Reproduced with permission of Caroline Gutmann.

But, if this had happened, who did it? And how? For that matter, how is it that a French obstetrician came to travel to the USSR and observe a birth using this innovative method in the final years of the Stalin era, arguably the most closed and repressive period in all of Soviet history? I knew that the Communist Party had enjoyed great popularity in postwar France. Did it play some role in the method's crossing of the Iron Curtain?

I did not even know exactly what the Lamaze method was. I associated it with natural childbirth, though I was unclear about whether they were one and the same. I knew that resistance to the use of pharmacological pain relief during labor had in recent decades fallen out of fashion. Most American women of my generation embraced epidural anesthesia to render childbirth painless. By contrast, the Lamaze method, to the best of my lay knowledge, emphasized the use of breathing, particularly panting, to manage labor pain. I gathered from random pop culture associations that this "hee, hee, hee, hoo" technique was in vogue in the late 1960s and 1970s, when second-wave feminism crested and women sought agency in labor and birth in opposition to the patriarchal obstetric establishment. In some murky combination of information and imagination, I linked the word "Lamaze" with the twinned ideas of feminist empowerment and the avoidance of obstetric anesthesia.

Discovering that the Lamaze method in fact originated in the USSR challenged this assumption and made me want to learn more. Soviet ideology rejected liberal, bourgeois feminism as a false consciousness. I was confident that nothing with Soviet origins could have been embedded in or have intrinsically embodied the ideals for which American feminists fought in the 1970s. The last thing on the mind of Joseph Stalin was women's liberation. Clearly, the method's meaning had undergone a significant makeover as it made its way from the Soviet Union to France, and then to the United States. Excavation of this process of transmission and transformation led to years of work in archives and libraries in Russia, Ukraine, France, Great Britain, and the United States to weave together this story.

What exactly is the Lamaze method, also known as psychoprophylaxis? In brief, it is a way of giving birth that attempts to manage labor pain primarily through psychological conditioning and without reliance on drugs. Psychoprophylaxis is premised on the belief that pain in labor is wholly psychogenic in origin, a claim that today sounds absurd to nearly everyone. But, in fact, the original promoters of psychoprophylaxis unreservedly asserted that labor pain originated in women's minds, not their bodies. And if the mind was the site for combating pain, psychology was the weapon. Psychoprophylaxis was grounded theoretically in Ivan Pavlov's concept of conditional response, and the belief that women could be conditioned through prenatal preparation to respond to labor's onset with profound relaxation and calm. Psychoprophylaxis required that, in the weeks prior to labor, women studied the physiology of labor and birth to dispel any anxiety they might have about what was going to happen when labor began. They used conscious relaxation to remove tension from the body. Patterned breathing, the method's hallmark, was intended as a distraction, preoccupying the brain and interfering with the perception of pain signals in the cerebral cortex. Focus on the breath also supposedly facilitated relaxation and, when necessary, helped women to resist the urge to push prematurely. Psychoprophylaxis became so integral to American childbearing that the use of this patterned breathing is no longer even linked to this particular method. For forty years, American television and film has depicted Lamaze breathing. *All in the Family*'s Gloria Stivic (1975) and *Friends*' Rachel Green (2002), to give but two examples, both used patterned breathing to manage labor pain, Rachel long after psychoprophylaxis had fallen out of fashion.

Psychoprophylaxis was an artifact of the era that produced it and reconstructing its history opens a window onto some of the defining intellectual currents of the twentieth century. Across Europe and North America, a web of intertwined and widely held beliefs about medicine, politics, women, and the family underpinned this approach to the pain of childbirth. Reigning ideas about female psychology, pronatalism, marriage, and motherhood inspired and legitimated the Lamaze method and readied the public to embrace it.

Early twentieth-century notions about psychology and the mind-body dynamic developed in two directions, both of which contributed to explanations of how psychoprophylaxis worked. Stressing the neurological system's role in human behavior, one stream of thought derived from the work of Ivan Pavlov; a second school emerged around Sigmund Freud. Pavlov's investigations into conditional and unconditional response were well known and respected around the globe, and earned him a Nobel Prize in 1904. Emphasizing the role of the central nervous system, this approach to human behavior became orthodoxy in Stalin's USSR. Pavlov's work challenged that of Freud, whose popularity spread across Europe and the Americas in the first decades of the twentieth century. Freud stressed the role of the subconscious and early childhood psychosexual experiences in the formation of the psyche and the development of mental disorders. With its epicenter in the United States, psychosomatic medicine married Freudian psychoanalytic concepts to the diagnosis and treatment of physical ailments.

In general, it can be asserted that faith in the mind's influence over the body—whether from a Pavlovian neuropsychological or Freudian psychosomatic perspective—was widespread and growing in the medical community and the general public in the first half of the twentieth century. Seeing women's bodies as particularly susceptible to the influence of weak and nervous minds, physicians were quick to attribute women's illnesses to psychogenic causes. It was a small step to the belief that pain in childbirth was in whole or in large part a product of female psychology and could therefore be conquered through psychotherapeutic intervention.

Freud's disciple Helene Deutsch crafted an influential psychoanalytic interpretation of female psychology in pregnancy and childbirth. Her study, *The Psychology of Women* (1945), proved to be profoundly influential on the proponents of the Lamaze method.[1] In Deutsch's view, women's personalities fall on a continuum, with the feminine woman at one end of the spectrum and the masculine woman at the other. During childbirth "the masculine-active type of woman... wants her delivery to be an active accomplishment on her part," but her distorted, unhealthy personality "results in complications of childbirth."[2] By contrast, passive-feminine women "blindly follow other people's instructions and, like children, are interested only in getting rid of their fear and being subjected to as little pain as possible."[3] Difficult pregnancies, long labors, and painful childbirth experiences indicated personality disorders and ambivalence toward motherhood, symptoms of profound childhood traumas, and stunted psychosexual development.[4] Deutsch characterizes a "normal, active delivery" as one in which a woman neither seeks to dominate her experience of birth in a masculine way, nor exhibits a feminine submission to the aid and intervention of the medical team.[5] Ideally, "even the most active woman should entirely subordinate herself to the inner forces—a passive, cooperative, patient endurance of the process is her only task."[6] The well-adjusted woman in labor actively engaged in her birth experience through her forbearance and compliance. Strongest in the United States but present in the United Kingdom and France as well, this psychoanalytic interpretation of female reproduction worked to reinforce physician authority and to undermine the agency of women, whose psychological state, particularly during pregnancy, labor, and birth, was thought to compromise their ability to recognize what was in their own best interests.

These transformations in how medical professionals and the general public understood women's personalities, and the role of the mind in pregnancy and birth, coalesced amid profound political and social change. Beginning in the late nineteenth century and intensifying in the first half of the twentieth, many in Britain and France agonized over declining birthrates, particularly relative to Germany. Even in countries where birthrates remained high, like Russia, or where robust immigration mitigated declining birthrates, like the United States, anxieties surfaced over whether the "right" people were having enough babies. Eugenicists championed curtailing, if necessary through forced sterilization, the birthrates of non-whites and of the poor and working classes; they promoted increased fecundity for white members of the middle and wealthy classes. Nazi atrocities discredited the most flagrantly eugenic social engineering proposals, but state concern with how many children were born and to whom persisted.

In the wake of World War II, Cold War imperatives permeated the case for pronatalism. In the USSR and the United States, government officials and social commentators drew a straight line between opposition to the enemy and an expanding birthrate. Having more babies and raising them in the right ideological spirit became signs of loyalty. Great Britain and France, too, participated in these Cold War pronatalist debates. Replenishing the population after devastating losses during World War II was of central importance to postwar governments, and the construction of ambitious social welfare schemes—like the National Health Service (NHS) in Britain and *Sécurité sociale*, France's medical and social welfare system— were intended in part to buttress the ability of citizens to bear and raise children. They also served to undermine support for domestic Communist parties by conceding to their core demands for social services for the poor and working classes. In the USSR, the regime continued to offer, as it had since the 1930s, financial supplements, more spacious housing, and other privileges to mothers with large families.

Postwar pronatalism went hand-in-glove with ideologies of companionate marriage and family togetherness. Coined by social scientists in 1924, the term "companionate marriage" was characterized by relatively greater democratic family decision-making, fewer children, and an emphasis on a satisfying emotional and sexual relationship between spouses.[7] By the 1940s and 1950s, companionate marriage was considered by middle-class Americans and Western Europeans to be the path to an emotionally and physically rewarding family life. Women's magazines in France, Great Britain, and the United States presented the nuclear family as the foundation of the postwar order. The progressive language of women's liberation and sexual emancipation that had followed World War I—when American and British women gained the right to vote, hemlines rose, corsets fell by the wayside, and the flapper took center stage—knew no equivalent in the post–World War II period. French women earned voting rights at the close of World War II, but the defining image of women to emerge in this era was that of domestic partners to wage-earning husbands. However much this image was mythical, it was nonetheless the reigning ideal of the day.[8] The media propagated the notion that men and women partnered to create a domestic oasis and wile away their newfound leisure hours with shared family activities. Drawing the father into a more active parenting role, a cult of "togetherness"—a term first used by *McCall's* magazine in 1954— made child-centered activities the focal point of the family's leisure time. This wholesome private life was understood as an extension of the Cold War, a domestic front for creating a stable, healthy citizenry capable of resisting the seductions of Communism.[9]

While companionate marriage and family togetherness constituted the foundation of domestic life, the postwar baby boom set the woman's role as mother into sharp relief. With roots in the Victorian romanticization of maternal love, the postwar cult of motherhood was shot through with paradoxes that the rise of Freudian psychology amplified. The popular media lauded women for their roles as wives and mothers, but cautioned the need to strike a balance between the two, lest husbands feel neglected. Emphasizing the mother's power and influence, students of Freud rooted personality formation in early childhood experiences and imbued the role of mother with individual and social significance. This fresh emphasis on the long-term consequences of early childhood experiences brought mothers potential acclaim for their influence, but it was also an opening to lay blame on them for any perceived personal or psychological problems that children developed later in life. Psychologists and advice columnists implored women to lavish love and care on their children, put them at the center of their attention, and find personal satisfaction in the role of mother. At the same time, they counseled mothers not to suffocate children with an overbearing and, for their sons, emasculating maternal presence. White, middle-class American mothers of the late 1940s and 1950s teetered on the fine line between proper, selfless, healthy mothering and what writer Philip Wylie denounced as stifling "momism."[10]

Inflected with Cold War overtones, these ideas about marriage and family shaped expectations for what constituted a desirable birth experience. Albeit in the minority, some midcentury women expressed a desire to give birth with a clear mind and a sensate body. They aspired to a more satisfying birth experience, with their husbands by their side, supporting them during labor and sharing with them the joy of bringing their child into the world. Concern among a small but growing number of physicians about the side effects on women and their babies of powerful anesthetics, analgesics, and sedatives further fueled the desire to find another way of managing pain in childbirth.

Set against this social, political, and ideological backdrop, telling the story of the Lamaze method requires crisscrossing the national borders of the Soviet Union, France, Great Britain, and the United States to understand why this approach gained traction, and how its practice changed in different times and places. It is an account in equal measure about medicine, politics, and gender, pieced together through the recovery of disparate voices: mostly male medical practitioners and mostly female childbirth educators; mothers and fathers; supporters and detractors. The first chapter offers a thumbnail historical sketch of the emergence of medicalized birth and the response to these developments put forward by British physician Grantly Dick-Read, who crafted the first psychological, non-pharmacological approach to obstetric pain to enjoy widespread dissemination, prefiguring the success of psychoprophylaxis. Building on this foundation, chapters two and three chronicle the launch of psychoprophylaxis in the USSR and France, respectively. Developed in Ukraine by psychotherapist I. Z. Vel'vovskii, psychoprophylaxis emerged in the late 1940s and, in 1951, became standard practice across the Soviet Union. In the late summer of 1951, psychoprophylaxis made its way to France with Dr. Lamaze, as chapter three describes. By the mid-1950s it had spread to nearly every corner of France, where the Communist Party and its allies played a prominent role in the method's popularization.

The second half of the book embraces a transnational perspective to understand the movement for psychoprophylaxis as it fanned out around the globe. Amid physician complaints of inefficacy and a shifting political climate, psychoprophylactic practice in the USSR dwindled after 1956. The French movement went through a period of crisis following Lamaze's death in 1957, but enjoyed a growing following over the 1960s. Meanwhile, in the United States, psychoprophylaxis gained ground with remarkable speed. In the 1970s feminist movements in the United States and France took markedly different stances toward the Lamaze method and what constituted an empowered birth experience. An epilogue casts a glance forward to the 1980s and beyond, reflecting on contemporary debates on American maternity care.

Psychoprophylaxis was just one way of birthing that emphasized and valued the rejection or minimal use of pharmacological pain relief. "Natural childbirth" is colloquially used to describe many different ways of giving birth without reliance on anesthetics and analgesics. I avoid the use of the term "natural childbirth" in this informal way for a number of reasons. First, the phrase masks a range of approaches that vary in ways big and small, but that share an antipathy toward the routine use of pharmacological pain relief in normal birth. Not long after psychoprophylaxis gained popularity in the United States, Denver obstetrician Robert Bradley developed his eponymous method, which was similar to psychoprophylaxis. Frédérick Leboyer's "birth without violence" and water birth, popularized by Michel Odent, both gained prominence in France in the 1970s before making their mark on the American way of birth. Despite shared roots with psychoprophylaxis, the use of hypnosis in childbirth, or hypnobirthing, has a distinct historical trajectory. These different ways of preparing for and giving birth have much in common with the Lamaze method, but are addressed in this book only as they intersect with psychoprophylaxis. To further complicate matters, the use of "natural childbirth" as an umbrella term to refer to these and other non-pharmacological methods of obstetric pain management makes for confusion with the work of Dick-Read, who called his particular approach Natural Childbirth. It is capitalized here where it refers specifically to Dick-Read's technique, which was developed in the 1920s and 1930s and popularized in the Anglophone world in the 1940s and 1950s. I also call it "the Read method," as it was described in the popular literature of the era.

The focus in this history of psychoprophylaxis is squarely on the mainline story, on the "typical" woman who was drawn to the method. In France, that meant mostly working class and Left-leaning women. In the United States, well-educated, married, white, middle- and upper-class women were the method's primary demographic base. Soviet women, by contrast, did not choose the use of psychoprophylaxis, but had it foisted upon them by a central government that was unable or unwilling to provide widespread access to other options for obstetric pain relief. It is in the Soviet context that women's voices are most difficult to hear. They break through occasionally in the perhaps unreliable paraphrases of their medical caregivers, but women rarely speak for themselves in the published and archival sources.[11] By contrast, women's testimonials in the form of letters, memoirs, hospital exit surveys, and newspaper and magazine articles from France and the United States are abundant, offering a much richer picture of the Lamaze method as a lived experience in those countries.

CHAPTER 1

✧

Medicalized Childbirth and Natural Childbirth

Labor is rarely so swift or spectacular as it appears on television or in movies, when the expectant mother doubles over in agony, her "waters break," and the amniotic fluid surrounding the baby releases in a dramatic (or comic) gush. Even before labor commences in earnest, the body readies itself. The cervix begins to efface, as tissue thins and stretches to allow for dilation, or the opening of the cervix. To permit the baby to pass through the vaginal canal, the cervix must dilate to 10 centimeters in diameter before birth. Some women can be partly effaced and dilated even weeks before labor truly begins. Known as the "bloody show," the expulsion of the thick mucus plug lodged during pregnancy at the opening of the cervix sometimes heralds labor's imminent onset. The establishment of uterine contractions at regular intervals signals active labor, which is divided into three stages. During the first stage, the cervix thins and dilates fully. The contractions that accompany this phase of labor range from mild, akin to menstrual cramps, to severe. Getting stronger, longer, and more frequent as labor progresses, contractions last from thirty to ninety seconds. The first stage can pass in a couple of hours, or it can last for more than a day. As the cervix opens from 8 to 10 centimeters dilation at the end of the first stage—a period known as transition and lasting about fifteen minutes—pain typically peaks, with contractions coming in rapid succession. When the mother-to-be reaches full dilation, she enters the second stage of labor, which usually passes far more quickly than the first. Within a period from fifteen minutes to two hours, the woman works with the uterine contractions to push out her baby. Though this is the phase of labor often depicted as most painful, because grunting or yelling may accompany the intense effort of pushing, many women find the second stage to be a great physical and psychological relief. In the final, third stage of labor, the new mother expels the placenta in ten to thirty minutes of usually painless, mild effort.

A clinical description of this universal biological process cannot capture the range of women's experiences of childbirth, which are always set in a social context. Birthing conditions vary enormously according to cultural practices, beliefs, and material circumstances, and these differences defy easy division between so-called developed and developing countries, Western and non-Western methods, or science and superstition. Such dichotomies fail to reflect the modern global circulation of ideas, complexities at the local level, or the way that values and assumptions are social, cultural, and historical products. For example, contemporary women in the Netherlands have access to hospitals and drugs when necessary, but many favor home birth without routine resort to anesthesia. They live in a culture of belief in the innate ability of healthy women's bodies to bear children without drugs or other major medical interventions. Most women in the United States—where hospital births are nearly universal and as many as three-quarters of birthing women make use of epidural anesthesia—have birth experiences determined by a set of beliefs, particularly regarding labor pain, that could hardly be more different from those of Dutch women. Even within the borders of a single nation-state, birth practices differ markedly according to race, ethnicity, age, income, location, level of education, and myriad other factors.[1]

The way many urban, middle-class women in the developed world give birth today is shaped by practices that arose primarily over the nineteenth and twentieth centuries. Wide-ranging changes in biomedicine, or what is casually—if imprecisely—referred to as Western medicine, revolutionized birth practices. Global patterns are discernible, even as national variations persist. One sees a clear and consistent trend toward the professionalization of maternity care and the shift of that care from home to hospital. In general, these changes came to the privileged classes in urban areas first, before spreading to rural regions and trickling down to less affluent citizens.

From the mid-nineteenth to the mid-twentieth century state regulators across Europe and North America came to define who was and was not qualified to attend women in childbirth. In the United States, the rise of educational requirements and certification for the care of women in child birth enabled physicians to drive midwives to the brink of extinction. By the middle of the twentieth century, general practitioners (GPs) found their position similarly threatened by obstetricians/gynecologists (ob/gyns), who claimed their specialized skills were an asset to women even in cases of normal birth.[2] In France, midwifery persisted, but physicians there, too, came to play a prominent role in maternity care. After the establishment in 1946 of *Sécurité sociale*, a law mandated that expectant women receive from a physician the certificate needed to access state-mandated maternity benefits. This requirement greatly increased the number of women attended by physicians. Professional French midwives persevered, but their numbers and their autonomy declined through the 1950s and 1960s.[3] As they elevated their qualifications in the face of new state requirements, British midwives in the early twentieth century succeeded in resisting the threat of physicians to their livelihood. Physicians found a following among some privileged women, but midwives in Great Britain maintained their role as caregivers to most women in pregnancy and birth.[4] Given financial and personnel limitations in the Soviet Union, there was never any question of a physician takeover of maternity care there, but the state over time professionalized midwifery. This shift proceeded slowly, and only in the decades after World War II did state certified midwifery care penetrate fully into the USSR's most remote regions.[5]

Whether in the care of physicians or midwives, women in the twentieth century increasingly left their homes to have their babies in hospitals. Notorious for unsanitary conditions and indifferent care, maternity wards had once been places where only urban charity cases gave birth. With the rise of the germ theory, incidents of postpartum infection, or puerperal fever, fell in both homes and hospitals. The advent of sulfa drugs in the 1930s, followed by the development of antibiotics and the refinement of blood transfusion techniques in the 1940s dealt a decisive blow to high rates of maternal mortality.[6] Hospitals came to be seen as safer, more sterile environments, and hospital birth expanded dramatically. Already in 1939, three-quarters of urban births and half of rural births in the United States took place in hospitals. In Great Britain in 1946, the year that the NHS was established, 54 percent of British women gave birth in the hospital; the number climbed to 64 percent by 1954, but stagnated for nearly a decade. Britain achieved parity with the nearly universal American practice of hospital birth with a jump to 91 percent by 1972.[7] In Paris, 92 percent of all births were in hospitals or clinics by 1939, with other French cities quickly catching up in the years after the war. Nationally, 53 percent of French women gave birth in 1952 in maternity wards, a figure that rose to 85 percent in 1962 and to over 98 percent by 1974.[8] In the USSR, laws in 1936 and 1944 evinced the regime's commitment to moving childbirth out of the home by mandating a dramatic expansion of the number of obstetric beds. As elsewhere in Europe, urban areas relatively quickly made this transition and rural areas lagged behind, but by the 1970s Soviet rates of birth in maternity wards matched those in France, Britain, and the United States.[9]

One of the most compelling reasons for women to seek in-hospital maternity care was to gain access to pharmacological pain relief. Pain in childbirth had been a source of misery for women since time immemorial. In Genesis 3:16, God punishes Eve, proclaiming that "in sorrow thou shall bring forth children," a passage that for centuries imbued childbirth pain with profound spiritual significance in Western culture and was taken by some to justify women's suffering in childbirth. Folk remedies and comfort measures, such as the use of belladonna and other botanicals for the pain of labor, eased suffering, but the development of anesthesia brought conquest of labor pain within the grasp of women in Europe and North America. Though ether was discovered in the fourteenth century, only in 1847 did Scottish physician James Young Simpson see its obstetric potential. Shortly thereafter he began to favor the use of chloroform, a relatively new anesthesia. In 1853 Dr. John Snow administered chloroform to Queen Victoria during the birth of her eighth child. Her delight with this miracle of modern medicine was a boon to the use of obstetric anesthesia, which spread rapidly among the wealthy. Across the Atlantic, similar changes were afoot, as Boston physician Walter Channing turned to the use of ether not long after Simpson's initial experiments. The vocal and enthusiastic endorsement of Henry Wadsworth Longfellow and his wife Fanny helped to spur ether's application in American obstetrics. In Russia, Polish-born physician Stanislav Klikovich first experimented in the 1880s with the use of nitrous oxide in obstetrics. Nitrous oxide found supporters at home and abroad, but political upheaval and economic hardship impeded its widespread use in Russia, where obstetric anesthesia of any sort would remain a rarity until the post-Soviet era. In the early twentieth century, affluent British and American women embraced the use of twilight sleep, or dämmerschlaf, to aid in labor and birth. Developed in Germany, twilight sleep tackled labor pain through the use of the analgesic morphine and the amnesic scopolamine. Morphine was not particularly effective in easing the pain of labor, and many continued to suffer physically, even if they had no memory of the pain upon waking.[10]

First upper- and then middle-class urban women led the charge for obstetric anesthesia. Writing in 1915, two American feminists advocating for twilight sleep speculated that not only could anesthesia liberate women from the harmful psychological effects of childbirth, but it could also transform women's personalities, and even their position in American politics and society. They wrote that, when obstetric anesthesia became more widely available, "we shall know the full extent how much [the pain of childbirth] accounts for the irritability, superficiality and instability alleged against women. We may find that it has been a potent factor in retarding their development to a position of equality with men."[11] Needless to say, the popularity of ether, chloroform, nitrous oxide, twilight sleep, and, later, the cornucopia of sedatives, analgesics, and anesthetics used in obstetrics did not revolutionize ideas about female psychology or women's role in society. Moreover, women's enthusiasm does not negate the significance of institutional and social pressures that pushed them toward the use of anesthesia in conjunction with an increasingly medicalized and pathologized vision of childbirth. For some women the desire to be "knocked out" offered escape from the alienating environment of the hospital. With no understanding of what was happening to them or what to expect, and no one to offer comfort or companionship, women retreated from their fears and from the brusque treatment of hospital staff into the relief of unconsciousness, a choice that can hardly be characterized as empowered.[12]

By the 1930s and 1940s the diversity of drugs available for obstetric pain relief translated into quite varied national practices. British women and their caregivers turned increasingly to nitrous oxide, which could be safely administered by a midwife in the hospital or in the laboring woman's home. Established in 1928, Britain's charitable National Birthday Trust Fund (NBTF) worked to expand the routine use of labor pain relief for poor and working-class women. Access to pain relief was understood by middle- and upper-class women active in the NBTF as a feminist and social justice cause, which they sought to further through the popularization of Dr. R. J. Minnitt's gas-and-air apparatus. Developed in 1933, this machine allowed the self-administration of nitrous oxide, mixed with air or oxygen, without fear of overdose.[13] Simple to use, safe, and cost effective, nitrous oxide offered "analgesia for the masses."[14] After 1936, British midwives were authorized to oversee the use of nitrous oxide, but stronger pain medications stayed strictly in the hands of physicians.[15] Nitrous oxide remains the drug of choice for many women in Britain. In the USSR, too, it was favored, but demand far outstripped supply. For hazy and complex reasons, nitrous oxide never gained a following in the United States, and is virtually unavailable today in American maternity wards.[16] Both French and American doctors instead favored powerful anesthetics over milder analgesics. Barbiturates and narcotics were used in various, often complex combinations according to protocols developed at each hospital. Tranquilizers helped women to "relax," in practice making them quieter, calmer, more compliant, and easier to manage in the context of the regimented hospital routine.[17]

Were the benefits of the physician's increasingly frequent attendance in childbirth, the relocation of birth to the hospital, and the popularization of obstetric anesthesia worth the loss of women's control over childbirth in the home, under a midwife's care? At the heart of this question is the issue of women's agency in birth. Though there is disagreement over degree, most historians concur that these changes adversely affected women's authority, irrespective of their active and enthusiastic embrace of change.[18] In their quest to achieve safety and comfort in birth, women supported its medicalization through a conscious, deliberate, and rational consumer choice. At the same time, in the name of women's and babies' well-being, modern obstetrics brought mothers under the control of professionalized caregivers—often male physicians—and medical institutions. Historian Judith Walzer Leavitt captures the social meaning of this medicalization when she observes that women went from being "brought to bed" amid friends and family in the comforting environment of the home, to being "alone among strangers" in the alienating modern hospital.[19]

Women expressed discontent with the care and treatment they received in maternity wards, even as they supported the medicalization of childbirth. Soviet maternity care was notoriously cruel, but in the West, too, women suffered from a harsh regimen designed for the convenience of the medical staff and not the care of the patient. Sparked by a 1957 letter to the editor of *Ladies' Home Journal* on "the tortures that go on in modern delivery rooms," readers flooded the American magazine's office with hundreds of testimonials that speak to the widespread discontent with medicalized birth practices.[20] Women were separated from their husbands, then left alone and without support. Many told of nurses forcibly holding their legs together to keep them from giving birth until the physician arrived. They feared that their children had suffered brain injuries as a result of such actions and felt that they themselves had been scarred psychologically by the experience.[21] In a typical commentary on the quality of hospital-based maternity care, a Mrs. W. S. B. wrote that "there seems to be a feeling that a woman in childbirth has brought her troubles on herself and so deserves no kindness. One moaning with pain from an operation is an object of sympathy. A woman moaning with pain in childbirth is just a nuisance."[22] Drugs were used to quiet these women, but many complained of unpleasant side effects, especially hallucinations that led them to be forcibly restrained as they thrashed about in terror.[23] Taken together, these letters—and similar testimonies from Britain and France, as well as the scanty evidence from the USSR—attest to frustration with conventional medicalized birth practices and the desire for an alternative.

DICK-READ AND THE INVENTION OF NATURAL CHILDBIRTH

Practically from the first whiff of obstetric anesthesia, concern over its use arose on a variety of grounds. Some religious leaders used the passage in Genesis to argue that God would not approve of drugs to alleviate the suffering that he had decreed was women's lot in life.[24] The use of ether and chloroform carried serious risks. A highly flammable and potentially explosive gas, ether threatened the lives of doctor and patient; both ether and chloroform had adverse side effects, and their fumes could overpower attendant caregivers. Women were often too drugged to birth their babies, necessitating forceps deliveries that could do injury to mother and child. Writing in the late 1940s, an American obstetrician observed that meddlesome, "ill-advised interference with pregnancy and labor," including the use of debilitating anesthetics and the consequent reliance on forceps, "has probably caused as much damage to mothers and babies as obstetric disease itself."[25] Women in a drug-induced haze also posed a potential physical hazard to themselves and others. Delivery tables had to be equipped with straps to restrain women who might inadvertently contaminate the sterile field, or who might in the midst of a hallucination struggle against or even attack the medical staff. And though it was beyond their control, women fretted over the indignity of such behavior. Some mothers experienced alienation from their babies, whom they had no recollection of birthing. Women were certainly glad to have relief from pain, but the drugs available through the 1960s left much to be desired for both maternity caregivers and their patients.

For many decades before Dick-Read developed his method of Natural Childbirth, medical men had sought a psychological alternative to the available obstetric pharmacopeia. Sharing a common faith in the mind's ability to conquer the body, positive thinking, suggestion, and hypnosis all have a place in the history of psychological pain relief in obstetrics, of which the Read method was but one chapter. The genealogy of Dick-Read's ideas traces back to at least late eighteenth- and early nineteenth-century Vienna, where Franz Anton Mesmer propounded the theory of animal magnetism, which posited the presence of invisible magnetic forces in the body that could be manipulated for therapeutic ends. Illness stemmed from the failure of these magnetic forces to flow properly, and a physician could intervene to redirect these forces with sweeping hand gestures. Mesmer suffered his profession's opprobrium for having exploited and manipulated his patients, but the hope remained that the mind-body connection had therapeutic value in the hands of a reputable physician. Nineteenth-century French neurologist Jean-Martin Charcot sought to delve deeper into the mind's power through his investigation into hypnosis's therapeutic application in hysteria cases. Given the era's popular and medical views linking gynecological problems with mental disorders, it is no coincidence that Charcot's work focused on women.[26] In the early twentieth century, Charcot's compatriot Dr. Emile Coué developed his eponymous method, also known as autosuggestion or positive thinking, which American Dale Carnegie helped to popularize. The Coué method entailed the repetition of the phrase "every day, in every way, I am getting better and better" in order to improve one's physical and psychological well-being.[27] Across Europe and the United States, the circulation of these ideas about a dynamic mind-body relationship—especially in women— laid the groundwork for the popularization of the Read method and, later, psychoprophylaxis.

The use of suggestion and hypnosis, or hypnosuggestion, to alleviate pain in childbirth first gained currency in the nineteenth century. Scottish physician James Braid, an opponent of Mesmerism and the coiner of the term "hypnosis," described the case of a woman whose pregnancy was threatened by complications. He informed her of his intent to induce labor, as a result allegedly triggering the onset of labor through an inadvertent use of suggestion. Braid's observation of this phenomenon indicated a powerful mind-body connection in childbirth. In the 1880s and 1890s reports of the effective use of hypnosis and suggestion in labor and birth appeared from Belgium, Britain, France, Switzerland, and elsewhere.[28] By 1922 approximately three thousand women had given birth under hypnosis, and it was in Germany and the Soviet Union that this method found its most vigorous support. Studies there pointed to the benefits of psychological approaches to obstetric anesthesia and highlighted, in contrast to pharmacological solutions, the lack of negative side effects.[29] But there were drawbacks, principally that effective preparation was time consuming for both doctor and patient. Patients had to meet for weeks or even months with the hypnotherapist in advance of labor. The use of suggestion before labor to reassure women that all would go well and that it would not be a painful process took less time, but also tended to have a weaker anesthetizing effect. Suggestion and hypnosis could be expensive, as expectant mothers needed access to medical professionals who were trained in these techniques. For most rural women, psychological pain relief in childbirth proved as inaccessible as pharmacological means due to a lack of qualified practitioners.

In a 1933 book Grantly Dick-Read, pictured in fig. 1.1, first proposed his alternative to the conventional, anesthetized, physician-supervised way of birth common among women of privilege in Britain, France, and the United States. Dick-Read offered an approach to childbirth that anticipated much of psychoprophylaxis. He called his technique Natural Childbirth, also known as the Read method.[30] In several books published over the next quarter-century, Dick-Read elaborated on his basic premise: fear lay at the root of pain in childbirth; through education and relaxation women

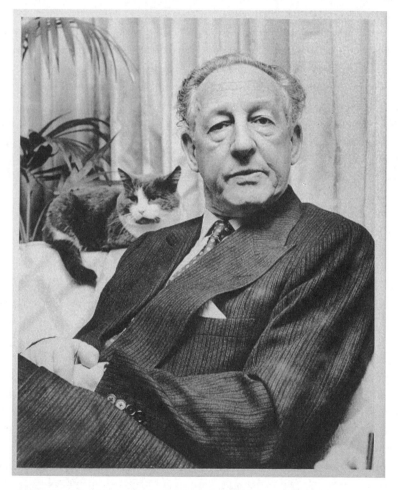

Figure 1.1: Grantly Dick-Read during his North American tour, 1957. Courtesy of Wellcome Library. Reproduced with permission of Pollinger Limited and The Estate of Grantly Dick-Read.

could give birth in comfort without resorting to anesthesia.[31] Dick-Read promised mothers not only a comfortable, fulfilling personal experience, but their husbands' respect, a deeper bond with their babies, and happier, healthier children. Though his impact was primarily in the Anglo-American context, Dick-Read's numerous books appeared in more than a dozen languages and inspired millions of women to seek a kind of birth experience that was atypical for urban, middle- and upper-class, white women in Europe and North America.

Dick-Read's major theoretical contribution to the debate over how women should best give birth was what he termed the Fear-Tension-Pain cycle. Fear, not physiology, caused labor pain. Relatives' and friends' horror stories stoked concerns. Physicians could inadvertently exacerbate a laboring woman's worries with a "wrong note, a mistaken word or a careless insinuation," transforming otherwise painless uterine contractions into agonizing pangs.[32] The glimpse of medical instruments, the mention of anesthetization, or an onlooker's excessive fretting could all trigger a woman's fears and, in turn, her physical suffering.[33] Dick-Read believed that as a natural, normal physiological function, akin to the expulsive capabilities of the bowels, childbirth could not have been designed in such a way as to be an inherently painful process. "Nature has not prescribed injury as an essential factor in the reproduction of the species," Dick-Read stressed.[34] Fear allegedly led to tension in the cervix, and, as if stating a self-evident truth, Dick-Read claimed that "all obstetricians know the effect of a tense cervix: pain, resistance at the outlet and the innumerable complications of a prolonged labor."[35] Women's minds, not their bodies, were at the root of pain in childbirth, and fear was "the greatest evil."[36]

Education and relaxation constituted the Read method's two-pronged attack on the Fear-Tension-Pain cycle. By the time a woman went into labor, a qualified medical professional "should have instructed her in such a way that no fear exists, that all the terrible stories of pain and the pictures of agony...are blotted out of her mind."[37] In the weeks prior to birth, women received detailed instruction in the physiology of pregnancy, labor and birth, nutrition, exercise, hygiene, and baby care from their physician, midwife, or qualified childbirth educator. Both in prenatal classes and at home, women trained for labor by practicing relaxation for thirty minutes a day. Cultivating an ability to note tension and release it prepared the expectant mother to do the same during labor.[38] Men did not accompany their wives to all sessions of the childbirth education course, but attended a few select classes during which they learned about the physical and emotional experience of pregnancy, what to expect during labor, and even some infant care and feeding.[39] With her husband at her side for support and armed with knowledge about what was happening, the woman greeted labor with joy rather than anxiety. Her calm, cheerful, and relaxed attitude was believed to be key to minimizing pain.

Dick-Read repeatedly asserted that he was opposed not to obstetric anesthesia, but to its routine use. Given his claim that childbirth was naturally painless and that pain could be managed through education and relaxation, the routine use of anesthesia was an absurdity to which, in Dick-Read's estimate, "Walt Disney could hardly do justice."[40] He insisted that the knowledge that analgesics and anesthetics were available, if needed, was often all that most women required.[41] He denounced the persistent and "damaging myth" that his method banned anesthesia.[42] Dick-Read certainly discouraged the use of pharmacological pain relief, believed it almost never to be necessary, and tried to coax his patients away from it, but he was unequivocal that "if the woman in labor desires it, it should be administered."[43] In his native Britain, Demerol, trilene, and nitrous oxide were widely used within the framework of the Read method, though in his own practice he avoided them.[44]

The particularly liberal use of Demerol, Nembutal, and other drugs among his American followers vexed Dick-Read.[45] One Iowa obstetrician observed that it was a "misconception that 'natural' childbirth means going through labor with no medication." He "did not believe anyone practicing obstetrics would let a woman suffer if a safe amount of drugs would help her."[46] For many American physicians and their patients, the great benefit of the Read method lay not in the elimination of pharmacological pain relief, but in its dramatic reduction.[47] In a book for expectant mothers, Yale University obstetrician Frederick Goodrich notes that, assuming labor proceeds without complication, the woman prepared in the Read method

> will need very little in the way of medication. Perhaps one injection during the first stage and a few inhalations of nitrous oxide in the second stage will be all that you require.... If you are desirous of being awake at the time your baby is born, do not feel that you are barred from having any drugs at all. As we have tried to bring out, the purpose of preparation for childbirth is to enable you to have a more satisfactory experience. The necessity for the use of drugs is incidental, as is consciousness at delivery. The essential point to remember is that by such preparation you will enjoy your experience to a greater extent.[48]

Goodrich links prenatal preparation in the Read method with a rewarding birth experience that might or might not encompass pharmacological pain relief, up to and including general anesthesia. He reflects both the medical culture in which he was enmeshed and the American inclination at the time to see the pain of labor as unendurable and undesirable for white women of privilege.

Goodrich and his colleagues did not foist medication on passive women. American women trained in the Read method in the 1940s and 1950s rejected a dogmatic stance against analgesia or anesthesia. Expressing neither disappointment nor a sense of failure for resorting to pharmacological pain relief, one new mother wrote to her childbirth educator that "my back ache was so terrific I was actually grateful" when ether was administered.[49] The openness of this mother, Goodrich, and other American proponents of the Read method to the full, if less heavy-handed, integration of sedatives, analgesics, and anesthetics is a far cry from Dick-Read's position of reluctant use or, for that matter, the wholesale rejection of drugs that some Americans came to champion in the 1970s.

For all Dick-Read's radicalism on the origins and management of obstetric pain, his beliefs were in step with reigning ideas about female psychology, gender relations, and pronatalism. Dick-Read and his disciples leaned on Freudianism to explain his theory of the psychogenic origin of labor pain. Prenatal classes purportedly resolved any underlying personality disorders and subconscious fears that sprang from a woman's abnormal psychosexual development in childhood. The supposed therapeutic value of childbirth preparation courses paved the way for a positive birth experience.[50] Childbirth itself could be a psychologically healing and personally rewarding event for a woman, as motherhood was her most important function in society and the family. Dick-Read described birth as "an ecstasy of accomplishment that only women who have had babies naturally [i.e., without anesthesia] appreciate."[51] Popular books and magazines touted the experience of an unanesthetized birth as "the supreme moment in a woman's life."[52] With this great achievement behind her, the mother could properly bond with her child and set the next generation on the path to healthy psychological development.

The Read method left unchallenged both the physician's and the husband's male authority, even as it touted women's agency. It was a paradox of the Read method that, to derive from childbirth a sense of strength and accomplishment, women had to defer wholly and unhesitatingly to the physician. Childbirth education classes encouraged women to see their role as active and critical to a successful delivery. At the same time, Dick-Read affirmed that his method enabled women "to carry out [the physician's] instructions."[53] Husbands partnered with their wives to share in the experience of becoming parents, but they also acted as agents of physician authority. Some hospitals allowed the husband who had received prenatal training to stay by his wife's side, where he provided support for her during labor, and also served as a conduit for the doctors' and nurses' communication to her. Husbands remained almost unseen in delivery rooms of this era, as, among other reasons, obstetricians worried about these men looking over their shoulders, questioning their decisions, or fainting at the sight of blood.

Like many privileged white men of his era, Dick-Read feared that the "right" women were not having enough babies. He believed fecundity among middle- and upper-class women was vital to the preservation of the British "race" and its "quality."[54] In what he saw as a terrible irony of modern life, the poor woman in a dodgy London quarter had a body well-suited to childbearing, but lacked the financial means to support a large family. The "cultured" woman of the middle and upper classes had money and education, but a body and psyche withered by "civilization."[55] The state, Dick-Read argued, should avert the nation's numerical decline and qualitative degeneration by encouraging middle- and upper-class women to fulfill what he believed to be their innate desire to reproduce and to have no less than four children, the "eugenic minimum."[56] He thought that joyful birth experiences would translate into women wanting more babies.[57] A happy delivery, he claimed, "leaves permanent marks upon the character of the child and the mother, the family life and therefore the nation."[58] Peace, prosperity, and social harmony awaited a more fecund society, for, as Dick-Read put it, "the man who has a 'full quiver' and adequate maintenance is a peace-loving worker whose presence in the community is an influence toward moderation and reason," a force against the evils of Communism and proletarian unrest.[59]

Whatever his ideological motives, Dick-Read tapped into a genuine desire for change among hundreds of maternity caregivers and thousands of childbearing couples. Though it was never the dominant way to give birth, Dick-Read's method found a particularly receptive audience in postwar America. His *Childbirth without Fear* was first published in the United States in 1944. In 1946 New Jersey obstetrician Blackwell Sawyer reported tremendous success in the first American study of the Read method.[60] By the late-1940s major studies of the method were underway at Yale University and Johns Hopkins University. Yale University's Herbert Thoms met Dick-Read when he came to the United States in 1947 under the aegis of New York City's Maternity Center Association (MCA) and became one of his most active and influential American proponents. Garnering attention in the press, the work of Thoms and the MCA went a long way toward spreading word about the Read method in the United States.[61] Groups of enthusiastic young mothers, nurses, and others banded together to form organizations, such as the Boston Association of Childbirth Educators

(BACE), Milwaukee's Natural Childbirth Association, and Seattle's Association for Childbirth Education, to meet burgeoning grassroots demand.[62]

Why did Natural Childbirth strike such a cord with Americans at this particular historical moment? The MCA's Hazel Corbin, an early and ardent advocate for the Read method, offers a compelling explanation in her observation of a link between young couples' ideals of a satisfying marital partnership and the pull of the Read method. Writing in 1950, Corbin argues that "the young men who have been to war, deprived of their normal family life, the young women who have... trundled... after their soldier husbands until they said 'goodbye' at some port of embarkation, know what lack of security means.... These young people now place a high value upon the homes they are setting up and the physical and emotional security they are trying to build for themselves." The rise of the Cold War threatened these aspirations. Among other trends, the turn to the Read method, which supported the collaboration of husband and wife in childbirth, is "without a doubt the result of a search for security in an unstable world; for it is the young married people who have been through the disorientating experience of war—eager for security, resistant to unreasonable regimentation—who are the consumers of maternity and pediatric care. They are looking for security when they have their babies and highly prize being together to share the great experience."[63] Couples defined security not strictly in terms of the physical safety of mother and child, but also as the emotional strength derived from togetherness. From where Corbin stood, at the helm of the leading US organization promoting the Read method, these questions—national security, personal security, and young couples' desire to be together during labor—were intertwined. On the heels of lengthy wartime separation and under the shadow of the atom bomb, couples did not want and had no need to endure separation during the most important moment of their married lives.

Corbin tied this desire for togetherness to another factor that had redefined the American obstetric scene in the mid-twentieth century: the rise of a consumer culture. The postwar American economy was changing in fundamental ways. Escaping World War II unscathed, American industry hummed. Blue- and white-collar workers enjoyed unprecedented wealth and buying power and a rising sense of self linked to consumption patterns. The postwar period also witnessed increasing numbers of consumers enrolling in employer-based health care plans, leading them to greater access to medical services and a readiness to demand customer satisfaction from doctors and hospitals. By paying toward insurance policies, or having their employers foot the bill as a benefit of their employment, Americans began to see themselves as medical consumers "entitled to care without the stigma of grudging charity" that had sometimes characterized hospital care prior to World War II.[64] They chose medical care "as they would the other services or commodities bought in the open market—whether it be an armchair or fresh fish."[65] In Britain and France, where the state provided universal health care, consumers felt no less empowered to demand the services they desired, including prenatal education.[66]

Evolving economic relations between medical providers and consumers only in part explain women's sense of authority and empowerment to ask for—and get—what they wanted in maternity care. Middle- and upper-class white women had since the early twentieth century been vocal in their demands about how they wanted to give birth, lobbying effectively in both the United States and Great Britain for expanded access to anesthesia. Women's rising level of education surely contributed to their growing sense of authority about the kind of birth they wanted and what they saw as dignified maternity care. Corbin observes that providing maternity services for well-educated mothers is "a challenge to the doctor and nurse" who "no longer hold a mystical power."[67] That maternity care providers chafed under the demands of well-educated medical consumers is evident in the words of one British physician who stated that, before World War II, "the profession was able to do much more good when the public had unquestioned confidence.... The less they know, the happier they are."[68] Doctors bemoaned their diminished authority, but those medical professionals who were receptive to the Read method attracted a patient following, benefitting financially from its popular appeal. Over the 1950s a growing number of hospitals responded to consumer demand by allowing advance tours of their facilities and permitting husbands to remain with their wives during labor. Rooming-in, which kept the newborn with the mother rather than in a hospital nursery, gave some hospitals an advantage in the marketplace. By 1959 the American College of Obstetricians and Gynecologists' *Manual of Standards* reflected these consumer demands by noting that these services, as well as prenatal preparation courses for expectant mothers and fathers, enjoyed great popularity.[69]

As the Read method won supporters, women began to share their birth stories with Dick-Read, their Natural Childbirth instructors, and their friends and relatives. In 1946 Dick-Read wrote that "a day rarely passes without a letter from someone expressing gratitude that such simple measures can give such satisfactory results."[70] In a typical letter, from 1950, an English mother wrote to Dick-Read that giving birth using his approach "was a great and wonderful experience" and "the happiest day of my life." Vocal in her advocacy for the method, "I am always telling people about your teaching."[71]

Word-of-mouth certainly figured prominently in the Read method's popularization. Though most GPs and ob/gyns in both the United Kingdom and the United States resisted the Read method, demand grew from below thanks to the high marks mothers gave it. One American hospital receptionist captured this popular enthusiasm when she observed that "mothers used to leave with their new babies [and] the doctors would crack at them, 'See you next year.' Most of the women would say, 'You will not!' Today, do you know what mothers answer? They say, 'I hope so. It was wonderful.'"[72]

Not all women trained in Natural Childbirth—so-called "Read mothers"—had the positive experience he believed was nearly universally attainable. Pursuing their objectives within the parameters of standard maternity care posed challenges, with women's efforts frequently thwarted. A 1949 letter from one New York City mother to her Natural Childbirth instructor paints a portrait of the typical midcentury urban, white, middle-class American birth experience and its implications for those who sought to use Dick-Read's alternative. Though Mrs. K. hoped to forgo any pain medication, her "birth was anything but natural."[73] Not long after her labor began, Mrs. K. was admitted to a Manhattan hospital. As was common in the United States in the 1940s, even for couples trained in the Read method, her husband stayed in the waiting room. She entered a labor room furnished with "a horrible iron bed, narrow, no pillow and a cross on the wall. It looked like a prison cell."[74] Her obstetrician, Dr. Brown, told the nurse that Mrs. K. was "one of Dr. Reed's [sic]," but that seemed to have no meaning for her care. Dick-Read advocated the steady companionship of a doctor, nurse, or spouse by the laboring woman's side; Mrs. K. was left alone for stretches that appeared to her to be "endless." Dr. Brown came eventually, did a pelvic exam, and, without a word, stepped out and then returned with "a little white pill." "You mustn't fight [this]. It will help you to sleep and relax," he told her. Under his gentle but firm insistence, and exhausted from her lengthy, lonely labor, she obediently took the pill, which knocked her out for several hours. Nearly a day after her admission, Mrs. K. had not fully advanced through the first stage of labor. Intent on hastening labor's progress, "somebody gave me an injection. I had absolutely no strength to resist or to ask or to do anything." Mrs. K. felt the intensity of her contractions increase exponentially. She began to push and "felt quite happy and relieved doing it.... I enjoyed myself." But then, despite her wishes, her doctor administered ether. "I remember turning away from it—but of course I was helpless." Dr. Brown delivered Mrs. K.'s son with the assistance of forceps, she later learned. Reflecting on her experience, Mrs. K. noted that Dr. Brown "is a perfect doctor for your body—but nothing for the soul." She felt cheated out of a desired experience and "will always wonder what exactly happened to me when I was unconscious." In an indictment of the medical profession, she asked her childbirth educator, "the next time I do want a doctor with soul—I wonder where I [will] find him?"[75]

Much of Mrs. K.'s description of her experience in an American hospital would have been familiar to urban, middle- and upper-class, white women in Britain and France. The aloof, noncommunicative doctor offered little in the way of bedside manner. His authority was unchallenged and it was all but unthinkable to resist compliance with what he determined to be in the patient's best interest. Rather than accompany Mrs. K. throughout her labor, neither Dr. Brown nor any member of the nursing staff offered effective emotional support, let alone constant companionship, while her husband was denied access to her. The physician's unchallenged authority enabled him to easily trump her desires for an unmedicated birth, as he cajoled and ultimately compelled her to take sedatives, uterine stimulants, and anesthesia. Despite her prenatal preparation and her aspirations, Mrs. K.'s efforts to assert herself and her vision for the birth she desired were undermined and dismissed.

***

It was this harsh, alienating, interventionist atmosphere that Dick-Read and his allies sought to revolutionize and they faced an uphill battle. The heart of the problem lay in the routine use of anesthetics that robbed women of their conscious, active participation in childbirth. Women found in the methods that Dick-Read advocated an appealing alternative to standard practices. But maternity services needed to undergo systemic change for women like Mrs. K. to get the kind of support and care neces-sary to achieve their goals. The rise of more woman-centered maternity care was still a distant dream in 1949, when Mrs. K. gave birth. Only in the 1970s and 1980s did such change come to maternity care in the United States, but it remains hotly contested whether those developments made a substantive, positive difference in women's childbearing experiences or were mere window-dressing designed to placate consumers without really threatening the medical establishment's authority and control.

Long before those struggles unfolded, while the Read method was still just getting off the ground in Great Britain and the United States, another, similar psychological approach to obstetric pain was taking shape in continental Europe. Developed in the USSR and rapidly earning a following in France, psychoprophylaxis overshadowed the Read method's modest inroads outside the Anglophone world. So quick was its rise that Dick-Read was left bewildered and bitter, clamoring with increasing shrill-ness as the 1950s progressed for the credit that he believed was his due.

CHAPTER 2

꙯

The Soviet Method, 1936–51

World War II was a catastrophe for the Soviet Union. Recent estimates put casualties at around twenty-seven million Soviet soldiers and civilians. Beyond the demographic cataclysm, the nation faced unfathomable physical devastation. Thousands of villages were wiped off the map; transport systems were in chaos; grain-producing areas had been scorched; factories, schools, and hospitals lay in ruins. The state had to launch the reconstruction project amid dire financial straits, limited human resources, and the rising specter of tensions with the United States. The Soviet government found itself in a bind: leaders hoped to buoy women's reproduction in an effort to recover from population losses, and they believed that alleviating the pain of labor would encourage women to have more children; at the same time, budgetary demands were great and resources strained to the limit. Even within the realm of women's and children's health, other issues were (rightly) seen as more pressing. With questions of maternal and infant death still to be conquered, alleviating obstetric pain seemed a luxury.[1]

Joseph Stalin's government had long seen a link between its economic agenda and women's reproductive function. Like other European nations devastated by demographic losses in World War I, the USSR feared inadequate population growth. To fuel industrialization and ensure national security, the country needed more workers and soldiers. Fast on the heels of famine in Ukraine, southern Russia, and Kazakhstan, in 1936 the Soviet government banned abortion—which had been legal since 1920—and launched a pronatalist campaign.[2] Soviet leaders sought to support increased fecundity through a variety of measures, including greater funding for maternal and child health, expanded child care services, and financial and material benefits for mothers of large families. Article 122 of the 1936 Soviet Constitution guaranteed "government protection of mother and child,...[and] an expansive system of birth centers, crèches, and kindergartens."[3] It was incumbent upon Soviet obstetricians and gynecologists to "raise considerably our scientific work to a level worthy of our wonderful socialist motherland."[4] From 1936 to 1940, nearly 2.5 million Soviet mothers benefited from a campaign to promote the routine use of anesthesia, especially nitrous oxide, in childbirth. An impressive number in absolute terms, this figure accounted for less than 10 percent of the USSR's more than thirty million births in this period.[5]

The Soviet government had neither the pharmaceutical industrial capacity nor the human resources to fulfill its promise of widespread access to obstetric anesthesia. By 1941, the year that the USSR entered World War II, medical institutions in the eastern Ukrainian city of Kharkov, for example, were "to a greater or lesser extent accustomed to the work of pain relief in childbirth," but the depth and breadth of that effort was far from satisfactory.[6] The central government's plan for 1941 called for the use of pain relief in 30 percent of rural Soviet births and 40 percent in cities with over fifty thousand inhabitants. The Russian Soviet Federated Socialist Republic (RSFSR) averaged a mere 20.9 percent. In rural areas, pain relief in childbirth was utilized in a "miniscule" number of cases.[7]

World War II destroyed the modest gains in obstetric anesthesia that were made during the interwar years. The question of pain relief in childbirth had, obviously, been far from a priority under German occupation, and almost nowhere was the war's impact more acute than in Ukraine, where the system for maternal and child health came crashing down.[8] According to the Ukrainian Ministry of Public Health (Minzdrav), the number of women in Kiev who received pain relief in childbirth plummeted from 47 percent before the war to 21 percent in 1944, when the Red Army liberated the city. In urban parts of Kharkov region (*oblast'*), 34 percent of birthing women benefited from pain relief in 1940, declining to a mere 3 percent in 1944. For the few rural areas across Ukraine for which there are wartime statistics, already modest numbers dwindled to near zero.[9] As Comrade Sverdlova from the Kharkov Medical-Sanitation Workers' Union noted in January 1945, conditions in medical facilities had "significantly improved" after liberation, but grave supply and personnel shortages persisted.[10]

In the immediate postwar era, central authorities were too overwhelmed to deal effectively with maternity care, leaving the Soviet Union's constituent republics on their own to address the problem. Ukraine's women's and children's health care system recovered unevenly. The number of obstetric beds available in Kiev rebounded from, in 1944, 30 percent of its prewar level to 84 percent in 1946. Kharkov region enjoyed a similarly rapid recovery, more than tripling its number of obstetric beds to reach 87 percent of prewar capacity by 1947. Ukraine's rural areas trailed far behind its cities. Many collective farms had no specialized birth facilities whatsoever, let alone the supplies or the staff to administer pharmaceutical pain relief. Where facilities existed, they were of questionable quality. For example, a collective farm in Kharkov region established a maternity clinic in 1949, but it had no electricity until 1954. Village women continued to prefer the local lay midwives and were only slowly coming to rely on the professional, state-trained midwives.[11]

In urban and rural areas alike, Soviet women gave birth in conditions that would have appalled urban, white, middle-class Western Europeans and Americans. Labor and delivery rooms accommodated multiple women at a time, and overburdened midwives treated their patients with brusque indifference. After giving birth, women spent their week-long lying-in period in large, noisy, Spartan wards, isolated from loved ones. Fearing the spread of germs, maternity clinics banned all family members—including fathers—from visits to the new mothers and their babies. Even basic services such as heating, hot water, and clean linens were sometimes lacking in these facilities.[12]

In the centralized, bureaucratized, and authoritarian Soviet context, edicts from above and not demand from below catalyzed change in maternity care, including in the arena of obstetric anesthesia. In mid-1947, officials in the Ukrainian Minzdrav's Department of Maternity Wards and Women's Clinics took the lead in broaching the question of obstetric pain relief by putting out a call for recommended measures as a step toward establishing a republic-wide standard practice. An effort to promote fecundity after the deaths of tens of millions of Soviet citizens surely was at the heart of this renewed concern. Even before the war had ended, a 1944 law laid the groundwork for the government's postwar pronatalist agenda, with support for single mothers and other benefits intended to boost reproduction. As in the interwar years, the desire to raise the birthrate was linked with a push to alleviate childbirth pain.[13] Ukraine's singularly catastrophic population losses and Kharkov's reputation as a national center for medical training and research combined to create the right environment for the development and promotion of both pharmacological and psychological innovation in obstetric pain relief.

On April 14, 1948, Ukraine's Department of Maternity Wards and Women's Clinics issued an "Instruction for Application of the Simplest

Methods of Pain Relief in Normal Birth" penned by Professor V. N. Khmelevskii.[14] These guidelines provided practitioners with what the Ukrainian government considered to be the best available, most practical methods for application in the widest number of clinical facilities, including those in understaffed, undersupplied rural areas. The Instruction offered several options for pain relief at each stage of labor. During labor's first stage, it advocated what came to be called the Khmelevskii method, a warm-water solution of glucose, calcium chlorate, ascorbic acid (vitamin C), and thiamin (vitamin B_1) drunk every two hours after the onset of labor pain. Khmelevskii also recommended an alternative formula, with mostly the same ingredients and the addition of aspirin, taken once or twice during the course of labor. If these gentle measures proved inadequate, the midwife could use cupping on the abdomen; apply ice to the lower belly; use a Kiparskii Stick, composed of menthol and paraffin, on the belly; give a cocoa butter–based suppository that combined the anesthetic properties of the botanical belladonna with opioid and non-opioid pharmaceutical analgesics; or inject a solution of magnesium sulfate (Epsom salt) and the opiate pantopon. For transition, the last and usually most painful part of the first phase of labor, the Instruction advised the local administration of Novocain in the vaginal area. Mistaking moans and grunts for signs of pain rather than effort, physicians might administer a light dose of ether during the pushing stage.[15]

The 1948 Instruction drew attention to the use of psychological techniques to enhance pharmacological measures of pain relief. Khmelevskii noted the need for every member of the staff, "from the janitor to the doctor, to treat [the laboring woman] in a singularly respectful, attentive, and tactful manner." Every institution should maintain a clean and calm atmosphere, which worked to "suggest a feeling of complete safety." Khmelevskii emphasized the importance of using suggestion to promote the expectant mother's sense of "vigor, calm, and security."[16] Though likely unfamiliar with the works of Dick-Read, Khmelevskii echoed his beliefs when warning of the dangers of a careless, negative word spoken by a physician or other member of the medical team. The medical staff had to maintain what was described as "the sterility of the word."[17] Just as the physical atmosphere required special care and attention in order to inhibit the spread of contagion, so, too, did the clinical environment demand caution with words, which could be as deleterious to patient outcome as germs. Above all, Khmelevskii maintained that it was crucial that the entire staff of the birth facility "deeply believed in the application of [recommended] pain relief measures and conveyed this faith to every woman in labor."[18]

YBP Library Services

MICHAELS, PAULA A., 1966-

LAMAZE: AN INTERNATIONAL HISTORY.

Cloth   240 P.
NEW YORK: OXFORD UNIVERSITY PRESS, 2014
SER: OXFORD STUDIES IN INTERNATIONAL HISTORY.

AUTH: MONASH UNIVERSITY. DISCUSSES HOW LAMAZE
METHOD TRAVELLED ACROSS BORDERS, 1940-1970S.
LCCN 2013042938
  ISBN 0199738645   **Library PO#** FIRM ORDERS

		List	29.95	USD
8395 NATIONAL UNIVERSITY LIBRAR		Disc	14.0%	
App. Date 12/03/14 SHHS	8214-08	Net	25.76	USD

SUBJ: NATURAL CHILDBIRTH--CROSS-CULTURAL STUDIES.

CLASS RG661   DEWEY# 618.45   LEVEL ADV-AC

YBP Library Services

MICHAELS, PAULA A., 1966

LAMAZE: AN INTERNATIONAL HISTORY.

Cloth   240 P.
NEW YORK: OXFORD UNIVERSITY PRESS, 2014
SER: OXFORD STUDIES IN INTERNATIONAL HISTORY.

AUTH: MONASH UNIVERSITY. DISCUSSES HOW LAMAZE
METHOD TRAVELLED ACROSS BORDERS, 1940-1970S.
  LCCN 2013042938
  ISBN 0199738645   **Library PO#** FIRM ORDERS

		List	29.95	USD
8395 NATIONAL UNIVERSITY LIBRAR		Disc	14.0%	
App. Date 12/03/14 SHHS	8214-08	Net	25.76	USD

SUBJ: NATURAL CHILDBIRTH--CROSS-CULTURAL STUDIES.

CLASS RG661   DEWEY# 618.45   LEVEL ADV-AC

Over the next two years, the 1948 Instruction was put into practice across Ukraine, with particularly slow progress in rural areas, where personnel and supply shortages were acute. Zhitomir officials, for example, claimed that in urban birth facilities medical practitioners utilized pain relief measures in a respectable 60 to 80 percent of births. By contrast, the region's smaller towns reported pain alleviation efforts in only 20 to 30 percent of cases.[19] The desire to curry favor with superiors may have led to inflated figures, but even so these statistics speak to great disparities between rural and urban areas. Regional health officials across Ukraine blamed inadequate staff and supplies for their inability to make greater headway in obstetric pain relief.[20] Administrators in Kharkov, for example, noted the shortage of staples like glucose and Epsom salt in nearly every medical facility in the city. Complaints surfaced that numerous regions lacked the essential ingredients for the Khmelevskii method, but no evidence suggests any meaningful response.[21]

Even where supplies existed, the Khmelevskii method frequently yielded disappointing clinical results. Negative evaluations arrived at Ukraine's Minzdrav offices coupled with requests for drugs other than those recommended in the 1948 Instruction. Regional officials admitted that pain "quite frequently surpassed the efficacy of the pain relief measures."[22] According to a typical 1949 report, 72 percent of births in Dnepropetrovsk were carried out using pain relief measures. Of these, only 18 percent enjoyed "complete pain relief," while fully 26 percent experienced "dubious [benefit] or the absence of effect."[23] The 1948 Instruction did not detail how medical personnel should evaluate the Khmelevskii method, but it is clear from extant records that maternity caregivers rarely elicited patient feedback. Only one report makes explicit reference to medical personnel seeking women's own evaluation of their experience.[24]

Evidence in late 1948 of a rise in back-alley abortions and a concomitant drop in the birthrate, described by central authorities as being of "crisis" proportions, perhaps indirectly fueled a renewed push for anesthesia in maternity care at the national level.[25] In June 1949, the USSR Minzdrav leadership received a report on the state of obstetric anesthesia endorsing nitrous oxide as the best option for pain relief in childbirth.[26] This method was native to Russia, making it a good choice in the nationalistic political atmosphere of the era. It also met many essential criteria: easy to administer, fairly effective, devoid of adverse effects on labor's progress, and low risk for mother and baby. Significantly, the report advocated its use in cases of normal birth, not just when complications required intervention. More than a few Soviet medical personnel expressed doubt about the necessity of the routine use of anesthesia in birth, but underfunding was really the primary hurdle to its more widespread adoption. Each birth using nitrous oxide cost approximately two rubles, a pittance in any one case, but a significant aggregate expense in a country where over two million births occurred annually. Maternity wards did not have the finances to pay for nitrous oxide, the machines to administer it, or the personnel to staff the machines. Funds were also needed to boost production of nitrous oxide, which was in critically short supply. Moreover, the Soviet-manufactured machine used to administer the gas had proven to be flawed. A more durable machine that was simpler to use and allowed for self-administration—like the gas-and-air machine widely available in Britain since the 1930s—was needed.[27]

Moscow endorsed the 1949 report's recommendation to expand the use of nitrous oxide in normal birth, but failed to tackle the underlying financial obstacles.[28] Minzdrav put forward new standards for best practices in obstetric anesthesia that emphasized the use of nitrous oxide.[29] Minister of Public Health E. I. Smirnov issued an order to expand the training of medical personnel in the obstetric application of anesthetics and analgesics, to repair existing nitrous oxide machines, to create a panel to study the problem of obstetric anesthesia, and to move forward with clinical trials of gas-and-air machine prototypes, five hundred of which were to be produced by the first quarter of 1950. Production of nitrous oxide was also supposed to grow, with the USSR's Central Pharmaceutical Administration ordered to produce five thousand canisters for obstetric use by the end of 1950. However, no indication was given as to where the financing was to come from for these initiatives. Much finger-pointing ensued over who was to blame for the lack of follow-through, all to no avail.[30] Medical professionals and government officials concurred about the value of nitrous oxide in maternity care, but faith in efficacy alone could not put the necessary supplies in the hands of caregivers. Without a dramatic expansion of funding for the Soviet Union's pharmaceutical industry, all state directives for obstetric pain relief had limited impact.

The slow progress made in alleviating pain in childbirth was part of a pattern of low-quality maternal and child health services in the USSR in the late 1940s and early 1950s. Ukrainian Minzdrav officials criticized maternity wards for failing to perform even the most routine care.[31] In an environment of dire need and severely limited funding, obstetric anesthesia constituted a marginal concern. More than passing reference to obstetric pain alleviation in textbooks and journals was rare.[32] Even after the fresh attention sparked by directives from Kiev and Moscow, the issue remained a low priority for public health officials. With high rates of maternal and infant mortality, poor professional qualifications among medical personnel, staffing shortages, and other pressing issues, the Soviet government of necessity put priorities and funds in the field of women's health elsewhere.

A NEW PSYCHOLOGICAL ALTERNATIVE: PSYCHOPROPHYLAXIS ON THE RISE, 1947–51

To circumvent the limited availability of pharmaceuticals, a handful of Soviet obstetricians were drawn in the late 1940s to psychological methods of pain relief, such as suggestion.[33] Devotees of psychological approaches were particularly numerous in Ukraine, and by 1950 physicians in several cities there were working on combined psychological and pharmacological treatments for labor pain. Despite success, hypnosis and suggestion were unlikely to gain wide currency because there was no simple, accessible way for psychotherapists to train large numbers of physicians and midwives in this technique.[34] Psychological methods also typically demanded ample caregiver-patient contact, both in the weeks prior to birth and during labor itself.

Like Grantly Dick-Read, Kharkov psychologist I. Z. Vel'vovskii, pictured in fig. 2.1, was dogged in his pursuit of a psychological remedy to the pain of childbirth.[35] Under the tutelage of renowned neuropsychologist K. I. Platonov, Vel'vovskii spent the 1920s and 1930s researching the use of suggestion and hypnosis as means of obstetric anesthesia until World War II forced him to put his research on hiatus while directing an evacuation hospital.[36] Picking up where he left off in his investigations, Vel'vovskii returned to his duties in Kharkov not long after the city's 1944 liberation, but grew increasingly doubtful that hypnosuggestion could ever prove practical on a national scale.

Vel'vovskii set out to develop a psychological approach to obstetric pain relief that was easy and "accessible to any rank-and-file doctor and any ordinary midwife, feasible in any [rural] birth facility."[37] He and his team put forward their case for psychoprophylaxis initially in an article published in the Soviet journal *Obstetrics and Gynecology* in late 1950 and, more fully, in a 1954 textbook intended for physicians. They defined psychoprophylaxis as "a system of measures aimed at preventing the appearance and development of labor pain and effected through influences exerted on the higher divisions of the central nervous system."[38] While vigilant for any physical complications that might cause pain, caregivers were to sustain a woman's positive outlook on childbirth and to cultivate in her the conviction that

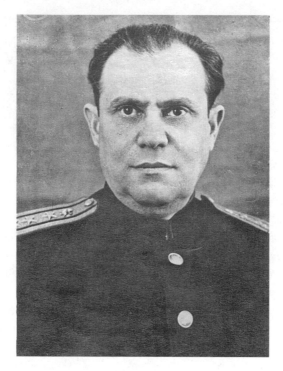

Figure 2.1: I. Z. Vel′vovskii, ca. mid-1940s. Courtesy of Department of Psychotherapy, KhMAPO.

labor would be painless. As with the use of hypnosuggestion, attendant medical personnel fought "influences by words whose meaning may serve to condition, provoke and reinforce pain sensations in labor."[39] Prenatal childbirth education classes removed any fears of the impending event, with psychotherapy to be used if anxieties persisted. Vel′vovskii explicitly distinguished psychoprophylaxis from hypnosis with his emphasis on the active, fully conscious participation of the laboring woman. Whereas hypnosis worked to suppress cortical function, psychoprophylaxis mobilized it in the elimination of pain.[40]

Vel′vovskii posited that a series of prenatal classes with expectant mothers rewired the cerebral cortex's reception of stimuli that had once been perceived as painful. After an initial, private physical exam and intake assessment, during which the physician gauged the patient's fears, a series of physician-led lessons began.[41] Women were grouped by their "general development" and "preparedness," code for sorting them along lines of class and educational background. Vel′vovskii encouraged physicians to separate first-time mothers from those who had given birth before.[42] Many women had negative memories of previous labors, leading them to expect pain and making them challenging cases for psychoprophylactic preparation. Establishing belief in the painless nature of childbirth for first-time mothers, Vel'vovskii argued, was easier.[43] A series of group sessions gave physicians an opportunity to impart knowledge to their patients and reinforce the idea that childbirth would be a painless experience. Like Dick-Read, Vel'vovskii insisted that "the expectant mother must be convinced that childbirth is a physiological act and, like any normal physiological act, it will be painless, that painless or slightly painful labor is the norm for which we must strive."[44] The second session with the patient—the first held in a group setting—offered a lecture on female anatomy and the physiological changes that accompanied pregnancy, including the three stages of labor and the natural painlessness of normal birth. The third and fourth sessions taught women to recognize the signs of labor's onset, detailed the process of dilation and effacement, and trained women in "pain prevention techniques."[45] These methods included many that would be familiar to anyone attending an American natural childbirth course in the 1960s and 1970s: patterned breathing, light massage, and the use of pressure points, especially on the lower back and hips. Laboring women were encouraged to walk around, time contractions, and stay alert during the first stage of labor to facilitate the process and track progress.[46] The fifth session provided guidance for the second stage of labor, including body positioning and bearing down during expulsion. Pain prevention during this stage meant teaching the expectant mother "how to strain well and properly. . . . The physician must make the pregnant woman understand that the ability to [bear down] properly helps at once to prevent pain and expedite labor." Fear distorted women's natural impulses, leading them "to try to suppress the urge for straining or to prevent proper straining, something which may prolong the course of labor."[47] Doctors, not the laboring women, knew how best to give birth, and it was their responsibility to teach patients how to do it.

In the final lesson of psychoprophylactic training, the state's demands and the physician's authority became fully transparent. This session was conducted at the maternity ward, where physicians oriented women to the ward's layout and facilities, detailed how admission would proceed, and explained the policies and procedures to expect when they arrived in labor. Emphasizing the need for a sterile environment, doctors explained how women would, upon admission, have their genitalia shaved, receive an enema, take a shower, and be given a vaginal examination, all standard practices at the time in the USSR and much of the West. Doctors advised expectant mothers "to be ready to fulfill the requirements of the maternity home personnel precisely and to be considerate of them." To be a good patient meant to be compliant and respectful of the doctors' and nurses' needs. Finally, the physician used that last meeting with the patient to praise Soviet power, explaining that "the solicitude of the maternity home medical personnel...is part of the state patronage of the mother. In analyzing the concern of the state and society for motherhood the physician should emotionally emphasize motherhood's high social virtues confirmed in the Soviet Union by the establishment of government awards—orders and medals—and honorary titles to mothers of many children."[48] The joy of motherhood meant gratitude toward the regime for the material support and social status it accorded mothers.[49] After this final lesson, women arrived at maternity wards "immunized to labor pain."[50]

Precisely when and how psychoprophylaxis emerged as a coherent curriculum, distinct from prenatal hypnosuggestion, is hard to establish. Throughout the 1947–50 period, reference is made in medical journals and public health records to hypnosis, suggestion, "psychotherapeutic pain relief," and psychoprophylaxis. Ample slippage in how these terms are applied makes it challenging to distinguish between the application of hypnosuggestion and the psychological method Vel'vovskii developed during 1948–49 in Kharkov. Terminological muddiness began to dissipate after a December 1949 conference, at which Vel'vovskii unveiled his "psychotherapeutic method" nationally. Leningrad obstetrician A. P. Nikolaev rechristened the approach "psychoprophylaxis," a term he hoped suggested the prevention of pain's initial development.[51] At the conference's closing session, Platonov noted that the method had been endorsed by the state and could move from an approach in isolated clinical facilities to a mass phenomenon. Within months of the 1949 conference, psychoprophylaxis had reportedly already spread to the republics of Uzbekistan and Georgia.[52]

Distinguishing psychoprophylaxis from other psychological approaches to obstetric pain already in circulation posed a challenge to its promoters. In 1951 psychotherapist M. I. Koganov questioned Vel'vovskii's claim to original authorship. Koganov complained to authorities in Moscow that he, in fact, had been working on a method much like psychoprophylaxis since 1935, had written a dissertation on the subject in 1941, and, after wartime delays, defended his dissertation in 1946. In early 1951 he published an article on "Anesthetization in Childbirth by Means of Suggestion without Advance Hypnotic Preparation."[53] The study employed the terminology of hypnosis and suggestion already long in circulation, but it indeed promoted some strategies similar to those Vel'vovskii and his collaborators recommended. Koganov's complaint triggered an investigation that kept Vel'vovskii and his team from having their work on psychoprophylaxis considered for the Stalin Prize, the country's highest honor in the arts and sciences. Some compelling but circumstantial evidence supported

Koganov's accusation. Platonov was on Koganov's dissertation committee and was familiar with his research. Vel'vovskii's collaborators V. Ploticher and K. Shugom had worked under Koganov's direction for four months in 1948 on psychological approaches to obstetric pain relief, yet his work was not credited in their publications with Vel'vovskii. The Scientific Medical Council (UMS) ultimately cleared Vel'vovskii of the plagiarism charge, noting that Koganov had remained wedded to a conventional use of suggestion, while Vel'vovskii's method moved in a fresh direction. The UMS highlighted Koganov's emphasis on suggestion without prior preparation, in contrast to the extensive prenatal instruction at the heart of Vel'vovskii's approach.[54]

Koganov's work was not the only challenge to Vel'vovskii's claim to originality. In a 1949 report to Ukraine's Deputy Minister of Public Health, Vel'vovskii asserted that "no one in the bourgeois countries is conducting" similar research, but his work bore an uncanny resemblance to that of Dick-Read.[55] Although Vel'vovskii's method emerged independently, it shared with the Read method common assumptions about fear and the naturally painless quality of childbirth, and both approaches sought a psychological remedy to pain. Despite considerable overlap in their theory and method, their explanations of the origin of and connection between fear and pain differed. Like Read advocates, psychoprophylaxis's supporters stressed that pain was not a biological inevitability, as is clear when Nikolaev states that "If the head is in any way responsible for labor pain, it is not the head of the fetus but that of the mother."[56] Compared to Dick-Read, Vel'vovskii offered a more elaborate theory of the cause of pain in childbirth, explained as the product of sociohistorical processes and treated with methods inspired by neuropsychology. Whereas Dick-Read emphasized the role of the individual psyche and the physical tension that fear created in the cervix, Vel'vovskii accentuated the impact of collective conditioning accumulated over millennia and distilled into the experience of each expectant mother. Art and literature, such as Leo Tolstoy's *War and Peace*, with its grim portrayal of childbirth, reinforced stories handed down from mother to daughter and woven into a culture's collective memory, what Soviet neuropsychologist M. B. Bekhterev, a contemporary of Pavlov, dubbed a "collective reflex."[57] The product of visual and verbal suggestions, this collective reflex made childbirth nearly universally painful. Labor's onset then triggered the individual conditional response of pain. Prenatal preparation had a potentially therapeutic effect, ridding women of this socially conditioned fear. In both preparatory lessons and during the course of labor and delivery, "physicians must normalize and reorganize the minds of women poisoned by erroneous ideas, cultivated over many centuries, that labor pain is inevitable."[58] Reeducation of expectant mothers could eliminate their experience of pain, while mass propaganda had the potential to erode the deep-seated social underpinnings of the historically conditioned, universal belief that pain naturally and unavoidably accompanied labor and birth.[59]

Dick-Read ventured no grand claims about collective reflexes or Pavlovian conditioning, though he similarly trumpeted the broad social, economic, and demographic implications of his method. Of immediate concern to him was the personal, private, individual experience. Central to his work was a belief in childbirth's profoundly mystical quality. He characterized the spiritual dimension of childbirth as "the greatest ultimate force" and the source of maternal love, with all the implications that carried for the next generation's psychological well-being.[60] For a secular scientist like Vel'vovskii, such rhetoric had no place in serious medical and psychological research. Even if Vel'vovskii had been inclined in that direction, expressing these sentiments would have been impossible in the atheist USSR.

Vel'vovskii pled his case for psychoprophylaxis in a climate where medicine and science were highly politicized. Scholarly research had to pass ideological muster. Especially after World War II, tensions with the West prompted researchers to demonstrate their patriotism by genuflecting before the Russian and Soviet scientists who preceded them and by rejecting innovations linked, however loosely, to Western bourgeois capitalism. Ideology's preeminence worked in some cases to elevate charlatans to positions of great power, with damaging consequences for Soviet science. The most notorious example was Trofim Lysenko, who promoted the unsubstantiated theory that acquired traits could be inherited; his influence held back development of the budding field of genetics in the USSR. Unlike Lysenko, Pavlov had earned his place in the pantheon of Soviet science, though homage to his work, too, was deployed for political ends. At the 1950 centennial celebration of Pavlov's birth, S. I. Vavilov, head of the USSR Academy of Sciences, ushered in an era in which Pavlov's work was applied in a wide range of scientific and medical arenas, both appropriate and inappropriate. Through his explication of the nervous system, Pavlov offered a materialist foundation for understanding the mind-body connection; his work would become the foundation for all Soviet psychology. Ritual kowtowing to Pavlovian physiology became an indispensable component of medical teaching, research, and writing, and Pavlov's ideas were integrated into the agendas of research institutions and the curricula of medical educational facilities.[61] Every department at the Kharkov Medical Institute conducted its own celebration of Pavlov's life and work, and offered an educational program about the relationship between its specialty and Pavlov's research.[62] Like Lysenkoism, orthodox Pavlovism impeded the development of certain areas of Soviet science for which its relevance was questionable. For neuropsychologists like Platonov and Vel'vovskii, Pavlov's influence on their thinking proved to be both of genuine merit and to political advantage.[63]

For the promotion of psychoprophylaxis, the timing of the Pavlov centennial celebrations in 1949–50 was fortuitous. Supporters of the method drew repeated, ostentatious attention to psychoprophylaxis's rationale in Pavlovian ideas about the physiological bases of pain. As Platonov elaborated, Pavlov's work on human physiology gave a material foundation to psychoprophylaxis and armed physicians and psychotherapists with the means to induce at will specific physiological responses in the human body under controlled conditions.[64] The emphasis on Pavlov is especially pronounced in Vel'vovskii's 1954 psychoprophylaxis textbook. Two of seventeen chapters are wholly devoted to Pavlov's investigations into pain, states of consciousness, and conditional reflexes, and other chapters make liberal reference to his work.[65]

While this reliance on Pavlov was in keeping with the political demands of the day, it also had an appropriate place in the theoretical justification for psychoprophylaxis. Historian John Bell suggests that the reference to Pavlov was largely an opportunistic rhetorical strategy used to promote psychoprophylaxis under the restrictive ideological conditions that governed Soviet science in the late Stalinist period. While frequent invocation of Pavlov's name and theories was essential to the method's success, proponents in fact deeply believed in its relevance. In the 1920s and 1930s, Platonov and Vel'vovskii drew on Pavlov's work in their writings on hypnosis and suggestion. By 1950, they had spent a quarter-century building on the implications of Pavlov's work for pain management during childbirth. Reference to Pavlov by the architects of psychoprophylaxis transcended rank careerism.[66]

However they justified their work theoretically, advocates for psychoprophylaxis appreciated the political propaganda value of an effective method of obstetric pain relief that was materially feasible on a mass scale. Soviet power, they claimed, deserved credit for making the issue of childbirth pain a priority. Nikolaev described the alleviation of women's pain during labor and birth as "one of the most important, most humane efforts of Soviet medicine."[67] Platonov enthused that "successes have been achieved, because none other than Soviet power pursued in such breadth and with an appreciation of the importance of the problem of pain relief in childbirth, and the liberation of women from suffering and strife."[68] Official discourse emphasized that "pain relief in the bourgeois countries is a privilege of the

rich; in the Soviet nation, all women, women workers and women collective farmers, enjoy the benefits of scientific achievements."[69] Women in the
West suffered because capitalist science served the almighty dollar, not the
masses, with pain relief given only to those who could pay.[70] Such claims
fit within a broader state strategy to present the Soviet government as a
benevolent protector of proletarian women. Psychoprophylaxis provided
evidence that the USSR, not the countries of the capitalist West, cared
more about women's well-being.

Making the political case for psychoprophylaxis was easier than persuading the medical community, which required careful study of the
method in accordance with professional research standards and conven-
tions. Appearing in 1950, Vel'vovskii and his collaborators' first published
assessment of psychoprophylaxis boasted an impressive success rate. With
an initial group of 562 expectant mothers prepared in psychoprophylaxis, Vel'vovskii claimed good to excellent results in 83 percent of cases.
Vel'vovskii scored women's performance as poor, fair, good, or excellent. In
cases of poor results, psychoprophylaxis offered no help, and, despite her
prenatal training, the laboring woman "conducted herself during the course
of labor as in a birth without pain relief."[71] A patient earned fair marks if
she exhibited some pain and unrest, a good grade if such complaints of pain
and restless behavior were minimal, and an excellent evaluation if "from
the beginning to end of labor the woman was active and demonstrated no
unease or pain."[72] Physicians made assessments based on the diagnosis of
any complications, the duration of each stage of labor, patient behavior and
demeanor, and the "woman's verbal account of her own sensations (complaints)."[73] The physician defined what information had value and assessed
its meaning. Women's testimonials earned only the negligible weight that
researchers accorded them.

Vel'vovskii and his collaborators advocated interviews with new mothers
after birth and during the seven- to ten-day lying-in period. They advised
obstetricians to judge these statements against their own observations
of laboring women's behavior to assess the efficacy of psychoprophylaxis.
Vel'vovskii stressed the need for "complete objectivity," which he saw as
grounded in physician observation, not patient testimony. Though the
woman "must be given a chance to describe her own sensations," he claimed
that "the appraisal of the [medical] personnel differs relatively rarely" from
that of the patient.[74] Vel'vovskii and his colleagues saw patient testimony
as a check on physicians' tendency to inflate success rates. They stressed
the importance of communication with the mother to make a valid and
accurate assessment of psychoprophylaxis, yet, as was the case in the West,
the power to evaluate and judge ultimately lay in the physician's hands.

How Soviet doctors evaluated psychoprophylaxis's success or failure was closely connected to physician expectations for patient behavior during labor and birth. What, exactly, were physicians looking for to rate psychoprophylaxis successful? Vel'vovskii and his colleagues expected Soviet women to exhibit discipline, defined as a calm and controlled demeanor, and a readiness to defer completely to the superior knowledge and experience of the medical staff.[75] These behaviors contrasted with those that the medical community rejected as inappropriate and undesirable. Women who showed restlessness, nervousness, or writhing were characterized as failures. Vel'vovskii and his team expressed particular disapproval of a woman in labor moaning, which they took as an indication that she was out of control, unable to communicate effectively with attendant medical personnel, and lost in an exaggerated, subjective experience of her pain.[76] The belief that psychoprophylaxis eliminated pain and that childbirth was naturally, normally painless left advocates for psychoprophylaxis with only women to blame for their screams. Unable or unwilling to admit the method's limitations, its promoters found many explanations for women's failures to experience pain relief, but the method itself was never at fault.

To illustrate and explain cases of failure in the application of psychoprophylaxis, Vel'vovskii and his coauthors offered detailed case studies of three first-time mothers. Comrade K., eighteen years old, served as an example of complete failure.[77] She complained of pain during her entire labor, but when instructed to undertake relief measures reportedly stated, "I don't need them." At another juncture, she lamented, "I have forgotten everything." During both the first and second stages of labor, she seemed restless and had "lost contact" with medical personnel, whose instructions she was unable to follow. In a subsequent interview, Comrade K. revealed that her husband had died unexpectedly a few days prior to the onset of labor. Twenty-two-year-old Comrade M. initially seemed headed for success. She was calm until she saw the bloody show, which frightened her. "The staff's explanation was poorly received, contact was lost, and pain relief measures ceased. Complaints of pain began. In that condition [Comrade M.] gave birth, becoming very agitated and complaining of pain the entire time." Comrade M.'s close relative had hemorrhaged to death after she gave birth, and, the authors argued, the sight of the bloody show triggered terror in Comrade M. Finally, twenty-six-year-old Comrade A. experienced no pain and went through her labor quite calmly. However, during her twenty-four-hour labor, she vomited repeatedly and with increasing frequency as labor progressed. Afterward, she was reported to have stated that "the vomiting—that was the worst, just like my mother said," which her doctors took to mean that the mother inadvertently induced Comrade

A.'s vomiting through suggestion.[78] In each of these cases, Vel'vovskii and his collaborators identified a preexisting trauma or fear that obstructed psychoprophylaxis's success. Vel'vovskii argued that, had the physician noted these psychological hurdles in advance, psychotherapy, in conjunction with psychoprophylactic training, could have rooted them out and paved the way for more successful outcomes.

How to judge outcomes and measure success cuts to the heart of questions of authority in the doctor-patient encounter. Women staked their claim to authority about their own bodily experience of pain during labor itself, through verbal and nonverbal cues about their comfort or discomfort communicated to the medical personnel. After delivery they reasserted this authority every time they told their birth stories during their lying-in period, when they shared rooms with several other new mothers in the maternity ward. If asked by medical personnel to assess their experiences, they again voiced their authoritative knowledge. At the same time, medical personnel chose whether or not to ask women to speak to these issues, decided what questions to ask, judged the value of the answers, and balanced women's evaluations against physician observations. In recording these evaluations for the state, medical personnel served as arbiters of women's experiences, writing up assessments for records to which patients had no access. These records then served as the foundation for medical studies and policy debates. No public venue existed in which Soviet women could express firsthand their experiences of childbirth. There was no free press to publish women's birth stories unencumbered by the state's censorial hand. To the extent that women's magazines turned to the issue of childbirth, they focused not on women's personal experiences in pregnancy, labor, and birth, but on the government's benevolent care of Soviet mothers.[79] No Soviet birth memoirs of the kind that had begun to appear in the West made their way into print. Although a Soviet baby boom was on, mothers' voices were absent from the public sphere, in stark contrast to the cases of Great Britain, France, and the United States. Beyond medical discourse, within networks of families and friends, women asserted their authoritative knowledge about their experiences, but their perspective barely left a trace on a public record crafted by medical professionals.

***

In an atmosphere of personnel and pharmaceutical supply shortages, psychoprophylaxis seemed like an ideal alternative. The fact that, as one 1950 report in Kharkov stressed, it "does not demand any financial expenditure, which makes it absolutely appropriate for pain relief on a mass scale," largely explains its rapid rise to national prominence.[80] On February 13, 1951, Soviet Minister of Public Health Smirnov issued Order No. 142, which commanded the constituent republics of the USSR to utilize psychoprophylaxis as the standard method of pain relief in all Soviet maternity wards. In inimitable Soviet style, psychoprophylaxis became the USSR's official, centrally dictated method of childbearing. Order No. 142 inaugurated a full-court press to spread psychoprophylaxis as far and as fast as possible. Within one month, the USSR Minzdrav was to carry out training sessions in all of the republic capitals and several additional major cities. By June 1, 1951, psychoprophylaxis was to be practiced in all Soviet birth facilities, while medical institutes were ordered to develop educational programs for training students and practicing obstetricians in psychoprophylaxis by the start of the new school year on the first of September.[81] Its impact would be limited as long as the focus remained on physicians, as midwives attended the vast majority of Soviet women. By the time attention shifted a few years later to training midwives to prepare mothers in psychoprophylaxis, the effort to promote the method was already losing momentum and meeting with resistance from skeptical maternity caregivers.

Psychoprophylaxis's value as propaganda abroad far outstripped its impact on maternity wards at home. In the context of the Cold War, Soviet authorities were quick to promote psychoprophylaxis as an example of progressive Soviet innovation that could benefit the world's working-class women. In June 1951 they sent Nikolaev to Paris to participate in the International Congress of Obstetrics and Gynecology, where he presented a paper on the work he, Vel'vovskii, and others were doing on psychoprophylaxis. In the audience that day sat Fernand Lamaze, a dapper, jovial, middle-aged Parisian obstetrician who ran a private practice and, since 1947, had headed the Maternité "Pierre-Rouquès," the maternity ward at the Metallurgists' Polyclinic, later known by the nickname "Les Bluets" after the street where it was located.[82] Tantalized by Nikolaev's talk, Lamaze was one of a dozen French doctors who traveled to the USSR in August 1951 for a three-week trip to gain familiarity with advances in Soviet public health and medicine. Along with French Communist Party (PCF) members of the National Commission of Communist Doctors, sympathetic but unaligned physicians like Lamaze toured medical facilities in Moscow, Leningrad, and Georgia. Lamaze pressed for an opportunity to go off the official itinerary and witness a birth using psychoprophylaxis. In despair over not having seen for himself this highly touted miracle of Soviet science, Lamaze threatened to denounce psychoprophylaxis as a sham and the trip as nothing more than a propaganda junket, or at least so the story goes. Soviet authorities relented, and two days before his return to France, Lamaze witnessed a thirty-five-year-old typist giving birth to her first child, "without pain and with joy," at Nikolaev's Leningrad clinic.[83] In a 1953 interview,

Lamaze reflected that the laboring woman's "uterine muscle seemed to work amid a body completely slack and relaxed, as if indifferent to the act of childbirth. There was not the least agony in her eyes, not one cry, not one drop of sweat beaded on her brow, not one grimace appeared on her face."[84] This scene overturned everything Lamaze knew about childbirth.

CHAPTER 3

༄

"Science Knows No Borders": Psychoprophylaxis in France, 1951–56

Inspired by what he saw at Nikolaev's clinic, Lamaze returned to France ready to spread word of psychoprophylaxis with missionary zeal. Promoted as *la méthode psychoprophylactique* (*MPP*) or, more commonly, as *l'accouchement sans douleur* (*l'ASD*), or "painless childbirth," the method that came to bear Lamaze's name in the United States was disseminated with remarkable rapidity across France, into neighboring European countries and beyond, making incursions into North Africa, the Middle East, and Latin America before the close of the 1950s.[1] Lamaze's charismatic personality and sense of mission played a key role in the method's rapid rise. Also crucial was early backing from Les Bluets' Communist administrators and their comrades at the Metallurgists' Workers Union, who recognized the propaganda value of Soviet psychoprophylaxis, and grassroots organizing by women on the Left. French Communists' embrace of psychoprophylaxis derived from an ideologically driven understanding of it as "a gift from the socialist fatherland, from Soviet science guided by Stalin's genius."[2]

The battle of the PCF for hearts and minds during the Cold War played a determinative role in the triumph of psychoprophylaxis at this particular time and place. In the USSR, material, personnel, and funding shortages all pushed central authorities toward the endorsement of a psychological, rather than pharmacological, solution to obstetric pain. In urban France, access to drugs was not a problem for those who could pay, though some obstetricians, including Lamaze, had reservations about their safety. Much like the Read method in Anglophone countries, psychoprophylaxis appealed to consumers who sought a painless birth experience but perhaps worried about reliance on available anesthetics, analgesics, and sedatives. Psychoprophylaxis promised a painless, satisfying experience of birth without resort to drugs that impaired women's faculties. But along with any perceived medical need and consumer desire, ideology contributed to the speed of the method's spread in France.

Women, particularly those affiliated with or sympathetic to the PCF, were in the vanguard of the French push for psychoprophylaxis. Beginning with the clientele of Lamaze's maternity ward at Les Bluets, working-class women welcomed psychoprophylaxis with enthusiasm. Lamaze and his team turned to women as the foot soldiers in their battle to spread the method, leaning in particular on the Union of French Women (*Union des Femmes Françaises*, or UFF), a women's organization allied with the PCF. Women spread the word about this new Soviet method of childbirth through published testimonials in leftist newspapers and journals, and by speaking to neighbors, friends, and relatives.

The mid-century French context in which psychoprophylaxis developed differed markedly from the Soviet one. Though less widely used than in Anglo-American obstetric practice, pharmacological pain relief was known and on the rise in urban postwar France. French women utilized a variety of anesthetics and analgesics selected on the basis of the obstetrician's personal preference. From the 1930s, urban France moved increasingly toward *l'accouchement dirigé*, what in today's parlance would be called "active management of labor," the use of pharmacological and other interventions to promote the progress of labor and to control pain. But utilizing anesthesia was not cheap and economic conditions in the immediate postwar years no doubt suppressed its popularization.[3]

Standard maternity care left much to be desired beyond a lack of universal access to pain medication. Reflecting in later years on her experience giving birth for the first time in 1949, Madame N. relates a story of gruff treatment, indifference to her pain, and abandonment at the hands of those charged with her care. Upon arrival at the maternity ward she was told that her labor was not well advanced, with delivery still a long way off. The nurses sent her husband home and ordered her to get in bed. They showed her where the bell was to ring them if she needed anything and indicated where the lamp was if she wanted some light. "If you have to vomit, here's the basin," a nurse barked, before leaving her to labor alone.[4] Without any prenatal education about pregnancy, labor, and birth, when her waters broke in the middle of the night she did not know what had happened and was frightened. Only in the early hours of the morning did the midwife appear, but "I had been alone during my whole labor and I had suffered a lot."[5] It is not surprising that Madame N. and others who had had similarly painful, lonely experiences sought something different for subsequent births.

Some medical professionals in postwar France showed a growing interest in making childbirth less painful and more humane. Writing in 1954, physicians Marc Rivière and Léo Chastrusse observed that, with the sharp decline of maternal mortality, "contemporary doctors seek to alleviate the last burden that weighs on childbirth. Making it painless became a legitimate and pressing objective."[6] As in Britain and the United States, the drawbacks of available drugs combined with growing maternal dissatisfaction to lead some obstetricians, Dr. Lamaze among them, to welcome new means of obstetric pain relief in France.

France's long-standing concern with mind-body medicine, most famously pursued by Charcot, contributed to the medical community's and nation's readiness to accept the efficacy of a psychological approach to labor pain management.[7] Like many young physicians at the dawn of the twentieth century, Fernand Lamaze may have pursued an interest in hypnotism and suggestion during his medical studies.[8] French Communist psychiatrists in the early years of the Cold War enthusiastically supported their ideological mentors in Moscow and embraced Pavlov's emphasis on the role of the nervous system and language as tools for the creation of conditional response.[9] Simultaneously, interest in psychoanalysis was slowly gaining momentum. Before World War II, French resistance to ideas generated beyond France's borders left Freudianism there underdeveloped compared to the rest of Western Europe. In 1914, Freud commented that "among European countries France has hitherto shown itself the least disposed to welcome psychoanalysis."[10] Feuds and organizational fragmentation wracked French psychoanalytic circles even as the field's reputation and reach expanded.[11] Psychosomatic medicine, popular in the United States in the postwar era, made modest advances in France over the course of the 1950s, gaining significant ground by the decade's end.

Psychoprophylaxis was not the first psychological approach to obstetric pain relief to arrive on French soil. Dick-Read's work had been known in France since he gave a lecture in Paris in 1938, and his method had been practiced in a few Paris maternity wards since 1949. Lamaze's knowledge of Dick-Read's work may have contributed to his openness to a psychological approach to labor pain management, even though he had remained skeptical about the Read method's efficacy.[12] Differences in tone may explain why Dick-Read's method failed to win more adherents. His work never displayed the scientific trappings that his colleagues expected from medical research. Soaring rhetoric backed up by little more than anecdotal evidence left Lamaze and other French obstetricians unconvinced.[13] By contrast, psychoprophylaxis's French and Soviet promoters made their ideas more persuasive by couching their findings in the widely respected work of Pavlov and presenting their results in the form of empirical statistics laid out in compelling tables, charts, and graphs.

France's preoccupation with its declining birthrate also primed the medical community, politicians, and the general public for the psychoprophylactic approach. Anxiety over France's precipitously declining birthrate came to the political foreground after defeat in the Franco-Prussian War (1870–71) and remained a cause for concern throughout the Third Republic (1870–1940), as exemplified by the 1930 pronatalist postcard in fig. 3.1. With wary eyes cast eastward to Germany, the French fretted over the connection between military strength and population growth.[14] Devastating losses during World War I exacerbated French fear of a dropping birthrate and a perceived degeneration of the population's quality. As elsewhere in Europe during the interwar era, France enacted legislative measures intended to encourage women to have larger families and become stay-at-home mothers. Beginning in 1920, the French government attempted to elevate the social status of mothers of large families by awarding medals for their patriotic service. Over the next two decades, punishments for abortion intensified, contraception was banned, and the state began to fund monetary subsidies to workers with children.[15] After France's swift fall to Nazi Germany, Vichy leader Marshal Pétain drove home his understanding of the link between national defense and population decline, famously attributing the loss to "too few children."[16] In 1945, Charles de Gaulle echoed Pétain when he called for French women to serve their country by bearing twelve million babies within a decade. A postwar baby boom did nothing to alleviate French fears of depopulation, and benefits for stay-at-home mothers and those with large families grew during the Fourth Republic (1946–58).[17] Only in the 1960s and 1970s, with the legalization of birth control (1967) and abortion (1975), did the national consensus on pronatalism give way to women's right to control their own bodies.[18]

Political and economic pressures from both the East and West fed demographic anxiety and were linked to security concerns in postwar France. American and West German pronatalist and familialist policies came bundled with anticommunist rhetoric, but in France these efforts transcended Cold War ideological boundaries. For much of the French public and political leadership in the 1950s, American military, economic, and cultural might appeared a far more imminent threat than Soviet invasion. Even conservative elements of French society worried about succumbing

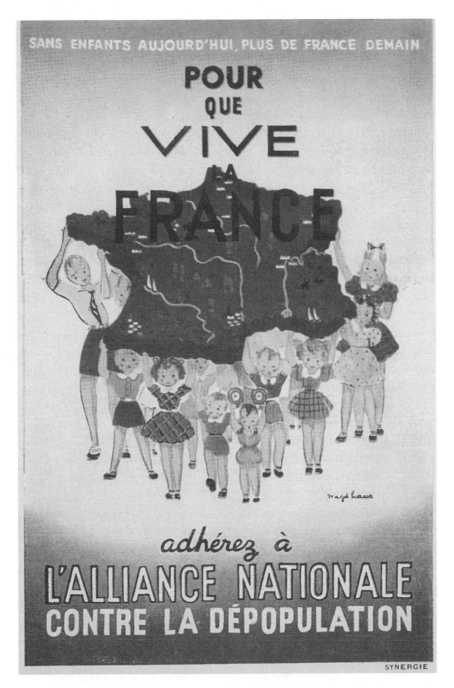

Figure 3.1: French postcard encouraging population growth. "If France is to live, join the National Alliance against Depopulation," 1930. Courtesy of Mary Evans Picture Library/ The Image Works.

to American economic and cultural domination.[19] Fears of a blooming trade deficit with the United States, the English bastardization of the French language, and the penetration of American consumerism caused alarm. For the Right, bearing more children and raising them in ways that sustained national pride and a distinct national identity became a means to stave off this American economic and cultural threat.

Leftist intellectuals and PCF loyalists shared the Right's antipathy toward the United States, while their political concerns over US militarism and virulent anticommunism compounded these cultural and economic worries. No less than the Right, the French Left embraced postwar pronatalist and familialist policies, endorsed as an antidote to neo-Malthusian fears of overpopulation by the poor and working class.[20] Such notions had a long history in France and the perception of them as Anglo-American imports did little to endear them to those on either the Left or the Right. The PCF greeted neo-Malthusianism as a tactic to undermine the numerical strength of the working class and the political power of the PCF. Rather than curb population growth among workers, the PCF advocated "the right to motherhood," guaranteed through the state's provision of social and financial resources to enable women of all classes to have as many children as they desired.[21] A baby boom, a national obsession with demographic decline, wariness about the effects of the available obstetric pharmacopeia, and openness to psychological approaches to pain management all served to make France circa 1951 the right place and time to receive a new, psychological approach to pain relief in childbirth. The PCF's close contacts with the Soviet Union allowed for the transmission of ideas, while showcasing the achievements of the Soviet worker's state played a decisive role in French Communists promoting this particular method.

When Lamaze returned to France from his 1951 Soviet sojourn, he immediately sought to establish the practice of psychoprophylaxis at the maternity ward under his direction. He reported at Les Bluets, pictured in fig. 3.2, that psychoprophylaxis had "drastically changed the conditions of childbirth in the Soviet Union." Trumpeting Soviet success at significantly reducing pain for roughly 80 to 90 percent of laboring women, Lamaze stressed that "there is nothing specifically Russian about this method. It... could be applied everywhere.... Childbirth will be only a source of happiness and joy when all the world's women know the enviable lot of their Soviet sisters."[22] Lamaze echoes leftist internationalism when emphasizing the method's universality and simultaneously making his case for its relevance for the French. He recruited fellow obstetrician Pierre Vellay and kinesiologist André Bourrel to establish a psychoprophylactic obstetric practice at Les Bluets. In February 1952, Les Bluets became the first

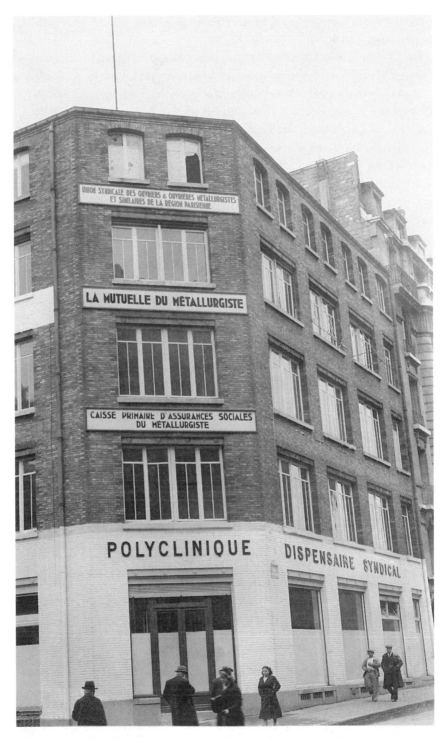

Figure 3.2: Metallurgists' Polyclinic, 1937. Courtesy of LAPI, Roger-Viollet/The Image Works.

maternity ward in the West to utilize this Soviet approach to childbirth preparation and birth.[23]

The immediate financial and organizational support that Lamaze received for psychoprophylaxis owed much to where and with whom he worked. The Union of Metallurgist Workers' Syndicates of the Paris Region (USTMRP, or simply USTM), a constituent member of the General Confederation of Labor (CGT), supported the Metallurgists' Polyclinic. PCF members ran the USTM and comprised much of its rank-and-file. The PCF was the party of France's working class in the 1950s, and, while not as powerful as it had been in the immediate postwar years, it remained an influential player in French politics and in the union movement. Never a PCF member, Lamaze allegedly had worked with Communists in the Resistance. After the war, he was sympathetic to their cause, but calling him a fellow traveler would overstate his loyalties. As his granddaughter later wrote, "he felt out of place with the Communists, though he worked with them."[24] Irrespective of the depth of Lamaze's political allegiance, Communist administrators at Les Bluets embraced his turn toward psychoprophylaxis with enthusiasm, touting the USSR as a beacon of progressive, humane medical advances and rallying support among working-class women.

Psychoprophylaxis linked Communist doctors, hospital administrators, and union officials with a worldwide movement based in the USSR. Communication and the exchange of medical knowledge flowed between the maternity staff at Les Bluets and obstetricians working on psychoprophylaxis in Bulgaria, Poland, Romania, and elsewhere in Eastern Europe during the early and mid-1950s. Such professional connections would have been all but unthinkable for an American physician at the time. In 1955, in the wake of France's defeat in the French Indochina War, Les Bluets' director and PCF member François Le Guay traveled to Vietnam as part of a leftist peace delegation.[25] While there he spoke to physicians about psychoprophylaxis and followed up on his visit by having Lamaze send a copy of a psychoprophylaxis educational film, as well as instructional materials and copies of his most recent article.[26] For the USSR, psychoprophylaxis supported the message that the Soviet Union was a world leader in medical innovation and the proponent of a more just medicine than the United States offered. France's Communist physicians sought to do their part to spread this narrative of Soviet benevolence at home and abroad.

Growing interest in psychoprophylaxis in France allowed the PCF and its Medical Commission to advertise the achievements of Soviet science and contrast them with the comparatively limited concessions on health and welfare made in France. Popular journals aimed at female consumers touted the Soviet Union as "a country where the present is, for us, an image of a possible future."[27] In late October 1953, Nikolaev came to France under the sponsorship of the France-USSR Association, a friendship society that also supported public talks by Lamaze and in other ways promoted psychoprophylaxis. Nikolaev attended a conference in Nice and gave a public lecture in Paris on the history of psychoprophylaxis.[28] Visits such as this one, possible between the United States and the USSR only after the conclusion of bilateral accords in 1958, sparked interest in Soviet science, society, and politics, bridging relations across the Iron Curtain.[29] Nikolaev's visit built on more than a year of press coverage on psychoprophylaxis. His personal appearance in France underscored the method's Soviet origins and ideological implications. His visit also deepened his personal ties with Lamaze, with whom he continued to correspond after his return to the USSR.[30] Vel'vovskii, too, corresponded with Lamaze and requested that he keep him abreast of developments in France, though he never visited Lamaze in Paris.[31]

Exchanges like Nikolaev's and Lamaze's were part of a larger scientific and cultural traffic between the two countries in the 1950s. The France-USSR Association fostered the kind of person-to-person diplomacy that led Lamaze to cross paths with Nikolaev. The PCF's popularity spurred broad interest in the USSR and the promotion of psychoprophylaxis was part of a wide range of information coming out of the Soviet Union and reaching the French public. The Moiseev Ballet toured France, while the troupe Comédie-Française went to Moscow. Week-long French film festivals in Moscow paralleled similar Soviet events in Paris. Soccer matches brought together Soviet and French teams.[32] The exchange of medical delegations and the publication of Soviet research in French medical journals and French research in Soviet journals were part and parcel of vibrant linkages between France and the USSR.

A FRENCH WAY OF PSYCHOPROPHYLAXIS

When Lamaze brought psychoprophylaxis back to Les Bluets, he did not simply replicate the work of Vel'vovskii, Nikolaev, and other Soviet promoters. He adapted both the theory and practice of psychoprophylaxis in subtle but important ways, believing that he could achieve better results through more detailed and prolonged prenatal instruction. He decided to begin lessons with expectant mothers not five or six weeks before their due date, as was typical in the USSR, but fully three months in advance of the baby's arrival. To facilitate instruction, Lamaze's team developed its own illustrative placards, which were "designed to disassociate the uterine contractions from the 'inevitable' pain."[33] The posters explained how a baby is typically positioned in the uterus at full term and how birth proceeds. An educational film produced at Les Bluets proved especially effective at easing women's fears.[34]

Lamaze's patients were to accomplish painless childbirth through the trained muscular relaxation and patterned breathing that he had observed in the USSR. Lessons offered at Les Bluets were similar to those taught in the USSR but lacked the explicit political agenda pursued in the final session of the Soviet course. Additional sessions added by Lamaze and his team explained in greater detail cortical function and conditional reflex. The lessons also acculturated women to biomedical terminology used during labor and delivery. The classroom offered women a crash course in basic obstetrics, as they and their caregivers thus learned to speak the same medicalized language. Mastery of vocabulary such as "dilation" and "effacement" enabled women to follow the course of their own labor in terms meaningful to their doctors and midwives. The staff at Les Bluets hoped that this additional instruction made women more confident and secure about childbirth.[35]

For French Communist psychiatrists, psychoprophylaxis's legitimation on the grounds of Pavlovian neuropsychology dovetailed with an anti-Freudian, pro-Pavlovian perspective. Vel'vovskii and his comrades had little need to debate Freudianism and politically could not do so inside the USSR, where Freud had been deemed persona non grata. But French physicians and psychologists sympathetic to the Soviet Union had to engage the psychoanalytic perspective that was gaining ground in France. For some on the Left, making the case against Freudian psychoanalysis and psychosomatic medicine was a path to denunciation of the United States, where these fields reigned supreme.[36] A 1953 article on Pavlov's work by PCF member and Les Bluets neuropsychiatrist René Angelergues captures this ideological dimension to the case for psychoprophylaxis. Angelergues denounces Freudianism as a tool of American exploitation and imperialism.[37] He juxtaposes Pavlov's materialist emphasis on the role of the neurological system to intangible "psychoanalytic myths," such as "the psyche" and "the personality."[38] Psychosomatic medicine was promoted first and foremost, and not coincidentally, by American psychoanalysts whom, Angelergues asserts, served as toadies for the US regime.[39]

Lamaze and his colleagues instead endorsed the Soviet cultural-historical explanation of labor pain's psychological origins. They accepted Vel'vovskii's assertion that pain in childbirth emerged from millennia of popular cultural and literary images, as well as the horror stories that girls grew up hearing from mothers, sisters, aunts, and grandmothers. Prenatal classes sought to undo these influences through both education and suggestion. Lamaze embraced the notion that this transformation transcended the individual and that "the essential goal of preparation is to break the link that has been created over generations between pain and childbirth."[40] Lamaze and his team sought nothing short of an end to the belief in childbirth as an intrinsically physiologically painful act.[41] Sounding much like Vel'vovskii, Lamaze asserted in a 1955 lecture to an audience of social workers that

> over centuries, the idea that suffering during childbirth was inevitable became deeply rooted. Feelings of fear, terror, and alarm became sentiments inseparable from childbirth.... Millions and millions of women found in a number of works a description of pathological, abnormal births, presented as normal births.... In these conditions, the normal physiological transmission of the cerebral cortex and of the sub-cortex are strained, debased, and perverted.... Childbirth, which is naturally a painless phenomenon, "was distorted." One must...not battle labor pain by means of pharmaceuticals...but struggle to destroy the idea of these pains.[42]

The experience of pain was real, but caused by an expectation, passed down through the generations to create a collective reflex. Break the hold of the notion that pain must accompany childbirth and birth could be restored to its naturally painless state.

The revolutionary potential of psychoprophylaxis hinged on faith in women's intellect and the physician's ability to harness it. This confidence in women's rationality was never highlighted in Soviet writings on the subject, and French medical men's belief in and admiration for women should not be overstated; it was for men like Lamaze, Vellay, and others to bring women's potential for rational thinking to the fore. Lamaze and Vellay retained the authority to judge the success or failure of a case on the basis of their observations of a woman's behavior, level of muscular relaxation, and facial expression during labor and birth. They maintained that the whole enterprise was "under the direction of the obstetrician," who was the unchallenged final arbiter of authority.[43] They expected laboring women to do exactly as a Madame Lefeuvre from Toulon did: "I listened attentively [to the doctor's instructions]. I would be obedient and would do exactly what he told me to do."[44] Characterizing this method at this point in time as a means of feminist empowerment clearly distorts the historical record.[45]

France's most significant innovation to Soviet psychoprophylaxis was a new role for the husband at his wife's side. In the USSR, Soviet men were banished from the maternity hospital. They paced and chain-smoked in front of the building's entrance, while their wives labored inside. Men remained separated from their wives and newborns for the week-long lying-in period, a practice that only began to change after the USSR's 1991 collapse. As a British nurse visiting the USSR in the 1960s stated, "all husbands can hope for is a glimpse of their wives from the window."[46] In France, as in the United States, the husband typically walked the halls and remained in waiting areas, joining his wife only after their baby's arrival. In the United States during the 1950s, pockets of change appeared as the Read method made inroads in American maternity wards, but on both sides of the Atlantic the father's exclusion from his child's birth remained the norm.[47]

An early student of psychoprophylaxis under Lamaze, Dr. Annie Rolland first hit upon the idea of elevating the husband to what came in the United States to be called the "labor coach." She served a rural population spread thinly over the mountainous terrain of the Pyrenees. Given the region's remoteness, it was imperative that the husbands be prepared to assist their wives until Rolland could reach them.[48] Like Dick-Read, Rolland argued that the benefits of giving the husband a more active role extended beyond pregnancy, labor, and birth, bringing the couple closer together and facili- tating the husband's more rapid bonding with the child.[49] For Rolland the husband was more than just the quiet observer that he was for Dick-Read, who expected husbands to hold their wives' hands, but not really do much more. Rolland engaged the husband as a full member of the birth team. To prepare for his role, he attended at least one or two of the prenatal classes. When the wife went into labor, the husband was to time contractions and help her to focus on her breathing and relaxation. Rolland shared her suc- cess with Lamaze, who recognized the benefits of it not only for the cou- ple's interpersonal relationship, but also for the working of the maternity ward. As fig. 3.3 seems to suggest, the husband's constant companionship soothed the laboring woman and eased the staff's burden. At times, the husband acted as an agent for and extension of the medical profession- als' authority, helping the maternity ward staff to manage the laboring woman's behavior and attitude. Seeing the advantages for all involved, Lamaze fully integrated the husband into psychoprophylactic practice at Les Bluets.[50]

In general, women found comfort in the presence of their husbands. They felt the shared experience helped them to maintain calm throughout labor and birth, and brought them greater closeness and mutual under- standing.[51] One woman, who gave birth using psychoprophylaxis in 1953, stated that, when her composure faltered, her husband "inspired" her to get back on track with the patterned breathing.[52] For Madame L., her

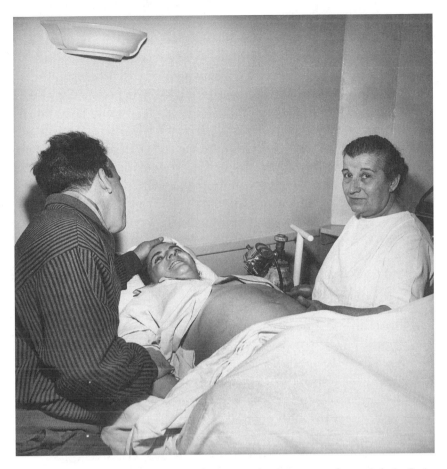

Figure 3.3: A husband at his wife's side during a birth using psychoprophylaxis, Paris, 1956. Courtesy of Roger-Viollet/The Image Works.

husband's presence above all else gave a sense of connection to him that had eluded her during her previous births, which had been marred by a feeling of "separation."[53] Similarly, Madame G. relished her husband's new-found appreciation for her. After the 1955 birth of their child with him by her side, he kissed her and said, "you are wonderful." "That is complete happiness," she attested.[54]

Husbands, too, felt grateful that they were able to play a role in their child's birth and experience closeness to their wives. Excluded from the labor and delivery rooms during his first child's birth, a Monsieur Juquin, "did not feel like I had really contributed to bringing my [first] child into the world. My wife had lived an enormous experience in the life of a couple without me. My child felt like a stranger to me. Of course, this impression did not last, but today I still have the feeling of having 'missed' something that could have been, that should have been important in our life together."[55] By contrast, Juquin found satisfaction in his second child's birth, which he shared at his wife's side. "Thanks to psychoprophylaxis, procreation is not a brief and fleeting act, but a prolonged creation through common effort," he reflected.[56] Psychoprophylaxis gave him a way to sustain involvement in his wife's experience of pregnancy, labor, and birth. A fully integrated partner to her every step of the way, he helped her to practice breathing and relaxation before, and then coached her through labor. Another man, whose wife gave birth at Les Bluets in 1955, attested that witnessing the birth of his child "will be one of the most moving memories of my life because...I was completely happy and in total harmony with my wife."[57] This greater marital intimacy purportedly extended to deeper involvement in childrearing and home life. A magazine article detailing a home birth attended by Rolland was accompanied by photos of a Monsieur Navarret bottle-feeding the baby and helping around the house.[58] Psychoprophylaxis supported a vision of companionate marriage as an enterprise that part-nered husband and wife in childrearing.

In France in the 1950s, few men chose to participate fully in their child's birth. Even among couples that underwent psychoprophylactic prepa-ration, there were those who preferred not to be together during birth. A 1955 magazine article describes how a Monsieur Belin assisted his wife "from an adjacent room." A photo depicts him looking through the glass pane set in the door to the delivery room.[59] Even if the man chose to keep his distance, however, the experience for the father-to-be changed with psychoprophylaxis. A 1953 photo of an expectant father nervously walking the halls came with a caption that conveyed his astonishment at the quiet that reigned at the maternity ward. "I can say that I didn't hear anything," he observed with awe.[60] The absence of cries from his wife's room brought him comfort, though he chose not to witness his child's birth.

BUT DOES IT WORK? FRENCH WOMEN'S TESTIMONIALS IN THE 1950S

Lamaze and his team placed unprecedented weight on patient testimony. Beyond any scientific merit to women's birth stories, psychoprophylaxis's proponents affirmed their propaganda value, with Vellay writing that "these reports, in their marvelous simplicity, are a source of great encour-agement and hope for women who have yet to give birth."[61] Women com-mitted their birth stories to paper within one week of their deliveries, usually submitting them before they were released from Les Bluets' maternity ward. Lamaze and Vellay asked women to describe, as journalist Louis Dalmas paraphrased it, "their initial skepticism, their surprises, and their joys."[62]

Women's birth stories seem, for all their problematic subjectivity, like an obvious and useful source. If one wants to know how much pain a woman experienced during labor and delivery, what better way than simply to ask her? But in the 1950s and well into the 1960s, across Europe and North America, the idea of asking women to assess their own experiences was met with skepticism. In France it was derided as unscientific. Lamaze and Vellay's decision to embrace women's testimonials as both a measure of efficacy and a tool of popular persuasion marks a shift to imbuing women's words with scientific validity and constitutes a major French innovation to psychoprophylaxis. Lamaze and Vellay appear to have been putting into practice the kind of leftist egalitarianism popular among the staff and patients at Les Bluets, where maternity ward personnel were encouraged to express their opinions irrespective of rank or seniority.[63] The solicitation of new mothers' birth stories extended that sense of equality, comradeship, and collaboration to the patients.

The single most pressing question that absorbed Lamaze, his team at Les Bluets, their patients, medical professionals, and the general public was what effect, if any, psychoprophylaxis had on the experience of pain. With rare exception, birth stories that appeared in the French press during the 1950s spoke to the method's efficacy in extremely positive, though nuanced, terms. Madame N., who gave birth in June 1952, described the pain as no worse than menstrual cramps, while Madame D. testified that she had experienced simply "a vaguely disagreeable feeling."[64] When asked by a skeptical friend, "so, you didn't feel anything?" one Lamaze patient raved, "No, on the contrary. I felt everything and it was wonderful!"[65] For Madame G., a couple of difficult moments during transition passed quickly and she maintained her composure and control throughout. Her rather clinical description of physical discomfort was coupled with an assessment of the important role of the staff in helping her to manage her emotions, which she described as one of "confusion, uncertainty, and fear, which was quickly dissipated by the voice of the doctor, who insisted that I relax and showed me a new breathing rhythm."[66] Madame G. does not deny physical discomfort or unpleasant emotions. In fact, by acknowledging them but minimizing their significance, she makes her case for the efficacy of psychoprophylaxis all the more compelling.

Testimonials trumpeted not only the alleviation of physical pain, but also a transformation of the psychological experience of labor and delivery.

Historian Sylvie Chaperon observes that "descriptions of smiling and relaxed women in labor were often too good to be true, but psychoprophylaxis took into consideration women's suffering and refused to accept it as inevitable. The laboring woman rediscovered her dignity."[67] A birth that women (and their caregivers) characterized as "calm," meaning one without screaming, yelling, or writhing, embodied the dignified birth experience they sought and is reflected in joyous, serene images such as fig. 3.4. No longer "something ugly and disgusting," labor became an opportunity for the woman to demonstrate dignity through her ability to use the power of her mind to conquer her physical sensations.[68] The inverse was also true: losing control correlated to a loss of dignity. Lamaze and Vellay quote Madame G.'s recollection of how at one moment during her labor she faltered: "I lost control of my breathing and a cry like that of a suffering animal escaped me, the kind of cry that marked a traditional birth."[69] Madame G. here suggests something uncivilized, wild, or irrational about such cries, a depiction that Lamaze and Vellay clearly shared. Rolland echoed this imagery, saying that a woman who uses psychoprophylaxis "acquires a superiority in no longer being a screaming beast by taking a conscious part in birth.... The woman attains greater dignity in the eyes of her husband, who sees and

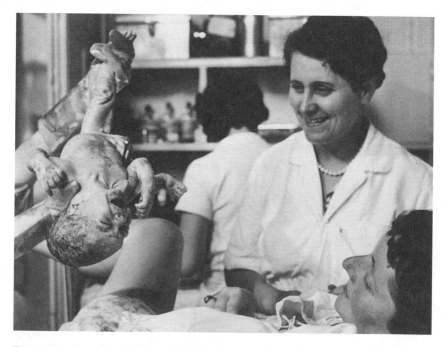

Figure 3.4: A psychoprophylactic birth, Saint-Denis Hospital, 1956. Courtesy of Janine Niepce/Roger-Viollet/The Image Works.

admires her effort."[70] A woman's self-respect here becomes something granted through her husband's gaze as a reward for her good performance, as seen and judged by him. There is nothing intrinsically undignified about the vocalization of labor pain, but clearly a powerful taboo existed against it in 1950s' France.

Dignity derived also from a woman's sense of active participation in labor and delivery. In the mere choice of psychoprophylaxis over a conventional birth, which at that time in France might or might not have included anesthetics or analgesics, women asserted an active role in their birth experience. This self-selecting group sought out something that they defined as more desirable, modern, and civilized. As one young mother explained, "I rejected subjecting myself to suffering like everyone else. It struck me that it was like leaving the Television Era for the Middle Ages."[71] Regardless of how well psychoprophylaxis worked for them, women found satisfaction in asserting their choice of this alternative approach to childbirth. Thirty-seven-year-old Madame L. C., who gave birth to her first child at Les Bluets in 1953, expressed these sentiments when stating that "personally, I am proud of not having been a hunk of passive and panic-stricken flesh, but a 'conscious and orderly' being."[72]

This opposition of a rational, active, modern vision of childbirth to an irrational, passive, backward one tapped into ideas that circulated implicitly and explicitly in French public discourse about female psychology—ideas that found legitimation in Freudian psychoanalytic theory and to which even ardent anti-Freudians subscribed to some extent. In this view, an intrinsic, biologically determined passivity defined female psychology, including during childbirth. However much satisfaction women might derive from childbirth as an accomplishment, birth as an active achievement was an illusion, as labor and birth proceeded as an involuntary reflex. A woman's main job in childbirth was simply to wait patiently for nature to take its course, neither relinquishing responsibility wholly to her physician, nor setting herself up for failure and disappointment by trying to control the process of labor. At first glance, psychoprophylaxis might appear in conflict with such ideas given the claims of activity and control that run through the medical and popular literature on this method. Its advocates asserted that it promised to allow "the woman to acquire a less passive attitude toward herself and a more active one toward the world," liberating her through the use of her intellect to control her breathing and to relax.[73] Rather than challenge popular notions of female psychology, psychoprophylaxis dovetailed with a Freudian vision of female passivity. Psychologically healthy participation in the birth of one's child meant the woman neither tried to dominate the experience through sheer will, nor relinquished control and responsibility to her medical attendants. The laboring woman balanced between active and passive impulses.[74] Above all, physicians and midwives demanded that women in labor demonstrate quiet compliance and obedience, seemingly passive traits, even as the discourse of psychoprophylaxis emphasized activity and authority. Women were ostensibly required to do nothing and to do so actively.

In fact, remaining calm, quiet, and even cheerful demanded enormous effort and focus amid the extraordinary physical and psychological challenge of childbearing. Women frequently remarked on the concentration required to maintain control and the pride they derived from their effort. Madame P., who gave birth in 1952 at Les Bluets, noted, for example, that she was "above all happy with having personally participated *actively* in the birth of my child."[75] For a second-time mother aged twenty-seven, "when the baby emerged, *I was calm and overflowing with joy....* I was assisting *myself in total lucidity*."[76] One woman from Lyon clearly felt empowered by the feeling that "with this method, during the twenty-four hours of childbirth, I controlled the course of my labor."[77] In psychoanalyst Helene Deutsch's formulation, these women were mistaken to think they really influenced the course of their own labors, but they could claim a sense of accomplishment through their demonstration of calm, cooperative comportment.

AUTHORITY AND AGENCY

The majority of women who felt that they had used psychoprophylaxis to their advantage exhibited an authoritative voice both in testimonials and through informal social networks. Lamaze himself promoted women's belief in their power when he solicited their testimonies and inscribed them with scientific and propagandistic value. The women whose voices made their way into the works of Lamaze and Vellay claimed for themselves the right and responsibility to convey the truth of their experiences.[78] The confident voice of women speaking from first-hand experience combined with their marshaling of a medical or quasi-medical vocabulary to make these testimonials at once both accessible and persuasive to women reading these accounts in popular magazines and books.[79]

Women make clear that, for all their self-realization and self-direction, they depended on the medical staff's positive reinforcement for their sense of control and competence. They were quick to credit the medical staff, especially their obstetricians, with their ability to maintain the placid visage required by psychoprophylaxis. The loss or maintenance of control frequently seems to turn on the absence or presence of supportive members of the medical team, whether midwife, nurse, or obstetrician.[80] Confidence and trust in the obstetrician was considered "an important element in the success" of psychoprophylaxis and women were grateful to childbirth educators and their obstetricians for their help.[81] Laboring with her third child, twenty-six-year-old Madame C. experienced some painful contractions when she was alone, but "when the midwife was nearby, everything was better."[82] As Les Bluets patient Madame G. attests, "the doctor returned [to the room], and *he again controlled the synchronization of my breathing* in such a way that subsequent contractions, even those that were stronger, did not cause me any pain."[83] Going well beyond the kind of support that Madame C. leaned on, Madame G. here effaces her own active role and emphasizes instead the obstetrician's sway over her, a depiction that tempers advocates' claims to the woman's control of her labor and birth.

In cases that either obstetricians or women themselves defined as failures, one sees again this deference to medical authority. Women were apt to blame themselves when they did not get the kind of pain relief from psychoprophylaxis that they expected. Testimonials about so called failed psychoprophylactic cases teem with regret and self-recrimination. In evaluating their birth experiences afterwards, women were quick to take responsibility for not having practiced the breathing and relaxation techniques enough at home, for not having attended enough of the lessons, or for failing to have faith in and rely upon the medical team.[84] One young mother, for example, regretted not having "followed the instructions perfectly not to falter, not to cry." Not only was she disappointed for herself, but she believed in "the effectiveness of this method[.] . . . I would have wanted to show myself worthy to the end, and reward the effort of those who taught and helped me."[85] For others, estimations of their own failings yielded feel ings of deep regret and even anger. No extant testimonials from Les Bluets in the 1950s call into question the method's efficacy or the staff's competence, compassion, or skills.

Informal mechanisms were likely more influential than published testimonials in persuading women of the benefits (and limits) of psychoprophylaxis. Women spoke to their friends, relatives, and neighbors, and word spread across France about psychoprophylaxis. One woman's positive experience could ignite interest in a broad circle around her. Rolland reported that in the village of Soues (Hautes-Pyrénées) where she practiced, women came to her and asked if she thought they "could do as well as their neighbors" using psychoprophylaxis. When discouraged by her doctor from using psychoprophylaxis, a woman reported later to Rolland that she had retorted "you know, doctor, everyone in the village has done it. Who do you think I am? The village idiot? Or that I don't care about my child?"[86] Rolland explains that in the intimate atmosphere of a village, "from the moment that one woman gives birth using psychoprophylaxis, everything changes. The other women have proof that it's possible, that it's true. . . . Very quickly, the women moved to a more active attitude: what their neighbor had succeeded at, they wanted to accomplish also."[87] Seeking a certain kind of birth experience, these women then became instrumental in coaxing the medical community along in its adoption of psychoprophy-laxis, as would be the case in the United States in the 1960s. Vellay asserted that, in fact, it was not medical professionals who made for psychoprophy-laxis's rapid expansion in the West, but "the essential fact that women very quickly understood its value."[88]

No organization proved more useful in providing women with a forum for spreading word of psychoprophylaxis than the UFF, with its weekly organ *Femmes françaises* and the monthly magazine *Heures claires des femmes françaises* acting as the primary means by which Les Bluets com-municated the development of psychoprophylaxis in France to women on the Left. Especially from 1954 to 1956, a flurry of articles on psy-choprophylaxis, like the 1957 cover story pictured in fig. 3.5, appeared next to the kinds of homemaking tips, recipes, and sewing patterns one might find in any women's magazine of the day. A mere month after Lamaze's return from the USSR, his experience was the cover story in *Femmes françaises*. Working closely with representatives of Les Bluets and the Metallurgists' Workers Union, the UFF launched a grassroots campaign for psychoprophylaxis. Lamaze himself described the UFF's role as "primary in the battle that we are engaged in" to promote psychoprophylaxis.[89]

The UFF in the mid-1950s went beyond the pages of its publications to stir interest in psychoprophylaxis at the provincial level and accelerate the method's expansion. Reports came in from every corner of France of women gathering in groups from ten or twenty up to several hundred to discuss the method and ways to promote it locally.[90] UFF chapters circulated letters and petitions demanding the release of government funds to support psychoprophylactic instruction, while at the same time pressing midwives and obstetricians to offer preparatory courses. In 1955 it sponsored a national Day of Psychoprophylaxis, with local chap-ters organizing educational events across France, while in Paris it held a conference that brought together physicians, midwives, and new moth-ers trained in psychoprophylaxis. The UFF also published a sixty-page, inexpensive, accessibly written brochure on psychoprophylaxis that

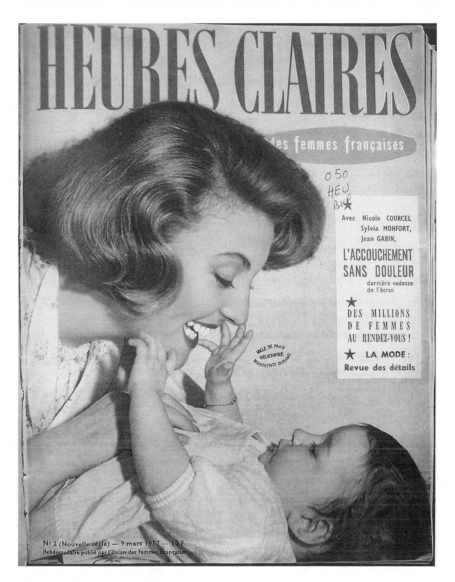

Figure 3.5: Cover, *Heures claires*, Mar. 9, 1957.

activists sold at local events organized to spread knowledge about the method.[91] The effort of UFF activists was vital to overcoming what one Les Bluets administrator characterized, perhaps exaggeratedly, as "the hostility of those who refused to accept the social and humanitarian progress [embodied in psychoprophylaxis] because it came from a socialist country."[92]

A NATIONAL AND INTERNATIONAL
MOVEMENT, 1954–56

By 1954, Les Bluets had become a national and international center for the promotion and development of psychoprophylaxis. Lamaze's professional reputation extended well beyond France's borders.[93] Les Bluets hosted interns from around the country and the world, expanding the ranks of medical cadres prepared to support psychoprophylactic births. As of March 1956, interns from all but ten of the ninety-five departments in metropolitan France had studied at the Metallurgists' Polyclinic. By the end of the year, 1,200 interns from forty-five countries had passed through Les Bluets' maternity ward.[94] Physicians and mothers-to-be wrote to Lamaze seeking advice and information.[95] Women who lived outside of Paris asked him for referrals or suggestions for how to spark interest in their communities and garner support from their local governments for psychoprophylaxis. Reports began to appear in the leftist press about provincial conferences on psychoprophylaxis and the increasing number of hospitals across the country offering courses in it.[96] In the earliest years, from 1951 to 1953, there was no mention of psychoprophylaxis outside of *Femmes françaises, Heures claire, l'Humanité*, and other PCF and UFF-sponsored organs. Beginning in 1954 and accelerating through 1956 and beyond, references to psychoprophylactic practice made their way into the mainstream press. Psychoprophylaxis moved out of Les Bluets' exclusive hands and stories, including critical ones, appeared in the center and right press. Lamaze struggled against some of the popularized discussions of psychoprophylaxis. Hoping to maintain accuracy, he tried to keep tight control over descriptions of the psychoprophylactic method and how it worked in the popular press, but it was a losing battle.[97]

Translation of this method to rural settings and to provincial areas of France, with their distinct regional identities, spurred diversification in the method's practice. Everywhere the method went it encountered conditions on the ground that affected its application. As Rolland's integration of the father into psychoprophylactic practice indicates, the method was not merely imported into the countryside, but remade to suit local conditions. In parts of the country where the use of anesthesia was more common, psychoprophylaxis may have received a cooler reception. From the Alsatian city of Mulhouse, Dr. Pierre Muller wrote to Lamaze in 1954, and, alluding to twilight sleep's German roots, stressed the challenge of working in an area that was "practically the birthplace" of obstetric anesthesia. Muller underscored not merely the medical community's support for pharmacological pain relief, but also the pressure from expectant mothers themselves. "A lot of Mulhousiennes were enchanted by the ability 'to be put to sleep,' to learn upon waking 'that it was all over,' and to see that their baby had been born while they slept.... This is to say that the population is strongly oriented toward a passive attitude and thus ill-prepared to adopt the active attitude needed to accomplish certain tasks in the course of pregnancy."[98] Whether or not Mulhouse's women were as unreceptive to psychoprophylaxis as Dr. Muller believed, he certainly perceived a lack of enthusiasm and attributed it to a unique, regional medical culture.[99]

Psychoprophylactic practice also faced challenges as it moved beyond metropolitan France. Interns from around the globe came to study with Lamaze, while others read his work and attempted to apply psychoprophylaxis without formal training. Vellay celebrated how psychoprophylaxis was "shared with humanity without consideration of race, religion, or ideology.... All women can succeed [at psychoprophylaxis]: the Western woman and the Oriental woman; woman of the North, as well as the Midi, white, yellow, or black; the intellectual and the manual laborer alike."[100] In his formulation, "science knows no borders."[101] This ecumenical view contrasted with Dick-Read's belief that by and large only urban, middle- and upper-class white women, victims of civilization's degenerative effects, suffered in childbirth. Such notions circulated in France, too, but Lamaze and his colleagues took pains to distance themselves from racist, classist assertions at odds with leftist politics.[102]

Whatever the personal beliefs of Lamaze and his colleagues, religious and ethnic identity impinged on how their students applied psychoprophylaxis at the local level and how they interpreted their results. Beginning in June 1953, Dr. Jean Larribère practiced psychoprophylaxis among Arab, Berber, and French women in Oran, Algeria, with great success, particularly with Arab women. Invoking the imperialist trope of the childlike, innocent savage, he credited the relative achievements of Arab women over European women to their supposed ignorance. In his eyes, Oran's Arab women lacked "the skepticism [that] still all too frequently plays a role among women of European origin."[103] With education came doubt in the method's efficacy for European women, while (in Larribère's estimate) naïve Arab women were more readily suggestible. Interestingly, Larribère did not seem to harbor the conviction that childbirth was painless for non-European women—a belief widely held among Westerners at that time—but he was quite ready to cast them as easy dupes.

***

Lamaze's success at spreading psychoprophylaxis was not without hurdles. Within France, there were those on the Right who resisted the promotion of a method of childbirth that originated in the USSR. For advocates of psychoprophylaxis in both France and the USSR, Grantly Dick-Read's Natural Childbirth was the fly in the ointment. Dick-Read bristled at the popularization of psychoprophylaxis over his method, and he found in France both long-time supporters and new converts interested in promoting to French women a non-Soviet alternative to psychoprophylaxis.

Psychoprophylaxis's Soviet developers faced no competitors inside the USSR, but had a different problem on their hands. How could they present their method as path-breaking when it surfaced in Kharkov only in 1948, a good fifteen years after Dick-Read's *Natural Childbirth* appeared in print? Psychoprophylaxis could hardly be the benevolent gift of progressive Soviet science to the world's proletarian women if it was developed by an English anticommunist with a penchant for Christian mysticism. Moreover, big changes were afoot inside the USSR. Stalin's death in 1953 created an opening for more honest, frank debate, including in the realm of science and medicine. For the promoters of psychoprophylaxis, this was not an entirely welcome shift, as it gave their opponents a chance to challenge the central government's endorsement of psychoprophylaxis as the Soviet Union's panacea to obstetric pain.

CHAPTER 4

ᴏᐚᴏ

"Passionate Controversies": Conflict and Change across Europe in the 1950s

Psychoprophylaxis was never static. It emerged out of a process of trial and error, feedback and refinement. Even before it left Vel'vovskii's Kharkov clinic, each encounter between patient and physician was, for all its shared characteristics, a unique, dynamic interaction. Once the method fanned out across the USSR and then to France and beyond, differentiation and innovation in the method's practice became pronounced. When Lamaze brought psychoprophylaxis to France, it entered a new, democratic environment where, in the mixed economy of the French medical system, women exerted agency as consumers and as citizens. France was also an atmosphere of more open professional debate in medicine and the site of a free press where popular and medical arguments could play out.

Dick-Read sought to compete with psychoprophylaxis for professional and popular support. He had spent his career struggling against the powers-that-be in British obstetrics, and he refused to let physicians on either side of the Iron Curtain deny him his due. His teachings, he claimed, had been "mutilated by [the] materialistic outlook" of psychoprophylaxis. "The Franco-Russian adoption of [my] methods," he complained, was nothing more than "a political stunt."[1] The more traction psychoprophylaxis gained across Europe, the more insistent Dick-Read became that "there was no Lamaze method. . . . It was only a political method of converting women [to communism] using [my] own ideas."[2] He did his best to sound the alarm against the red menace stalking Europe's maternity wards, but his rants fell mostly on deaf ears.

Medical and political arguments in the West over psychoprophylaxis reverberated inside the USSR, compounding upheavals already rocking that country following Stalin's death. Hampered by physician and patient skepticism, the campaign for psychoprophylaxis got off to a shaky start and never made a significant impact on Soviet maternity care. By 1954 support had begun to wane and central mandates met with only half-hearted implementation. Advocates for psychoprophylaxis inside the USSR watched and reacted to developments in France and Great Britain. They reflected on the applicability of experiences there for their own work, and they responded to Dick-Read's denunciations of them as frauds and plagiarists. Vel'vovskii continued to fight for his method, but by the close of the 1950s psychoprophylactic practice inside the USSR had been reduced to little more than a footnote in Soviet obstetrics.

DRAWING A LINE WITH THE READ METHOD

Only after psychoprophylaxis arrived in France did the question of its relationship to the Read method arise, as Lamaze and Vellay could not help but see the similarities between the two approaches. Psychoprophylaxis put greater emphasis on patterned breathing techniques, and the Read method included some light calisthenics, but the techniques diverged only in small ways.[3] If there was a meaningful distinction in practice, and one that Soviet and French partisans for psychoprophylaxis hit upon as critical, it was in their attitude toward the laboring woman's mind-body relationship. To enable the body to do its work without pain in labor, Dick-Read sought "an alienation of the mind from any active interest in the uterine function."[4] This dissociation contrasted with psychoprophylaxis's emphasis on mental presence and full, attentive engagement. Sound recordings of Dick-Read and of Vellay, each attending a birth, highlight the differences in their approaches and their personalities. When listening to Dick-Read's 1957 record, one is struck by the laboring woman's docile, disengaged demeanor. His patient, Mrs. Usill, appears to talk about what is happening to her body, especially during the first stage of labor, as if she is observing it from outside, and Dick-Read greets her assessments with equal dispassion. A 1955 sound recording of Vellay attending the psychoprophylactic birth of Madame Crémieux paints a strikingly different picture. Like the woman in Dick-Read's record, Crémieux is pleasant and cheerful. However, when contractions come she appears not detached, but deeply focused, and when the time arrives to push, Vellay cheers her on with gusto.[5] At the time, observers might have chalked Dick-Read's and Vellay's two styles up to divergent British and French national characters.[6] But the differences in atmosphere in the labor room reflected ideas embedded in these methods about whether a detached or engaged mind yielded the optimal physical results. As scholar Jenny Kitzinger pithily phrased it years later, the psychoprophylactic approach distinguished itself from the Read method by seeking "victory over the body rather than surrender to it."[7]

Recognizing that the similarities outweighed the differences, Vellay reached out to Dick-Read within a few weeks of Lamaze's return from the USSR in 1951. Vellay asked whether Dick-Read would be willing to extend to him the rights to translate *Childbirth without Fear*. He made no mention of Lamaze's recent trip to the USSR and his exposure there to a similar approach to obstetric pain. Dick-Read responded matter-of-factly that a French translation was already underway, but he appreciated Vellay's interest.[8] That exchange appears to be the sole direct communication between Dick-Read and the obstetric team at Les Bluets.

In a January 1952 article, the first on psychoprophylaxis to appear in a French medical journal, Lamaze and Vellay acknowledged Dick-Read's work and argued that his method was basically one and the same as that which Lamaze had observed in the USSR. They noted their faith in Dick-Read's Fear-Tension-Pain cycle. Like him, they asserted that education and relaxation, not drugs, were the keys to liberating women from pain in childbirth.[9] In another article later that year, they described training in relaxation and breathing that differed from that of Dick-Read, but that was not altogether unrelated. French psychoanalyst Léon Chertok concurred, characterizing the differences between psychoprophylaxis and the Read method as "minimal."[10] Only in later years, perhaps partly in response to Dick-Read's belligerence, did supporters of psychoprophylaxis become more dogmatic, drawing a firmer line between the two approaches.[11]

Despite the small differences in tone and emphases, debate between partisans for psychoprophylaxis and for the Read method sparked what Chertok called "passionate controversies" in Europe in the first decade after Lamaze's Soviet trip.[12] Publicity generated by Lamaze's efforts stirred interest in Dick-Read's work. The Read method had been practiced for years in a few select French venues, most notably Paris's Saint-Antoine Hospital. The first French translation of Dick-Read's *Childbirth without Fear* appeared in 1953, nearly a decade after its publication in English, and the timing seems unquestionably linked to growing French interest in psychoprophylaxis.[13] Unfortunately for advocates of psychoprophylaxis, Dick-Read (or his publisher) translated the title as *L'accouchement sans douleur* (Childbirth without Pain), rather than *L'accouchement sans crainte* (Childbirth without Fear). The latter phrase would have been an accurate, literal translation of Dick-Read's title; the former was the French term for any form of obstetric pain relief, though over time it would become a synonym for psychoprophylaxis. The clarifying phrase *l'accouchement naturel* (natural childbirth) appeared only in the book's subtitle. Dick-Read also published a series of articles in the French magazine *Votre santé* using the title "L'accouchement sans douleur."[14] These terminological choices opened the floodgates to both deliberate and inadvertent confusion between the two approaches in publications other than those controlled by the UFF, PCF, and CGT.[15] In medical journals and popular women's magazines the line between psychoprophylaxis and the Read method was perpetually blurred.[16] Whether the conflation of the two methods outside leftist publications was deliberate or not, it had the cumulative effect of blunting the pro-Soviet propaganda value of the term *accouchement sans douleur* for the PCF.[17] In a 1956 UFF magazine, Lamaze's colleague Roger Hersilie insisted that the difference between psychoprophylaxis and the Read method was "not just a semantic squabble or a question of terminology.... Some think and say that these are just linguistic subtleties and byzantine quarrels. Nothing could be less true."[18] Unquestionably, Dick-Read and his supporters tried to capitalize on the growing interest in psychoprophylaxis to promote the Read method, and it is clear from Hersilie's tone that such tactics were wearing thin on psychoprophylaxis's advocates.[19]

The ideological motivations of those writing in support of the Read method are not as transparent as those of psychoprophylaxis's leftist supporters. For most of them ideology had no place in these debates. Beyond Dick-Read's own vocal anticommunism, advocates for his method offer no direct testimony that links the method with an explicit political agenda, but on rare occasions they drop subtle hints. For example, in his endorsement of the Read method, Dr. Pierre Theil writes that psychoprophylaxis put less emphasis on building a woman's "personal confidence" than the Read method, implying that a practice born out of Soviet collectivism undervalued the individual.[20] But hinting at a nefarious ideological agenda may very well not have been Theil's intent, and one needs to be cautious not to ascribe political motives where none may have existed.

When Lamaze brought psychoprophylaxis to France, it ignited genuine, grassroots consumer support that Dick-Read had not been able to spark outside the Anglophone world. Why did his method fare poorly relative to psychoprophylaxis in continental Europe? His writings had clear appeal beyond their initial audience. By 1950, the year before psychoprophylaxis arrived in France, Dick-Read's work had been translated for popular and professional audiences into Arabic, Danish, Dutch, French, Italian, and Swedish.[21] The spread of psychoprophylaxis, however, boosted interest in the Read method, though the former garnered the lion's share of attention. French fears of American domination may have worked against acceptance of the Read method. The strength of the Anglo-American alliance perhaps linked the Brit implicitly to the United States, for which so many French in the 1950s had mixed feelings. At a time when the French were beginning to look for a path between the American and Soviet camps, Dick-Read's virulent anticommunist rhetoric and high praise for his American followers not only inflamed opponents on the Left, but may also have alienated potential adherents of a more centrist or apolitical orientation. No doubt of greater significance, Lamaze and his supporters had a clear advantage with their ability to tap into UFF and PCF networks to promote psychoprophylaxis. Dick-Read had no comparable, ready-made organizational structure to lead the charge and that may have been decisive in the French medical community's and public's embrace of psychoprophylaxis over the Read method.

From the time he learned about Soviet psychoprophylaxis and its French followers in 1952 until his death in 1959, Dick-Read fought an ever-escalating, increasingly shrill and largely futile battle to win recognition for his life's work as the first and best psychological approach to obstetric pain. In February 1952, within weeks of the first baby being born using psychoprophylaxis in Lamaze's Paris clinic, Dick-Read heard from a Swiss colleague about "the Grantly Dick-Read method as practiced in the Soviet Union." He was informed that a Kiev obstetrician name Lur'e, "is the leader of this work, but as you expect from the Soviet Union the [British] origin...is suppressed."[22] The Ukrainian Soviet Socialist Republic's Chief Obstetrician-Gynecologist, A. Iu. Lur'e, had worked in the field of obstetric pain management since the 1930s and was indeed active in the spread of psychoprophylaxis, though not "the leader." Dick-Read wrote to Lur'e, sending him copies of his writings in English and German through the Soviet embassy in South Africa, where Dick-Read was living at the time. Hopeful that his prior contribution to the field would be recognized, Dick-Read waited for a response from Kiev, but none ever came.[23]

Dick-Read's fight against psychoprophylaxis came to his own backyard when, getting wind of developments in the USSR and France, British leftists sought to spread word of the method in Great Britain. In November 1953, Lamaze traveled to London, where he gave a talk on psychoprophylaxis sponsored by the Medical Section of the Society for Cultural Relations with the USSR, a Soviet-British friendship organization.[24] Coverage of psychoprophylaxis in Britain's *The Daily Worker* stoked interest in Lamaze's visit.[25] The following year, a group of British nurses traveled to Paris to observe first-hand Lamaze's method. A footnote to an article on the nurses' experience remarks in passing that "relaxation was also one of the essentials in the painless childbirth system of Dr. Grantly Dick Read, the famous British pioneer of 'natural'childbirth."[26] Barely acknowledging his contribution and making no mention of the distinctions between the two methods, this article surely infuriated Dick-Read. Seeing the Soviet method as, at most, a "slight modification" to his own approach and "coming in to the market...some twenty years after my own publication," Dick-Read chaffed at the presentation of psychoprophylaxis as either a new or improved way of giving birth.[27] That professional colleagues inside his native Britain had begun to speak of psychoprophylaxis and Natural Childbirth in one breath rankled after decades spent championing his approach with little recognition or support.[28]

Over time Dick-Read became increasingly frustrated by his marginalization on the Continent, and his accusations grew more pointed. Initially he may have been willing to accept that the Soviet developers of psychoprophylaxis independently arrived at a similar method, but by 1955 Dick-Read moved toward denouncing Vel'vovskii and other Soviet researchers as plagiarists. In a letter to a Japanese colleague, he fumed that "the Soviet method is, of course, my method and they had all my books sent to them. There is very little doubt that their procedures were adopted from the information they have obtained in recent years."[29] He repeatedly claimed that Vel'vovskii and his French followers were plagiarists who had appropriated "this teaching since my books were received in Russia, and since that time passages, phrases as well as directions for the clinical use of my theory have been quoted by them in lectures and at conferences in other countries."[30] Titled "Russians Pirate Painless Childbirth," a 1956 British newspaper article claims that "there is evidence that Dr. [Dick-]Read's books reached Russia long before doctors there began to talk of 'the Pavlovian method' of 'painless childbirth.'"[31] The article fails to specify what that evidence was, but one suspects that it was only Dick-Read's own baseless assertions. By 1952, when he sent Lur'e copies of his book, psychoprophylaxis was already national policy in the USSR. His plagiarism claim defies the published and the archival record, including his own correspondence; all the evidence suggests that the Soviet developers of psychoprophylaxis arrived at their method independently. Anger and frustration appear to have compromised his memory of the sequence of events or clouded his judgment about hurling unsubstantiated accusations against colleagues.

Dick-Read's dogmatism led him to rebuff the overtures of those who sought to facilitate reconciliation with Lamaze. After visiting Lamaze's Paris clinic in 1955, Lisbon obstetrician J. Seabra-Dinis wrote to Dick-Read in the hopes of brokering a peace between the two camps. He attempted to persuade Dick-Read that a truce with Lamaze would yield "mutual benefits."[32] In response, Dick-Read offered up a laundry list of the petty slights he had suffered at the hands of psychoprophylaxis's supporters, including the fact that when he had spoken recently in Paris "Lamaze did not turn up." He asserted that, from what he had heard from those who traveled to the USSR and Paris to witness the application of psychoprophylaxis, "the majority of ways the work is being carried out [is] entirely on my principles, but they tend to treat their patients with a more regimented violence than I do," suggesting some kind of authoritarian, repressive streak in Soviet psychoprophylaxis.[33] Seabra-Dinis responded by encouraging Dick-Read to write to Lamaze so the two could clear the air and discuss their shared interests. Dick-Read shot back that no overture from him would be forthcoming. In Dick-Read's view, it was for Lamaze as the newer practitioner to approach him as a veteran colleague.[34] In all fairness, Dick-Read had a point, but for reasons unknown, other than Vellay's 1951 letter to Dick-Read, neither Lamaze nor anyone from his team appears to have approached Dick-Read. To have done so might very well have been for naught. Nothing short of Lamaze's unequivocal condemnation of the Soviet method as plagiarism and a communist plot was likely to have satisfied Dick-Read.

Dick-Read's refusal to see any validity to or benefit from psychoprophylaxis drove a wedge between him and the British women who supported his work. A group of activists had in 1956 started the Natural Childbirth Association (today, the National Childbirth Trust, or NCT) to promote Dick-Read's work. Their priority was to get women access to the most up-to-date information on non-pharmacological means of pain management, and they were reluctant to be dragged into doctrinal disputes. Dick-Read's polemics did not interest them, nor did they wish to offend the man whose work they revered and promoted. At a May 1959 NCT meeting, Dick-Read denounced psychoprophylaxis as "nonsense and the [different patterns of] breathing merely frills." One board member, a Mrs. Parsons, had the temerity to inquire of Dick-Read what they should do to assist women who came to them after previously having been trained in psychoprophylaxis and what she described as its "lighter type of breathing. Did he then think it wrong for them to have help from the Trust?" Dick-Read sniped that "those wishing for Lamaze should be put in touch with the Sigerist Society," an organization for physicians interested in bringing a Marxist perspective to bear on issues of medicine and health.[35] The NCT board of directors remained unconvinced that ideology had a place in this discussion. A Mrs. Hunter quipped that "the time has not come when we must look for red devils under the accouchement couch."[36] Childbirth activists clearly cared more about pain relief than red baiting, and by 1960, the NCT turned away from the Read method and fully committed to promoting psychoprophylaxis.[37]

At the invitation of French advocates for psychoprophylaxis, the Catholic Church weighed in on these debates about the diverse psychological approaches to obstetric pain. Christians in general and Catholics in particular were interested in the question of labor pain relief for two reasons. First, the Bible enjoined women to "bring forth children in pain," which raised concern that relieving labor pain might conflict with church doctrine. Second, the Church emphasized procreation, which obstetric pain relief might encourage.[38] Catholic women and their obstetricians sought to take advantage of psychoprophylaxis and the Read method with the pope's blessing.[39] Pope Pius XII expressed support for these developments when, in January 1956, he issued a proclamation that clarified the Church's position on obstetric pain relief measures. Pius XII argued that, in contrast to twilight sleep or hypnosis, which robbed women of their conscious participation in childbirth, psychoprophylaxis and the Read method only diminished or eliminated pain.[40] The pope, in Vellay's words, "liberated the Catholic woman."[41] For Lamaze, the decree was "an important event. Its repercussions are infinite."[42] The announcement of the pope's approval triggered a flurry of press coverage around the globe, particularly in Europe, North Africa, and South America.[43]

While the pope authorized Catholic women to embrace psychological approaches to obstetric pain relief, he frustrated supporters in Lamaze's and Dick-Read's camps with his refusal to express a preference for one method over the other. His proclamation refers throughout to both psychoprophylaxis and the Read method, which he praised in equal measure. He described the Read method as "an analogous technique" to psychoprophylaxis "in a number of ways," even as he recognized a dissonance between Soviet materialism and the more "philosophical and metaphysical" approach of Dick-Read. Psychoprophylaxis raised alarm for some because of its origins in the godless Soviet Union, but the pope made explicit that approval of psychoprophylaxis did not translate into acceptance of a communist world view. "Even a materialist researcher can make a real and valuable scientific discovery, but this contribution does not constitute in any way an argument for his materialist ideas."[44] Given his emphasis on the spiritual aspect of childbirth, it must have peeved Dick-Read that the pontiff did not accord his method a more privileged position in the debate over psychological approaches to obstetric pain relief. Certainly press coverage in Britain and the United States of the papal decree was for Dick-Read a mixed blessing, giving attention to his work but also elevating the profile of psychoprophylaxis.[45]

Catholic mothers welcomed the pope's endorsement and doctrinal disputes over psychoprophylaxis and the Read method on medical and ideological grounds were of no significance to them. As a Madame Le Flem, who had given birth to her second child at Les Bluets, stated following the pope's approval of psychoprophylaxis, "all Catholics are happy about it."[46] For other Catholic women, the pope's words merely validated a method they had already embraced. In a 2010 interview, Geneviève Grattesat, editor of the leftist Catholic newspaper La Quinzaine, stated that the pope's endorsement was of no real consequence, as progressive Catholic women, enthusiastic supporters of psychoprophylaxis from the start, had been working for its expansion for several years already.[47] The pope had entered this debate late from Grattesat's perspective, but his edict put an end to any lingering objections from local religious authorities.[48] With the pope's decree, "most of the wind was taken out of the sails" of religious and political opponents to psychoprophylaxis.[49]

SEISMIC SHIFTS IN THE USSR

Inside the USSR, psychoprophylaxis had faced a road no less bumpy, despite endorsement at the highest levels of Soviet power. Limited growth and disappointing clinical results followed an initial push for Vel'vovskii's method. Pain relief in childbirth remained out of reach for most of the USSR's women. Less than half of births in the RSFSR benefited from any form of pain relief, psychoprophylaxis included, from 1951 to 1954. Statistics from urban areas at first appear more positive, but closer inspection of, for example, the city of Stalingrad, reveals a complicated picture. From 1951 through early 1952, the centrally dictated campaign for psychoprophylaxis drove a 28 percent increase in the overall use of pain relief in childbirth. Psychoprophylaxis accounted for this expanded access and also for a decline by two-thirds in the use of pharmacological anesthetics and analgesics.[50] Medical practitioners in Stalingrad substituted psychoprophylaxis for drugs, either because the drugs were no longer necessary or because psychoprophylaxis was a convenient excuse to refuse women access to pharmaceuticals that were in short supply. Some evidence points indirectly to the latter explanation. A Kharkov study asserted that few women experienced the "painless" labor promised by psychoprophylaxis's most ardent advocates, but the majority found the pain "tolerable."[51] If a woman could bear the pain of labor through psychoprophylaxis, then care-givers may have been stingier with scarce drugs.[52]

A variety of factors hampered the Soviet drive for psychoprophylaxis. As of 1953, most rural midwives remained untrained in psychoprophylaxis and unqualified to instruct their patients in the method. Ethno-linguistic diversity posed further problems in the USSR's periphery. In Ukraine's Transcarpathian region, a language barrier cordoned off the ethnic Hungarian minority from Russian- and Ukrainian-speaking medical pro-fessionals.[53] Finding medical caregivers who spoke the local language in Turkmenistan was similarly an obstacle, while customary childbearing practices there added another layer of complexity. Turkmen women sub-scribed to a cultural prohibition against the outward expression of labor pain; to scream or cry threatened to invite the evil eye, they believed. Turkmen women's reticence posed a challenge to the evaluation of psy-choprophylaxis's efficacy, as their quiet demeanor made it impossible to assess the impact of prenatal preparation based on observation of their comportment.[54]

Stalin's death in March 1953 brought a new era of economic, politi-cal, and cultural reform in the fields of science and medicine, with efforts to reassert the primacy of methodological rigor and sound practice over ideological imperatives. Certainly, there were false starts and reversals in the process of de-Stalinization, but there was also a real opportunity for change. Over the course of 1954 and 1955, amid this refreshing if tenta-tive atmosphere of what came to be called the Thaw, medical and public health officials initiated several reforms to psychoprophylactic practice in response to unsatisfactory conditions on the ground. In the hope that a shorter prenatal preparation course might shore up attendance, the num-ber of class sessions was trimmed. Long waits to see their caregivers had discouraged women from pursuing psychoprophylactic training or even seeking regular prenatal care. Doubting psychoprophylaxis's value, expect-ant mothers were reluctant—at least, according to some medical practi-tioners—to squander precious time attending preparatory classes, and ill-timed class sessions conflicted with women's work schedules.[55] One doctor reported that his efforts at a collective farm to convince women of psychoprophylaxis's value met with ridicule. "They did not believe in the method. They were convinced that their grandmothers and mothers had given birth in pain and they, of course, would give birth in pain. Many refused instruction, citing a lack of time," which this physician believed was merely a cover for their absence of faith in the method.[56] Authorities cut the required number of classes from six to as few as four, optimistic that they could raise compliance.[57]

To further address low attendance, as well as to lighten the workload of overburdened caregivers, medical administrators began to promote the practice of "express preparation." One physician reported a new mother telling him that the whole of her prenatal preparation consisted of being instructed only "to breathe deeply and massage my belly when I went into labor."[58] Offering women only a single lesson, or even a few furtive instructions while in the throes of labor after arriving at the maternity ward, express preparation saved time and money for everyone, even if its benefits were dubious.[59]

Staff shortages, particularly of physicians, were a frequently cited obstacle to better outcomes and inspired another early modification to Soviet psychoprophylactic practice. At a 1955 midwifery conference in Kharkov, Lur'e announced that across Ukraine, responsibility for teaching psychoprophylactic preparatory courses was to shift to midwives, a strategy rolled out nationally the following year. Lur'e claimed that the closer, more intimate relationship of midwives to their patients made them more effective instructors than doctors.[60] Physicians' skepticism of psychoprophylaxis's efficacy undermined their willingness to invest much time in patient training, sometimes offering, much like in express preparation, little more than "a few words about painless childbirth, or in passing [saying] something about the need to breathe deeply during labor."[61] Transferring responsibility for instruction from physicians to midwives reflected the declining fortunes of psychoprophylaxis. Local and regional medical leaders and public health administrators were less willing to commit resources to the promotion of psychoprophylaxis, and pressure to do so was not forthcoming from Moscow. Like physicians, midwives too were stretched thin, and burdening them with additional responsibilities did not necessarily raise the quality or availability of instruction.[62] The resultant poorer outcomes from hasty or shoddy preparation in turn reinforced the widespread belief that psychoprophylaxis was ineffective at combatting pain.

Many physicians held fast to their faith in pharmacological means of pain management, and, not long after Stalin's death, professional criticism of psychoprophylaxis began to appear for the first time. One Soviet obstetrician in 1953 cautioned that psychoprophylaxis "is not always effective," particularly in cases of long labors. Moreover, "psychoprophylaxis should not lead us to neglect work on other methods of pain relief," including belladonna, Novocain, and a range of other botanical and pharmaceutical options.[63] P. A. Beloshapko, USSR Minzdrav's chief obstetrician-gynecologist, and A. M. Foi, chair of the Saratov Medical Institute's Department of Obstetrics and Gynecology, advocated the combined use of psychoprophylaxis with pharmacological pain relief when necessary, especially in combination with uterine stimulants to speed labor.[64] Nikolaev had since the mid-1930s worked on this kind of active management of labor and remained a strong advocate.[65] His promotion of psychoprophylaxis in no way compromised his faith in and support for pharmaceuticals.

Amid lackluster performance and waning interest, in February 1956, a few weeks after the pope's decree, over two hundred obstetricians, psychologists, neurologists, midwives, and public health administrators gathered in Kiev for a four-day, national conference on psychoprophylaxis.[66] The conference was an opportunity to take stock on the fifth anniversary of USSR Ministry of Public Health's Order no. 142, which had established psychoprophylaxis as a national practice. The Thaw imbued the Kiev conference, held just weeks before Nikita Khrushchev gave his famous Secret Speech denouncing Stalin, with a spirit of reform. Participants engaged in open, vigorous, and authentic debate to a degree that had been uncharacteristic of the previous quarter-century. The central problem for discussion was "what kind of action [psychoprophylaxis] exerts—anesthetization or discipline. The laboring woman behaves calmly because she experiences less pain, or because she has learned to behave more calmly?"[67] Arguments largely pitted psychologists against physicians. Vel'vovskii and other psychologists continued to tout the value of psychoprophylaxis as a tool for pain relief. Obstetricians, however, were vocal in their skepticism. They appreciated that the method helped women to remain quiet and cooperative, but doubted it significantly alleviated pain.

There was at the 1956 conference overwhelming support for a turn to pharmacological pain relief, predicated on a rejection of Vel'vovskii's contention that obstetric pain was principally psychogenic in origin. The director of research at the Institute for Protection of Maternity and Childhood in Kharkov, V. I. Konstantinov, argued most forcefully against Vel'vovskii's claims. He acknowledged that childbirth was not always painful, but when pain was present, he insisted, it was a normal, physiological phenomenon and drugs offered a simple, effective response.[68] If psychoprophylaxis adequately managed pain, that was good news, but it was no panacea. Most physicians believed that ultimately, resort to drugs was useful in most cases.[69] As Lur'e stated simply, "the combination [of psychoprophylaxis] with the use of narcotics seems to me will largely resolve the problem of pain relief in childbirth."[70] Among the drugs recommended for use in obstetric pain management were a variety of opioid narcotics and nitrous oxide. Despite consensus among physicians that drugs had a major role to play in normal birth, no progress could be made without a dramatic infusion of investment in the pharmaceutical industry, and that capital was not forthcoming. Pharmacological pain relief could not become the gold standard for care when the drug industry could not keep pace with demand and an acute shortage of medical personnel trained in the administration of anesthesia only compounded the problem.[71]

With claims about the natural painlessness of childbirth and the ability of psychoprophylaxis to relieve pain under attack, proponents argued that there were a number of benefits to which the method could still lay claim. Slim evidence supported their assertions that psychoprophylaxis improved oxygen supply to mother and baby, strengthened contractions, reduced incidence of postpartum hemorrhage, decreased infant mortality, and minimized perineal tearing. Some claimed that the mother's milk came in sooner and more abundantly, and that she recuperated from labor and could return to work more quickly thanks to psychoprophylaxis. Speakers at the Kiev conference frequently touted shortened labors as a benefit, which was attributed to the method's ability to ease women's fears and help them to relax. Vel'vovskii drew attention to a Dr. Turkin's evidence that psychoprophylaxis facilitated labor's progress by making contractions stronger, and their intervals shorter and more regular compared to those of women who were untrained in psychoprophylaxis.[72]

Given their shaky medical evidence, it is unsurprising that Vel'vovskii and his supporters tried to buttress their case for psychoprophylaxis with political arguments. A. A. Terekhova, RSFSR Minzdrav's chief obstetrician-gynecologist, stated that "obstetric anesthesia in our country became one of the links in the advanced system of Soviet public health due to the perpetual care of the Communist Party and the Soviet state for humankind."[73] Lur'e lauded psychoprophylaxis as "the greatest achievement of our era."[74] Others warmly referred to it as "our Soviet method," and claimed it was nothing short of "the greatest revolutionary act."[75] It was asserted that, thanks to the state's concern, the changes to obstetric care had been so profound that now "Soviet women demand a different kind of birth and we cannot return to the old methods."[76] Such a remark suggests burgeoning grassroots pressures and a responsive clinical care climate, but no evidence supports the view that either pressure from below existed for psychoprophylaxis or that, if it did, it exerted any kind of influence.

Physicians and psychologists at the Kiev conference reached consensus on one question: psychoprophylaxis had benefit for patient comportment and the atmosphere in the maternity ward. Konstantinov supported psychoprophylaxis's continued use despite his skepticism that it alleviated pain. Psychoprophylaxis's contribution, he argued, derived from the role it played in alleviating fear.[77] He endorsed its continued application to ensure a calm, controlled environment in Soviet maternity wards, what many speakers at the conference characterized as a more "cultured" atmosphere.[78]

Several conference participants described how psychoprophylaxis served "to discipline the laboring woman," by which physicians and midwives meant that the method enabled her to refrain from outwardly expressing pain.[79] Medical professionals agreed that even if women were still in pain, psychoprophylaxis was beneficial because it made them easier to manage. Screaming, crying, and writhing ceased. Quiet reigned in the maternity ward and the staff's routine went on without disruption. If there was concern, as there was in the West, for giving women a birth experience that they would find dignified, that consideration went unstated in Soviet professional debates about the value of psychoprophylaxis. Peace and quiet for the benefit of the staff was the primary consideration.

Despite disappointment at psychoprophylaxis's ability to relieve pain, its success abroad was a source of pride at home. Psychoprophylaxis had since 1951 brought the Soviet Union worldwide attention. China, Czechoslovakia, and other countries in the communist world pursued independent research on psychoprophylaxis.[80] But it was the method's growing popularization in France that earned particular praise at the Kiev conference. Nikolaev invoked Lamaze's accomplishments and French reception of psychoprophylaxis, speaking with authority as the individual who had introduced Lamaze to psychoprophylaxis at his Leningrad clinic. USSR Deputy Minister of Public Health P. L. Shupik lauded Lamaze's efforts and Colette Jeanson's 1954 book on psychoprophylaxis, the first to appear in French on the subject.[81] He took a jab at Dick-Read, contrasting Soviet psychoprophylaxis's success in France with the limited impact of the Read method, which he exaggeratedly claimed to have "not found wide dissemination even in his native England."[82]

Soviet obstetricians and psychologists watched developments in the West with an eye toward their own maternity care practices. Lamaze's efforts to experiment with and improve psychoprophylaxis were noted at the 1956 conference with particular interest. Nikolaev observed that Lamaze had increased the number of preparatory lessons from six to as many as ten, at just the moment when Soviet officials had trimmed their number to four. He dubbed this longer preparatory course the "Lamaze method," likely the first recorded use of this term. Nikolaev questioned the reduction in the number of lessons.[83] Material disparities between the USSR and France made French innovations seem unobtainable to Soviet observers, but they were watching, reflecting on, and drawing conclusions about Western psychoprophylactic practice, open to learning from their French disciples.

Lamaze and Vellay's use of patient testimony as evidence for the efficacy of psychoprophylaxis proved influential with a few Soviet investigators and was arguably the most important way that French work in this field resonated inside the USSR. A senior researcher from the USSR Minzdrav's Institute for Obstetrics and Gynecology, V. N. Shishkova, described at the Kiev conference how she and her colleagues surveyed over four hundred women who had given birth using psychoprophylaxis. Like Lamaze and Vellay, Shishkova's team interviewed the women in the days immediately following birth. In practice, Shishkova did not use these interviews to any great effect. She neither quoted them extensively nor drew any surprising conclusions from them, but the significance of her approach lay in its demonstration of Lamaze and Vellay's influence inside the USSR. Vel'vovskii also embraced this methodology and, even though neither of them credit their French colleagues explicitly, the imprint of Lamaze and Vellay seems unmistakable, as it was all but unheard of in Soviet medical research at the time to draw on patient testimony as evidence. By the time Vel'vovskii's new research appeared in 1957, however, it was too late for it to have much impact; the push for psychoprophylaxis had passed and his new work garnered little attention.[84]

In the wake of the 1956 conference, Soviet psychoprophylactic practice went into a period of precipitous decline. It continued to be applied in some facilities, but its ascendency as a centrally dictated national movement was over. Despite the method's fall from favor with authorities in Moscow, a few supporters continued to research and promote psychoprophylaxis. In the post-1956 era, the sole major innovation in the Soviet practice of psychoprophylaxis was the integration of prenatal exercises similar to those advocated by Dick-Read and his colleague, physical therapist Helen Heardman, and illustrated in fig. 4.1.[85] At the Kiev conference Nikolaev and Vel'vovskii endorsed recommendations by Shishkova and others to introduce prenatal exercises into psychoprophylactic training. Light calisthenics had not previously been a part of Vel'vovskii's plan. Like the hints of Lamaze's influence, clues to the provenance of these elements of psychoprophylactic practice are fragmentary and indirect, but exercise was a core part of the Natural Childbirth curriculum and it seems likely that Soviet researchers owed some credit to Dick-Read.[86]

Physical therapy was incorporated into psychoprophylactic training incrementally over the late 1950s. Advocates claimed that more physically fit women had lower incidence of failure-to-progress, hemorrhage, and other complication in birth.[87] This innovation was seen as important enough to warrant a change in the method's name around 1959 from psychoprophylaxis to "psychophysioprophylaxis" or "physiopsychoprophylaxis," reflecting a new fusion of physical and psychological conditioning.[88] By 1963 it was an integral part of prenatal preparation and postpartum

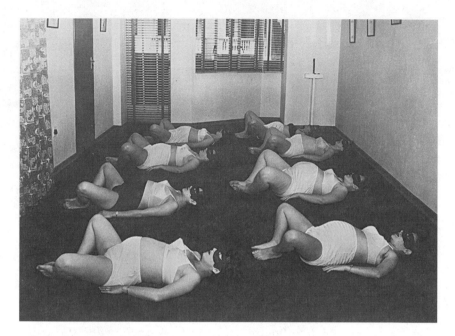

Figure 4.1: Women doing prenatal exercises as part of preparation in the Read method, 1955. Wellcome Library. Reproduced with permission of Pollinger Limited and The Estate of Grantly Dick-Read.

recovery, at least on paper. It took time for these new elements to seep into clinical practice across the USSR. For example, midwives in the Leningrad region only claimed to combine physical therapy with psychoprophylactic prenatal training in 1966.[89] Even then, no evidence points to the teaching or clinical practice of psychoprophylaxis anywhere in the USSR in a meaningful way. Practice existed largely on paper, with reports to central authorities boasting that plans had been fulfilled, but instruction in practice ranged from inconsistent to nonexistent.

Soviet authors credit the integration of exercises not to Dick-Read but to the homegrown work of two Soviet doctors, S. A. Iagunov and L. N. Startseva. Their 1959 article claims that Iagunov's obstetric application of the principles of physical therapy dates to 1955. In fact, Iagunov's interest in exercise during pregnancy can be traced back to at least 1938, as is evident in fig. 4.2, but it was only in the middle of the 1950s that he linked these exercises to psychoprophylactic preparation. In 1938 he was in all likelihood unfamiliar with Dick-Read's work, but this was probably no longer the case in 1955, when he began a new push for the incorporation of exercise into prenatal education. Repeatedly cited by subsequent authors as the source of this purportedly Soviet innovation, his 1959 article with

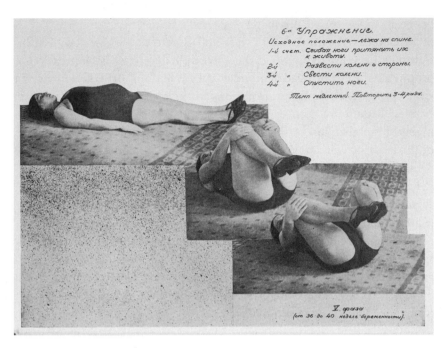

Figure 4.2: S. A. Iagunov, *Fizkul'tura vo vremia beremennosti (Exercise during Pregnancy)*, 1938.

Startseva advocates a few minutes of walking, followed by some very simple stretches and exercises, like leg lifts and arm raises, done standing, seated, and lying down.[90] As pregnancy advanced, the exercises became increasingly limited and after the fourth month included only movements done lying on a bed or the floor. By the end of the 1960s, the exercises for later in pregnancy included more varied and mildly more vigorous calisthenics. Innovations in psychoprophylactic practice were disseminated through prenatal courses and via articles in popular Soviet magazines like *Zdorov'e (Health)*.[91]

Not only did Soviet researchers and officials refuse to credit Dick-Read or Heardman for the exercises integrated into psychoprophylactic practice, but they also worked hard to denigrate the Read method in a variety of ways. An article on Natural Childbirth by an Australian obstetrician appeared in 1957 in *Obstetrics and Gynecology*, the leading Soviet journal in the field. In a note at the article's end, journal editors emphasized the dissimilarities between psychoprophylaxis and the Read method, the roots of psychoprophylaxis in Soviet work on hypnosis in childbirth dating from the 1920s, and the problems with the Read approach, including his advocacy of the father's presence during labor and delivery, which they believed compromised the maternity ward's sterile environment.[92] Much of a chapter of Vel'vovskii's 1957 doctoral dissertation is devoted to countering Western arguments that there was slim difference between psychoprophylaxis and the Read method.[93] Vel'vovskii and others emphasized that, despite Dick-Read's protestations to the contrary, the Read method entailed little more than hypnosuggestion.[94] Whereas psychoprophylaxis involved mobilization of the cerebral cortex and the active participation of the laboring woman, Vel'vovskii described the Read method as one that demanded profound passivity in the form of "a deep hypnotic state."[95] Vel'vovskii and others stressed that, in contrast to sophisticated Soviet arguments about Pavlovian neuropsychology, Dick-Read offered no persuasive theoretical explanation for his technique. Like their French comrades, Soviet critics took Dick-Read to task for his lack of rigorous scientific method and for his frequent lapses into mystical Christianity. They castigated him for the unsound premise that European women could give birth painlessly if they brought themselves to a more natural state, closer to that of the world's so-called primitive peoples.[96]

CONSOLIDATION AND STRUGGLE IN FRENCH PSYCHOPROPHYLACTIC PRACTICE, 1956–59

Changes in the USSR reverberated in France, where the tension between the Read method and psychoprophylaxis played out in legislative battles to secure funding for childbirth education through *Sécurité sociale*, France's system of medical and other social benefits. In March 1953, a group of communists in the National Assembly proposed a new law to support the "teaching and development of the method of painless childbirth by psychoprophylaxis."[97] The proposal's sponsors emphasized the method's Soviet origins, the Soviet state's support of psychoprophylaxis as national policy, and the linkage to Pavlov's work. Communists in the National Assembly met with less success than in the Paris municipal government, which authorized reimbursement to expectant mothers for childbirth education classes beginning in December 1953.[98] Angelergues claimed that neither human nor financial resources really stood in the way of national funding. At issue was ideological opposition among politicians in the National Assembly "less concerned with the wellbeing of women than with their class objectives, seeing in [psychoprophylaxis] a dangerous penetration of the 'red peril.'"[99] In 1955 Deputy Jean Frugier, a member of the Gaullist party Rally of the French People (Rassemblement du People Français, or RPF), attempted to revamp the PCF's proposal in a way that disentangled advocacy of childbirth preparation from the communist cause.[100] After a lengthy discussion of the Read method, his report proposed that "the National Assembly invite the government to take all steps to develop and disseminate the teaching and practice of *psychosomatic methods*."[101] Frugier's choice of terminology merits attention. He embraced the very term that Angelergues had denounced in 1953 as an antimaterialist American weapon of class warfare. Glossing the distinction between Dick-Read's method and the Soviet approach promoted in France by Lamaze, Frugier hijacked the PCF's proposal and severed the linkage between childbirth preparation and the Left's agenda. His proposal failed, but on July 11, 1956, the National Assembly adopted a new PCF proposal to reimburse psychoprophylactic preparatory courses through *Sécurité sociale*.[102] That decision marked the dawn of a new era for psychoprophylaxis in France, an epoch of accelerated integration into mainstream medical practice.

Controversy diminished but did not end with the government's endorsement of funding for prenatal preparation. Nationalism clearly lay at the root of a 1957 effort to promote kinesiologist Fernande Harlin's 1951 book as an original, native contribution to the practice of childbirth preparation. Her instructions on "how to give birth without fear, in a minimum of time, with a minimum of pain, and to quickly find strength and beauty in the most modern of methods" clearly derived in large part from Dick-Read's work.[103] Harlin's approach differs only in terms of inflection, with an emphasis on calisthenics that outstrips Dick-Read's. One Charles Devemy wrote to Les Bluets' maternity ward in May 1957, to draw the staff's "attention to *the French psychosomatic method of childbirth preparation*.... It is unnecessary to try to apply in our country foreign methods that are recognized as incomplete in comparison to those *developed in France*."[104] The author enclosed a summary of the published proceedings from the 1956 Kiev conference on psychoprophylaxis, including remarks about psychoprophylaxis as an often ineffective treatment of labor pain.[105] Given the limitations of psychoprophylaxis now acknowledged by Soviet researchers themselves, Devemy argued that there was no reason to endorse it over a method at least as effective and of French origin—even if the authenticity of that genealogy was suspect. For Devemy, neither the British Read method nor Soviet psychoprophylaxis could answer the needs of French women.

Dick-Read himself soldiered on in his fight against the promotion of psychoprophylaxis in France. In March 1957, he raised a ruckus over a new French documentary film. At the encouragement of his French colleagues François Lepage and Geneviève Langevin-Droguet, who had been practicing the Read method at their Paris clinic since 1949, Dick-Read agreed to appear in and narrate the introduction to a documentary that he believed was about the Read method.[106] To Dick-Read's horror, the film presented his work as a mere precursor to Soviet advances and seemed to legitimate claims that psychoprophylaxis had superseded the Read method. Director Éric Duvivier complied with Dick-Read's demand that his introduction be cut from the film. Expressing his disappointment and sense of betrayal to Lepage, Dick-Read wrote:

> I do not know to what extent you are acquainted with the activities of Lamaze and his group in France or to what extent you feel hostility or agreement with their behavior but, in simple facts, it is a piece of disgraceful plagiarism that the communist organization is using in a subtle way for propaganda of the most important type. There is no such thing as the Russian obstetric method. . . . I have preferred to believe that [Duvivier] was unaware of the trap into which he had walked and the insidious evil of these people who utilized motherhood as a means of spreading their evil doctrines.[107]

Lepage thought Dick-Read's tirade absurd and did not hesitate to tell him so. "As for your accusation against us that we are propagandizing for the Soviet method and its political objectives, let me tell you that that's ludicrous."[108] But for Dick-Read, this matter was serious indeed. Childbirth had become, to his grave concern, "a political weapon," a front in the Cold War.[109]

In April 1957 Dick-Read confronted in person the French proponents of psychoprophylaxis. The French Society of Psychosomatic Medicine organized a one-day conference on "psychological methods of obstetric anesthesia." Presentations addressed a range of issues, with papers by several ardent Dick-Read supporters.[110] Despite the presence of his partisans, Dick-Read felt embattled. From the moment he received his invitation, Dick-Read was disgruntled with the conference organizers, who referred to him and Vel'vovskii as "the two fathers of this method." He underlined this phrase on his invitation letter, vexed that his Natural Childbirth and Vel'vovskii's psychoprophylaxis were presented as one and the same.[111] When he returned from what was apparently an unpleasant experience at the Paris conference, Dick-Read wrote to organizer Chertok to complain, lamenting that debates there had been "more a matter of ideology than a matter of scientific truth and observation."[112]

Dick-Read's efforts to thwart the expansion of psychoprophylaxis failed, but Lamaze's untimely death in March 1957 shook Les Bluets and triggered a series of events that changed the method's practice and political implications. Two versions of the events surrounding Lamaze's death came to light in subsequent weeks. According to the USTM, the metallurgists' workers union that funded Les Bluets, the maternity ward's cost overruns needed to be addressed. USTM leaders reasoned that because psychoprophylaxis in France had begun to gain momentum and was receiving state funding, Les Bluets' maternity ward could pull back from its leading role in the promotion of psychoprophylaxis. Specifically, to balance the budget, the USTM recommended an end to internships for doctors and midwives to train in psychoprophylaxis, as well as a range of personnel changes to cut expenses. The most significant proposed changes to staff included letting go of André Bourrel, who had worked on Lamaze's team from the beginning, and shifting his responsibility for instructing expectant mothers in psychoprophylaxis onto the midwives. Les Bluets' administration and staff resisted the USTM recommendations and resented union interference with matters of patient care. Les Bluets' director Le Guay countered the USTM proposal with the suggestion that the remainder of the polyclinic's services simply subsidize the work of the maternity ward, which had brought Les Bluets international renown.[113]

Lamaze had in Le Guay an advocate for Les Bluets' psychoprophylaxis program, but their combined efforts to sway the USTM proved inadequate. USTM officials proceeded to impose their plan on Les Bluets despite the lack of support from the polyclinic's staff and administration. As Pierre Vellay later described it, "on the evening of March 5, 1957, Lamaze was called into a meeting with the metal workers. This was a pure formality. The decision had already been made to order a restructuring of the hospital staff and to dismiss most of [Lamaze's] closest colleagues."[114] Among the casualties that evening was not only Bourrel, but Le Guay himself, who was forced to tender his resignation. Lamaze left the meeting distraught and defeated. Early the next morning, he suffered a fatal heart attack.

Many of Lamaze's supporters believed the upheaval immediately preceding his death contributed directly to his demise. Le Guay, Vellay, and others lay responsibility for Lamaze's heart attack at the doorstep of the USTM and, indirectly, the PCF. In a letter to USTM head André Lunet, Dr. Jean Dalsace—Lamaze's longtime friend, Vellay's father-in-law, and a lifelong PCF member—suggested that the fact that Lamaze's death came just hours after a confrontation with the USTM "speaks to the responsibility that you have in his death. . . . I consider it my duty as a man, a friend, and a Communist to lay this before your conscience."[115] Writing on behalf of Lamaze's widow, Vellay asked the USTM not to hold any kind of memorial service on Lamaze's behalf, "considering that the events of recent weeks are not without influence on the tragic death of her husband."[116]

As the story of Lamaze's death and accusations of the USTM's role in precipitating his heart attack made their way into the press, a more complicated picture of the union's motivations to shore up Les Bluets' finances began to take shape. The PCF organ *L'Humanité* published a front-page notice of Lamaze's death and a lengthy tribute to his work accompanied by a statement from the PCF's Central Committee.[117] The following day, the weekly magazine *L'Express* told a different story of Lamaze's death with a short obituary asserting that not only was the maternity ward's budget the source of a heated argument between Lamaze and union officials on the eve of his death, but that the USTM "had viciously attacked the methods of Dr. Lamaze." The notice closed with the suggestion that Lamaze and Le Guay had fallen out of favor with the USTM's communist leadership for taking a public stand against the Soviet invasion of Hungary in the fall of 1956.[118] On March 11 the conservative *Le Figaro* fired with an article on Lamaze's death entitled "Communist Indecency," decrying that Lamaze and his colleagues had been "under the most virulent attack from union representatives" for budgetary overruns. The article repeated the suggestion that the true motives lay with Le Guay's open denunciation of the Hungarian invasion.[119] Accusations in *L'Express* and *Le Figaro* themselves became news, reported on March 12 in *Le Monde*. Despite his forced resignation, Le Guay publicly fell on his sword. He defended the USTM with letters to *Le Figaro* and *L'Express* insisting that Stalinist discipline played no role in his dismissal and rejecting the characterization of Lamaze as a victim of PCF politics.[120] Le Guay had no stomach for making budgetary matters, ideological conflicts, or personnel decisions fodder for scandal in the centrist and right-wing press. By contrast, Jean Dalsace quit the Communist Party in public disgust.[121]

USTM leaders found that Lamaze's death provided an opportune moment for staff changes at Les Bluets and Lamaze's psychoprophylaxis team rapidly disbanded. The naming of PCF loyalist Hersilie, not Vellay, to head the maternity ward triggered a rash of departures, including that of Vellay himself.[122] In her resignation letter, midwife R. Rouat, a PCF member and longtime colleague of Lamaze, cited among her reasons for quitting the selection of Hersilie over Vellay as Lamaze's replacement. She characterized Hersilie as "professionally divisive" and his appointment as "the usurpation of a post that rightfully belongs to Dr. Vellay," who was universally seen among the staff as Lamaze's heir apparent.[123] Amid USTM's belt-tightening measures, Lamaze's collaborators fled an atmosphere that obstetric intern Claude Bazin characterized as one of "mistrust and insecurity, creating a moral climate that had quickly become intolerable."[124] Bazin's and Rouat's comments point to the deep rift between staff and administration at Les Bluets' maternity ward, and between Les Bluets and its USTM patrons after Lamaze's death.

Les Bluets' maternity ward continued to provide psychoprophylactic training for expectant mothers, but as the 1950s drew to a close, it became only one among many French institutions, most with no ties to the PCF or CGT, that utilized psychoprophylaxis. The Left fragmented in the wake of growing disillusionment with the USSR, and the linkage between psychoprophylaxis and a single, clear political agenda frayed. Fleeing Stalinist diehards among the USTM leadership and Les Bluets' hospital administration, members of Lamaze's former team left not just the institution, but also the communist ideological fold. Even Angelergues, the articulate French interpreter of Pavlovian neuropsychology as applied to psychoprophylaxis, backed off his rigid anti-Freudianism and began to incorporate psychoanalytic perspectives into his understanding of psychoprophylaxis.[125]

Despite the disorder and tensions at Les Bluets and on the Left, Lamaze's ambition to spread psychoprophylaxis across France and around the globe was realized. By 1961 a remarkable 30 percent of French women chose to use psychoprophylaxis during labor.[126] L'Humanité claimed that as of 1962, between 40 and 50 percent of French births took place using psychoprophylaxis, though this figure may more accurately reflect the number of women who received training, rather than how many utilized it during labor and birth.[127] Intrigues regarding Les Bluets' personnel and administration perhaps slowed the spread of psychoprophylaxis, pointing to how communist infighting, as well as Left-Right tensions, played a role in the trajectory of psychoprophylaxis in France.

* * *

In June 1959, Dick-Read died at the age of sixty-nine. He had lived his life dedicated to improving safety and satisfaction in childbirth, scorned by most of his colleagues for what he advocated and beloved by women around the globe for his efforts on their behalf. At the memorial service held at the Royal Parish Church of St. Martin-in-the-Field, Yale University professor Lawrence Z. Freedman emphasized that "millions of mothers and thousands of doctors and midwives in all parts of the world are in his debt. . . . Because of his idea, women may be spared fear while they are freed in spirit for he never forgot that mankind has goals and dreams and wishes beyond the relief of physical pain."[128] For all his triumphs, Dick-Read lost his quixotic battle to prove that he, and only he, held the key to a dignified birth experience and that Soviet psychoprophylaxis was little more than a poor imitation. Within a few years of Dick-Read's death, psychoprophylaxis's reach would be greater than ever, and Lamaze would gain posthumous fame in the United States. The rise of what was popularized in the United States as the Lamaze method, in fact, built on networks that had been active in the movement for Dick-Read's Natural Childbirth. Americans who had promoted the Read method in the 1950s began to turn in increasing number to psychoprophylaxis, joined by a new generation of women seeking to give birth "awake and aware."[129]

CHAPTER 5

༫ᘯᘲ

Lamaze Goes Global, 1957–67

Unlike in Europe, Dick-Read had no rivals in the United States in the 1950s. The lack of US-Soviet contact and virulent anti-Soviet sentiment in America insulated the United States from the movement for psychoprophylaxis. Few American medical practitioners or consumers knew of Vel'vovskii or Lamaze. The pope's 1956 decree made news in the United States, and one Swiss obstetrician practiced psychoprophylaxis briefly in Cleveland in the mid-1950s, but to no significant professional recognition or popular fanfare.[1]

As the 1950s wore on, murmurings surfaced about something similar to the Read method coming out of the Soviet Union and France. As BACE's first childbirth educator, Justine Kelliher, later recollected, "ideas variously described as natural childbirth, Grantly Dick-Read method, trained childbirth, prepared childbirth, cooperative childbirth, family-centered obstetrics, or psychoprophylaxis" began to circulate.[2] Like European mothers, the women Kelliher worked with were not concerned with political squabbles or methodological dogmatism, and once the Read method was no longer the only psychological approach to childbirth pain, the obvious question became whether it was the most effective one. Growing awareness of psychoprophylaxis fostered a rising "feeling that, although Dr. [Dick-] Read was the pioneer... his advocated methods have been improved upon," rendering his work "outdated."[3] Dick-Read's emphasis on the spiritual quality of birth also put off areligious consumers and medical professionals who could not "get rhapsodic about giving birth" and preferred the more down-to-earth explanations of psychoprophylaxis.[4] Dick-Read's work seemed to some a relic of another time, and they sought an approach to childbearing that hewed more closely to the secular, scientific zeitgeist.

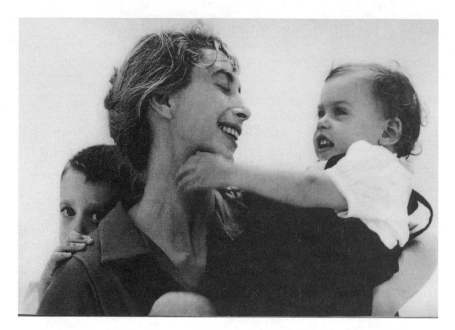

Figure 5.1: Marjorie Karmel with her children, Pepe (left) and Marianne, ca. 1959. Courtesy of Alex Karmel.

In 1955 Marjorie Karmel, pictured in fig 5.1, was a young, American, sometime actress living with her husband Alex, a writer, in Paris. Expecting her first child, the plucky and bright Karmel made her way to Fernand Lamaze's office at his posh private obstetric practice. He introduced Karmel to the psychoprophylactic method of childbirth, and she began to prepare with Blanche Cohen, who had been training Lamaze's private patients since 1953. Cohen and Lamaze saw Karmel through a strenuous but satisfying birth experience that left her thrilled with psychoprophylaxis and inspired to repeat the experience in the future. When she returned to New York and awaited her second child, she could not find an obstetrician who was knowledgeable about psychoprophylaxis. Wanting to spread the good word to her compatriots, she wrote *Thank You, Dr. Lamaze*, a memoir of her childbirth experience.[5] After reading her book, Dick-Read offered tepid praise for Karmel's "light hearted good humor," but denounced the book's "slight vulgarity" and cautioned his NCT supporters against its use in their natural childbirth courses.[6] Despite Dick-Read's warning, Karmel's engaging style won the day, throwing open the doors of the English-speaking world to psychoprophylaxis. Karmel's book helped to make "Lamaze" a household name.

With the publication of Karmel's book, we can properly begin to call psychoprophylaxis "the Lamaze method," an iteration of a psychological approach to obstetric pain relief that had roots in the USSR, underwent revision in France, and then found yet another incarnation in the United States, where its development continued.[7] At this moment, too, around 1960, the phrase "natural childbirth" began to be used in a generic sense, meaning not only the Read method ("Natural Childbirth" as a proper noun), but any combination of strategies intended to minimize medical intervention in childbirth, particularly in terms of pharmacological pain relief. Dick-Read and Lamaze each had their devotees, but in practice the two approaches intermingled and hybridized, as they already had in the USSR, France, and elsewhere. In American parlance, psychoprophylaxis, the Lamaze method, and natural childbirth became synonymous, and from this juncture forward I use them interchangeably, as they were at the time.

While accurate numbers about what percentage of women sought to give birth with minimal anesthetization do not exist, one critic of the method described natural childbirth in 1962 as "the most-dropped phrase among America's pregnant women today."[8] Karmel's work struck a chord with expectant mothers who were hungry for information about childbirth and interested in having a less medicalized birth experience.[9] One young mother who read Karmel's book shortly after it appeared described it as "joyous" in its celebration of birth and, in the way it captured the thrill of Paris in the 1950s, "as evocative of its era as, say, *On the Road*."[10] Another early reader for whom Karmel's words resonated was Elisabeth Bing, pictured in fig. 5.2, a physical therapist who had been working with expectant and new mothers since the 1930s and preparing women in the Read method since the 1940s. Employed as a childbirth educator at New York City's Mount Sinai Hospital, Bing first heard about psychoprophylaxis in 1958. Shortly after, she read Karmel's article in *Harper's Bazaar* about her experience with psychoprophylaxis. She initially took offense at what she read as Karmel's critique of the Read method, but she found Karmel's 1959 book to be inspirational.[11] As Bing recalled decades later, "I said, 'Yes, this is it!' as soon as I read it," and she immediately arranged to meet Karmel.[12]

In February 1960 Karmel and Bing teamed up with obstetrician Benjamin Segal to launch the American Society for Psychoprophylaxis in Obstetrics (ASPO), now known as Lamaze International, "dedicated to the Lamaze-Pavlov Method of Childbirth without Pain."[13] Their own paths to and interest in psychoprophylaxis dictated ASPO's tripartite structure, bringing together physicians, paraprofessionals such as childbirth educators, physical therapists and obstetric nurses, and expectant and new mothers. Despite aiming their efforts at professionals and consumers, the

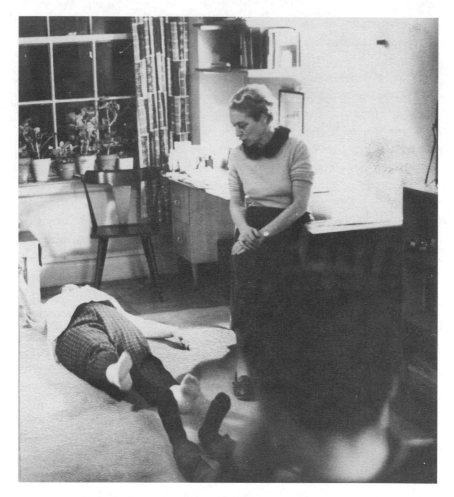

Figure 5.2: Elisabeth Bing conducting conditional relaxation exercises with a group of students in her New York City apartment, 1960. Courtesy of Laura Ellen.

organization saw winning over physicians as key to the method's popularization and legitimation. This privileging of physician authority and influence found expression in ASPO's bylaws, which initially gave only physicians voting rights as "full members," while nurses and childbirth educators were nonvoting "associate members." Expectant mothers and other laypeople could join as "supporting members."[14]

Hard work and dedication coupled with consumer desire to yield impressive growth for ASPO. By the end of 1961, less than two years after its founding, the New York–based organization had cultivated ties with burgeoning local groups across the country and began to liaise with promoters of psychoprophylaxis around the globe. Bing, Karmel, and Dr. Alfred Tanz collaborated on a training manual, popularly known as the "Red Manual," endorsed by ASPO and recommended to all expectant mothers who were interested in birthing using the Lamaze method. Though their reach was broad and their agenda ambitious, ASPO's ranks were spread thin in those early days. At the end of 1962, there were only sixteen full members among New York City's physicians and a mere eight associate members; another hundred individuals had expressed interest in joining. There was one member each in California, Massachusetts, and Michigan, but ASPO had established relationships with several American organizations and hospitals.[15]

ASPO's founders went on the offensive to spread word of psychoprophylaxis and to distinguish it from the Read method, taking their message to the airwaves. Shortly after ASPO's founding, New York City radio station WBAI presented a ninety-minute program on psychoprophylaxis featuring Bing and Karmel. The broadcast traced the method's Soviet and French origins, with a clear accent placed on the method's development in the hands of Lamaze.[16] Bing gave credit to Dick-Read and his American disciple Herbert Thoms for their work on Natural Childbirth, but said that "they did not comprehend the mechanism of de conditioning and conditioning" upon which the Lamaze method built its success.[17] Using clear and accessible layman's terms, Bing explained Pavlov's theory of conditional response and its relationship to psychoprophylaxis in childbirth. She emphasized the mother's active and participatory role in the birthing of her own child and stressed that breathing, massage, and other techniques eased or eliminated pain and shortened labor. Bing's and Karmel's words resonated with listeners, including one who was moved to write to the station with praise for the program: "I sat glued to the radio, excited by the presentation, almost joining in the discussion myself. It was such a marvelously adult program, so humanly and scientifically handled—I wish all parents and particularly mothers to be might have listened in."[18] When Pierre Vellay came to the United States for a 1963 tour (see fig. 5.3), ASPO's leaders again turned to WBAI to promote their efforts. In a program titled "Thank You, Dr. Vellay," he was interviewed along with ASPO chairman Dr. Heinz Luschinsky, a couple who had recently used psychoprophylaxis with success, and an expectant mother and father preparing for their baby's birth. That interview came on the heels of a CBS television program on the Lamaze method that broadcast excerpts from Vellay's childbirth education film *Naissance*.[19] Media appearances like these promoted the Lamaze method and associated psychoprophylaxis in the popular imagination with France, rather than the USSR.

As word spread about a new, psychological approach to obstetric pain, psychoprophylaxis came under the increasing scrutiny of critics. Hostility

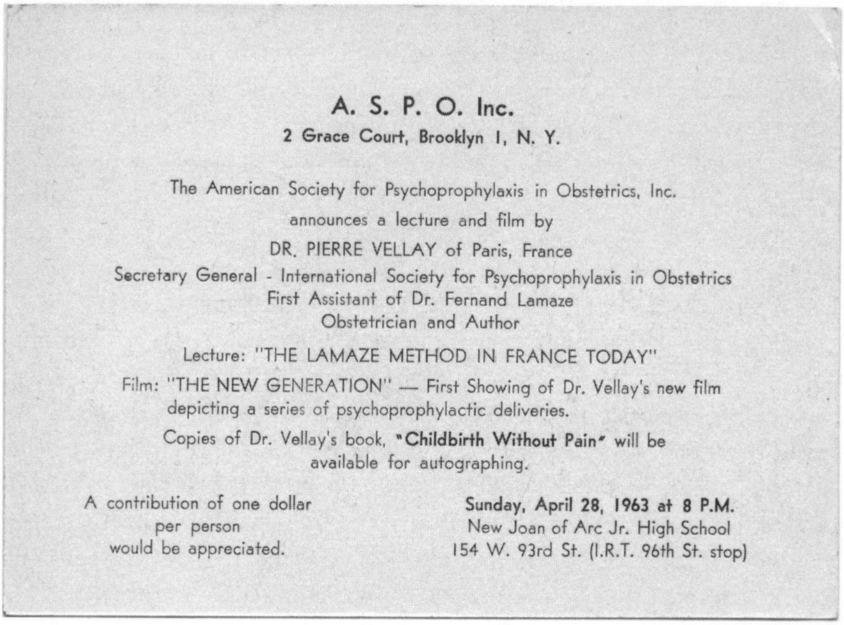

A. S. P. O. Inc.

2 Grace Court, Brooklyn 1, N. Y.

The American Society for Psychoprophylaxis in Obstetrics, Inc.

announces a lecture and film by

DR. PIERRE VELLAY of Paris, France

Secretary General - International Society for Psychoprophylaxis in Obstetrics
First Assistant of Dr. Fernand Lamaze
Obstetrician and Author

Lecture: "THE LAMAZE METHOD IN FRANCE TODAY"

Film: "THE NEW GENERATION" — First Showing of Dr. Vellay's new film
depicting a series of psychoprophylactic deliveries.

Copies of Dr. Vellay's book, **"Childbirth Without Pain"** will be
available for autographing.

A contribution of one dollar	**Sunday, April 28, 1963 at 8 P.M.**
per person	New Joan of Arc Jr. High School
would be appreciated.	154 W. 93rd St. (I.R.T. 96th St. stop)

Figure 5.3: Invitation to lecture by Pierre Vellay and a screening of his film *The New Generation* in New York City, 1963. Courtesy of the Schlesinger Library, Radcliffe Institute, Harvard University.

toward the Read method had already found expression in medical literature and the popular press.[20] ASPO leaders strove to distinguish the Lamaze method from the Read method, but opponents tended to tar them both with a single brush. A 1962 book, an excerpt of which appeared in *McCall's* magazine, sparked controversy with its vitriolic critique or, rather, caricature, of natural childbirth. Obstetrician Waldo Fielding partnered with his sister-in-law, journalist and young mother Lois Benjamin, to make the case against the whole compendium of practices associated with the Lamaze and Read methods. The authors condemned the effort to avoid anesthetization, resist routine episiotomies, install the husband at his wife's side during labor and birth, and have the newborn room-in with the mother. They disputed the very premise of natural childbirth as a satisfying, dignified experience. Rather than a moment of elation, unanesthetized birth was "a kind of ordeal by fire," inflated out of proportion to "a supreme physical and spiritual testing ground, rather than what it really is—a preamble to motherhood."[21] Other opponents similarly denounced natural childbirth for promoting an "unwholesome" preoccupation with the experience of childbirth, rather than a focus on mothering.[22]

Critics depicted Dick-Read's partisans as zealots and cultists, and called into question advocates' mental health. Encouraging frail or mentally weak women's desires to give birth with little or no pharmacological pain relief could precipitate a psychological crisis, they argued. Women "are convinced that to endure childbirth without the sedation of so much as an aspirin will, by some nebulous psychologic process, inspire" a closer bond with their babies and allow them to achieve "that precious lodestone of the female sex: true femininity."[23] A 1961 *Harper's Bazaar* article against natural childbirth invoked the language and authority of Freudianism to make its case that the adherent "anticipates that the lifelong wound she feels—the wound of womanhood, of not having been a boy—will be paradoxically healed by having a child." The author then stereotyped the woman who was interested in natural childbirth as "the fairly aggressive, masculine-oriented, nonconservative woman."[24] Fielding and Benjamin reiterate these arguments about women seeking "psychic masculinity" through natural childbirth and go so far as to assert that not only are "disturbed women...often attracted to natural childbirth," but they also "are the very women who are likely to be the most intensely enthusiastic volunteers."[25] When the woman in labor either experiences more pain than she anticipated or, in the face of that suffering turns to anesthesia, her birth experience becomes a trauma from which, Fielding and Benjamin, among others, claim she does not soon recover.

Their case against natural childbirth on physiological grounds was made in similarly stark terms. Critics put forward the baseless claim that any physician who promoted the Read or Lamaze method "abdicates his responsibility for deciding whether and when to administer drugs to a patient who is in no condition—and is not qualified—to make such decisions."[26] In a particularly tortured line of logical reasoning, they asserted that mother and baby were in jeopardy because, "if an emergency arises in a 'natural' delivery, it is complicated by the fact that the mother is not well sedated or under anesthesia." With the woman prone to panic amid the hubbub, the doctor "loses precious minutes because his patient is awake and frightened. If she cannot be made to respond quickly to a hastily applied anesthetic, he may not be able to interfere rapidly enough to bring both her and her child safely through the crisis."[27] In other words, irrespective of the risks associated with anesthesia, women were best off routinely, prophylactically anesthetized on the remote chance that an emergency might require it. Readers, including potential mothers, were to draw a straight and frightening line between the choice of natural childbirth and serious harm, even death, to a woman or her baby.

Opponents used red-baiting to discredit psychoprophylaxis as antithetical to American psychology and national character. Psychoprophylaxis
met with some initial opposition within the medical community because
the idea of Pavlovian psychological conditioning "had not appealed to our
American ideals of individual freedom, selfhood and independent choice."[28]
Fielding and Benjamin argued that "neither the Western obstetrical world
nor the Western woman's mind is geared for such a regimented system."[29]
American women allegedly were psychologically so different, so resistant
to the supposed collectivist orientation of Pavlovian conditioning, as to
render them poor subjects for psychoprophylactic preparation. Further,
humane American hospitals, with their supposed emphasis on patient
care, could not mimic the purported totalitarian environments of Soviet
maternity wards. "In a regimented society, such as the Soviet Union, hospital routine can be strictly disciplined, rigidly supervised and kept totally
devoid of distracting human elements, as the state decrees. But in our society such absolute control over disturbances and distractions," as is necessary for the success of psychoprophylaxis, "is virtually impossible."[30] There
is no question that most American women received gentler treatment than
Soviet maternity patients, but charges of inhumane, authoritarian regimentation could certainly be laid against American hospitals. The significance of such comments lies not in their accuracy, but in their challenge to
this way of giving birth on Cold War ideological grounds.

ASPO leaders were sensitive to the Cold War context in which they
sought to promote psychoprophylaxis. While it was certainly known, particularly among medical professionals, that the Lamaze method came from
the USSR, ASPO activists did not emphasize this fact, as Bing reflects in
her memoir, "given how Americans were feeling about Russians" in the
1950s and 1960s.[31] They did not hide the Soviet roots of psychoprophylaxis, but stressed instead that the method was further developed and
enhanced in France. Obstetrician David A. Meyer, for example, asserted
in 1961 that he prepared women in psychoprophylaxis "as developed by
the late Dr. Fernand Lamaze," implicitly distancing his approach from
that used in the USSR, to which he omitted any reference.[32] Similarly, an
article in a leading nursing journal claimed that psychoprophylactic practice "in the United States, while based on the same assumptions, has come
to be very different from the Soviet approach, largely due to the work of
the late Dr. Fernand Lamaze."[33] When Vellay toured the United States in
1963, he told an audience at Boston Lying-In Hospital that psychoprophylaxis "respects the individuality of women," perhaps to assuage concerns
about any connection between psychoprophylaxis and Soviet collectivism.[34] By the middle of the 1960s, ASPO dropped reference to Pavlov

from the organization's letterhead and publication masthead, promoting itself as "dedicated to the Lamaze Method of Family-Centered Childbirth Education," rather than "the Lamaze-Pavlov Method."[35] Not only were links to the USSR suspect, but Pavlov's association with salivating dogs did nothing to entice prospective clients.

ASPO mobilized to counter various lines of attack against its cause in those early days. ASPO leaders well understood the deleterious effect of anti–natural childbirth propaganda and fired back at Fielding and Benjamin with a letter-writing campaign to *McCall's* and a treatise of their own. When *McCall's* refused to publish a rebuttal article, the organization self-published a response written by ASPO treasurer Dr. Jean Anderson with ASPO board members Luschinsky, Segal, and Tanz.[36] ASPO's rebuttal tried to set the record straight by detailing how the Lamaze method worked, reiterating faith in the authority of obstetricians as the final decision-makers in the labor and delivery rooms, reaffirming the commitment of the obstetricians to a sweeping array of medical interventions when indicated, and rebutting Fielding and Benjamin's specific claims about the physical and psychological advantages of an anesthetized birth experience.[37]

ASPO activists attempted to defend the Lamaze method from attack in part by distinguishing it from the Read method, which they depicted as having been superseded by psychoprophylaxis. While Waldo and Fielding noted no meaningful differences, advocates for the Lamaze method critiqued Natural Childbirth and distanced psychoprophylaxis from it. When Dr. Wagner Bridger of the Albert Einstein School of Medicine's Department of Psychiatry gave a talk in February 1961 to ASPO members on conditional response and the Lamaze method, he acknowledged the similarities among psychoprophylaxis, hypnosuggestion, and Natural Childbirth, but he emphasized the grounding of psychoprophylaxis in Pavlovian conditioning, which, he claimed, enhanced its efficacy.[38] A former advocate for the Read method, Bing similarly underscored the limits of the Read method and the ways in which psychoprophylaxis had advanced beyond the foundation laid by Dick-Read. The Read method, asserted Bing, "has its limitations. Somehow, the suggested exercises, the particular breathing and relaxation as practiced have not altogether achieved their objective."[39] Invoking the same arguments made previously in the USSR and France, Tanz stressed that "with the Read approach, the patient is directed toward passivity and relaxation, but the Lamaze [mother] is active and alert throughout," a distinction that Dick-Read and his supporters certainly contested.[40]

To win support among medical professionals, ASPO leaders needed to back up their claims with empirical evidence that their colleagues would recognize as legitimate. Only systematic scientific study could offer that kind of persuasive power. To gather statistical evidence on the success rates of psychoprophylaxis, Segal turned to an evaluation form developed by Lamaze, who had modeled his on one that Vel'vovskii had crafted in the late 1940s. Physician reports on patient success and failure, principally in terms of pain management, were to be the foundation for demonstrating psychoprophylaxis's efficacy to the medical community. All patients were prepared in the Lamaze method, and obstetricians filled out the forms within hours or, at most, a few days of delivery. Segal completed the majority of them, though a handful of other doctors participated as well. Obstetricians noted information about the length of each stage of labor; the behavior of the patient during these stages; what techniques, if any, were used to manage pain; and what role the husband played during labor and/or delivery.[41]

These obstetrician reports offer a window into physicians' expectations for what psychoprophylactic training was to accomplish, especially with respect to patient comportment. In the column for describing patient behavior at each stage of labor, the suggested choices were "good, fair, uncontrolled." Juxtaposed with "uncontrolled," "good" implied obedient, calm, and controlled, or perhaps controllable, that is, by the obstetrician. Mrs. D., for example, was "calm" upon her admission to the hospital in 1963. Segal described her behavior during labor as "good," and her delivery with the assistance of forceps was deemed to be a successful application of psychoprophylaxis. Credit went to Mrs. D. only in part, as "intensive support by husband and physician" played a major role, in Segal's estimate. Segal described another patient, Mrs. E., as "excellent throughout.... The patient is generally well contained and controlled. Has rational attitude toward [the] situation; took advantage of necessary anesthesia with calm." For Mrs. E. a good performance meant deference to the doctor's judgment about the need for anesthesia. On Mrs. E.'s views about this course of action the record is silent. Physician reports suggest that American obstetricians shared the value that European doctors put on psychoprophylaxis as a means to impart—as Soviet obstetricians liked to put it—discipline. The laboring woman who willingly and quietly relinquished control of the process to her obstetrician, while playing an active role in assisting him to deliver her baby, was characterized as successful.

ASPO physicians clearly were pleased for the woman who had an experience that she deemed to be satisfying and dignified, but they were uncomfortable, intolerant, and judgmental of the patient who was vocal about her pain. Segal described the case of Mrs. C., who had a baby boy in 1961, as a "complete failure." Mrs. C. purportedly arrived at the hospital "excited." When Segal appeared early in labor's first stage, her behavior had deteriorated to what he described as "poor." She was given analgesics when her cervix was at 2 and 8 centimeters dilation, but was "restless" and "anxious." In Segal's estimate, even before Mrs. C. went into labor, problems were evident in her "inordinate sense of 'everything is all right' with no questions for the obstetrician, creating a cloak of safety in the [Lamaze] method." Mrs. C.'s "emotional insecurity (complete ten-finger nail biting)" made failure predictable. Segal assessed Mrs. C.'s display of pain as out of proportion, "with tossing about, restlessness and moaning—long before any average patient trained or untrained would or might so respond even with obstetric abnormality." She failed to listen to her obstetrician's instructions, pushing in the second stage "frantically and with groaning."[42] Segal judged Mrs. C.'s neuroses and denial, not any limitations inherent in the Lamaze method, the culprit in what he saw as her undignified, uncooperative, and undisciplined comportment.

At first glance, these early obstetrician reports seem to support the idea that the Lamaze method may have given women a more satisfying experience, but it left unchallenged the obstetrician's authority over birth, especially as practiced through the 1960s. As sociologist Barbara Katz-Rothman explains, ASPO "substituted psychological for pharmacological control of pain. While the difference between consciousness and unconsciousness may be all the difference in the world for the mother, from the point of view of the institution that single factor is relatively minor.... [Psychoprophylaxis] certainly poses no threat to the control of birth by obstetricians."[43] Physicians remained the gatekeepers of access to (or avoidance of) pharmacological pain relief and other interventions. They stood in omniscient judgment of women's performance, taking for themselves considerable credit for successes and laying blame for failure on their patients.

The testimony of one of Segal's earliest Lamaze patients complicates an overly simplistic narrative about the Lamaze method that defines it as either empowering to women or merely another misogynistic tool for obstetric control. Mrs. L. gave birth in New York City's Beth Israel Hospital in March 1960. Her labor was definitely not the "childbirth without pain" described in the prenatal classes that Mrs. L. attended in Bing's West Side apartment. Labor advanced slowly, and, as the day wore on, her contractions became more intense and her tolerance wore thin. Thinking she could endure no more, as she entered the transition phase she demanded to be "knocked out." Segal put her off, and, after he held a brief, hushed conversation with the rest of the obstetric team about fetal distress, Mrs. L. was rushed to the delivery room as she approached full dilation. "I want you to breathe," he told her as she lay on the delivery table. She recalled thinking at that moment: "that son-of-a-bitch, he's so into [psychoprophylaxis], he's going to make me do this even though I don't want this anymore." Mrs. L., however, did as she was told, deciding it was best to defer to Segal's authority and show genuine effort before again demanding anesthetization. Mrs. L. later reflected that, to her great surprise, "I start following him, doing what he says and I'm not feeling any pain!"[44] Segal's well-trained eye could see by the tautness of Mrs. L.'s abdomen when a contraction began. He guided her through it and she was able to "stay on top of" the sensation. To hear Mrs. L. tell it, her daughter's birth, accomplished with the assistance of forceps, was a collaborative effort, with doctor and patient working as a team. After more than fifty years, Mrs. L.'s respect and appreciation remains palpable when she says that, "He was wonderful and very caring. He was there for me."[45] Segal was very much in charge in that delivery room, but Mrs. L. was neither passive nor disempowered. She put herself unreservedly into his hands and to dismiss her choices as unenlightened deference to masculine, medical authority would be to underestimate her. Yielding to his expertise and skills enabled her to have precisely the kind of birth she sought. Her birth story upends easy assumptions about what constitutes an empowered birth experience and points to the messiness of authoritative knowledge and agency in practice.

In the mid-1960s psychologist Deborah Tanzer drew unprecedented attention to the value and complexity of American women's evaluation of their personal experience with natural childbirth. Unlike Segal's physician reports, which refract women's behavior, physical experience, and emotional state through the doctors' eyes, Tanzer grounds her analysis in the direct testimony of mothers themselves as they looked both forward to and back on their childbirth experience. Tanzer conducted three in-depth interviews, before and after birth, with forty-one women. Her informants included women prepared in natural childbirth, mostly the Lamaze method, as well as a control group that experienced conventional, anesthetized childbirth. Subjects were identified with the assistance of several obstetricians in private practice, including Segal and others active in ASPO.[46]

Her research points to a number of benefits to natural childbirth training, and helped to define the image of who sought natural childbirth and why. A student of famed psychologist Abraham Maslow, Tanzer applied to natural childbirth his notion of "peak experience," a transcendent, ecstatic, almost indescribable elation.[47] Her research indicated that prenatal preparation courses and the presence of the husband were essential to a woman's reflection on childbirth as a peak experience. She found that women who attended prenatal courses generally relied less on anesthetics and analgesics during labor, and understood their experiences as more rewarding and satisfying. Women described the feeling of natural childbirth as "fantastic," "marvelous," "exciting," and "thrilling."[48] These words contrast sharply with the reflection of women in the control group who received various drugs during labor and then were rendered unconscious for delivery using ether. Tanzer explains that they "do not describe a happy experience. They describe screaming, yelling, pain, moaning, fear and hostility," characteristics of the undignified, unsatisfying, undesirable birth experience that women prepared in psychoprophylaxis sought to avoid.[49] For the women who pursued natural childbirth, there may have been some pain, but no suffering. Echoing the most grandiose claims of Dick-Read, Vel'vovskii, and Lamaze, Tanzer asserts that, in cases without complications, women trained in natural childbirth had little or no discomfort whatsoever.[50] Considerations of pain were overshadowed by "feelings of work, activity, concentration, and confidence," which dominated their reflections on their childbirth experiences.[51] Disseminated through a widely read article in *Psychology Today* and in a popular book, Tanzer's research offered women a joyful image of what might await them after childbirth preparation: satisfaction, dignity, and minimal or no pain. She set a high bar for how women later reflected on their own experiences with psychoprophylaxis.[52]

A GLOBAL CONVERSATION

ASPO-supported research initiatives, like Segal's drive to gather obstetrician reports and Tanzer's exploration of the psychological benefits of natural childbirth preparation, were one way that the organization sought to represent the growing American movement for psychoprophylaxis to a worldwide community of medical professionals who were engaged in the method's promotion. When the Soviet Union turned away from psychoprophylaxis after 1956, the movement's capital migrated westward to Paris. Following Lamaze's death in 1957, it fell to his disciples, first among them Vellay, to continue this work at home and abroad, including in the United States. Physicians and childbirth educators who were active in ASPO traveled to Europe to exchange information and experiences about psychoprophylaxis with their colleagues from Great Britain, France, Italy, and elsewhere. In the fall of 1960, just months after ASPO's founding, Segal journeyed to Paris, where he met with Vellay. He toured Les Bluets' maternity ward, then under the direction of Roger Hersilie, who also headed the French Society for Obstetric Psychoprophylaxis (SFPO). Segal used his visit to build ties between ASPO and SFPO, and to purchase educational materials on psychoprophylaxis, such as several copies of a phonographic recording of a psychoprophylactic birth, an instructional film, and a series of slides for classroom use.[53]

Luschinsky represented ASPO at the First International Congress of Psychosomatic Medicine and Maternity, held in Paris in July 1962. Founded in 1958, the International Society for Psychoprophylaxis in Obstetrics, which sponsored the congress, united physicians, childbirth educators, and psychologists around the globe, and published a professional journal to which Americans began to contribute regularly.[54] The 1962 congress included a celebration, held at the United Nations Educational, Scientific and Cultural Organization (UNESCO) headquarters, of the tenth anniversary of psychoprophylaxis in France. Over four hundred representatives came from twenty-five countries, including virtually all of the leading figures in the field: Nikolaev from the USSR; Vellay, Hersilie, Chertok, and many others from France; American Read enthusiasts Corbin and Goodrich; Czechoslovakia's Miroslav Vojta; Italy's Piero Malcovati.[55] Anthropologist Margaret Mead served as an honorary congress president, along with Vel'vovskii and Herbert Thoms.[56] Doctors from both sides of the Iron Curtain exchanged information and observations during the formal sessions and talked over casual meals in Parisian homes and restaurants. The congress proved to be an exciting opportunity for international conversation and debate. American psychologist Niles Newton witnessed a Soviet obstetrician heatedly debate a group of Western European psychoanalysts over Freudian ideas about mother-infant bonding. Capping off the argument, a British physician "congratulated his Russian obstetrical colleague, saying that few obstetricians could have so effectively held their own with a group of psychoanalysts." Newton noted that, "contrary to the expectations of some Westerners, the Russians did not present a monolithic propaganda front."[57] She expressed surprise at the value Soviet doctors placed on anesthesia and analgesia as a supplement to psychoprophylaxis, a shift that French observers of Soviet obstetrics had identified back in 1956. Latecomers to the movement for psychoprophylaxis, American participants at the congress enjoyed an opportunity to finally learn firsthand from their Soviet professional colleagues.

In the spring of 1963, Vellay arrived in the United States for a tour under the joint sponsorship of ASPO and the Cultural Relations Department of France's Ministry of Foreign Affairs. The trip began in New York City, with speaking engagements in Boston, Washington, Baltimore, Detroit, St. Louis, Portland, San Francisco, Houston, and Jackson, Mississippi. In each city he met with activists for natural childbirth and family-centered maternity care (FCMC), which encouraged the father's presence during labor and promoted rooming-in. ASPO affiliates and members of the Milwaukee-based

International Childbirth Education Association (ICEA) feted Vellay as he crossed the country.[58] Vellay saw much that was praiseworthy in the United States. "The technical perfection of the American hospitals we visited, of the medical centers we saw, even in smaller towns, would make our old Europe blanche with envy." Nonetheless, Vellay believed that "the impeccable technical accomplishments of American obstetrics call for psychoprophylaxis as a correlate," a message that he trumpeted everywhere he went. His American colleagues often insisted that their patients demanded anesthesia, but Vellay was confident that American women just needed to learn that there was an alternative means of pain relief available. With proper information, the American woman "will immediately sense the value of the method which respects the personality of the woman, the emotional bond of the couple and the affective link of parents to child."[59] Nurses and physical therapists played a vanguard role in the development of psychoprophylaxis in the United States, and Vellay's trip brought him into contact with many leading figures in childbirth education, including Bing, Detroit's Flora Hommel, and San Jose's Mabel Fitzhugh. Physicians were a harder sell, and Vellay did more than preach to the choir on his tour. His ideas met a cold reception in Houston, where physicians who knew little about natural childbirth and relied heavily on anesthesia boasted to him of their success with prophylactic forceps delivery in 100 percent of their cases.[60]

It was apparent to Vellay that Americans, with their strong ideas about the value of drugs in the practice of obstetrics, readily fused psychoprophylaxis with the active management of labor: pharmaceutical interventions to stimulate contractions, numb the body, and relax the mind. In the 1950s, American Read advocates turned to the liberal use of anesthetics, analgesics, and sedatives in the conduct of what they nonetheless touted as natural childbirth. Like Vel'vovskii, Lamaze, and Dick-Read, early ASPO leaders believed that drugs were appropriate when necessary, but their role would be greatly reduced—not eliminated—through proper prenatal preparation. They objected not to the use of analgesics and anesthetics, but to their routine administration without consideration of the patient's ability to manage her pain without these aids. In practice, women trained in the Lamaze method typically used far less pain medication than untrained women, but even their much-diminished application contradicts popular notions today about what distinguishes natural childbirth from conventional, medicalized birth. At this point in time the definition of the method did not hinge on the absence of anesthetics, analgesics, or sedatives. For many American women and their physicians in the early and mid-1960s, a little Demerol or morphine to take the edge off pain and tension did not stand in the way of claiming success in achieving a "natural" birth.[61]

In their classic text on the Lamaze method, the Red Manual, Bing, Karmel, and Tanz stated the official position of ASPO toward anesthetics and analgesics:

> While the overuse and misuse of these helpful aids should legitimately be condemned, on no account should women develop the attitude that all use of drugs is harmful.... [The childbirth educator] may explain that once the doctor understands what the woman is trying to accomplish through her preparation she may count on him to restrict his use of drugs to the minimum that he considers necessary.... [The instructor] should point out that anesthesia is not a crutch or a means of shirking the work of labor.[62]

With these words, the Red Manual conveyed to its readers a mixed message. On the one hand, women should not shy away from using drugs if they, or, more accurately, their doctors, thought it was necessary. On the other hand, they had to be careful not to turn to it because they were too lazy or weak to do the hard work of childbirth. The trick was to know whether resort to pharmacological pain relief was a need or a desire. Bing, Karmel, and Tanz left it to physicians to make that determination.

The American depiction of natural childbirth as dogmatically opposed to drugs originated in two sources. First, opponents like Fielding and Benjamin caricatured the relationship between pain medication and support for natural childbirth, misrepresenting in stark, black-and-white terms a more nuanced stance. Second, despite ASPO's efforts to tamp down expectations, American mothers tended to "look upon childbirth in terms of *either* drugs *or* natural childbirth," as one British Lamaze activist noted with curiosity during her 1963 visit.[63] In the wake of the thalidomide scandal, as the knowledge spread beyond the medical community to the general population that medication quickly crossed the placenta from mother to fetus, women became more hesitant consumers of drugs during pregnancy. They carried these same concerns into labor and birth, contributing to a rising reluctance to turn to pharmacological pain relief.[64] But the view of drugs, especially pain medication, as anathematic to natural childbirth was not what psychoprophylaxis's US promoters officially endorsed, even if their depiction of anesthetics and analgesics as a crutch encouraged it.

In Europe lively debate over the place of drugs in psychoprophylactic practice characterized the conversation among obstetricians and psychologists in the 1960s. In the wake of the 1956 Kiev conference, Soviet obstetricians supported the integration of anesthetics and analgesics during labor and birth, though pharmaceutical production continued to fall short. Following a 1961 visit to the USSR, French natural childbirth advocate Armand Notter noted a Soviet turn toward active management of labor through the use of drugs like oxytocin to stimulate and strengthen uterine contractions, and nitrous oxide and Demerol to ease pain and tension. Notter observed that Nikolaev, a leader in the campaign for Soviet psychoprophylaxis, had come to support the routine obstetric application of a variety of uterine stimulants, anesthetics, analgesics, and sedatives.[65] Nikolaev's view on the place of pharmaceuticals in obstetrics is clear in an interview he gave in France in 1962, when he said that he "supports the use of certain drugs designed to stimulate labor and suppress fear."[66] Nikolaev's remarks are consistent with Soviet statistics, which point to an increased use of drugs in labor and birth. The vast majority of Soviet women received their maternity care from midwives who had minimal access to even the mildest pain relief medication, but the minority of women in the care of obstetricians found a new emphasis on the use of drugs for pain. Even in Kharkov, birthplace of psychoprophylaxis, a 1962 report confirmed that obstetricians "devote significantly more attention…to pharmacological pain relief."[67] In the case of women unable to complete psychoprophylactic preparation, Soviet obstetricians turned even more liberally to codeine, nitrous oxide, and Novocain when available, as well as naturopathic remedies like belladonna.[68]

In France, too, drugs came to play a more prominent role in combination with psychoprophylaxis. In the early 1960s, psychoprophylaxis was "at a new stage of development, as new problems appeared, emerging from clinical experience and requiring an appropriate theoretical response," as psychiatrist Bernard Muldworf wrote at the time.[69] According to one study conducted in Paris, approximately one in four women trained in psychoprophylaxis turned to pain medication during the course of labor and birth. Vellay endorsed active management of labor as compatible with psychoprophylaxis. Even in cases that progressed normally, Vellay advocated the use of Sparteine to strengthen contractions. He also turned to Promethazine, marketed in France under the brand name Phenergan, an antihistamine that has a strong sedative effect.[70] Obstetrician Albert Ayoub, a proponent of psychoprophylaxis who had trained under Lamaze at Les Bluets and practiced in Damascus, counseled that, for the woman who demanded pharmacological pain relief, he tried "to adapt to each case in light of the psychological patterns of each woman."[71] Among his favorite choices was Demerol, popular with American physicians as well. That the USSR had turned toward the integration of psychoprophylaxis within a program of active management of labor may have played some role in the new direction in France. Greater contact with their American colleagues, keen enthusiasts for faster, less painful labor through drugs, may have had a hand in it as well.[72] Above all, the mainstreaming of psychoprophylaxis, which was in the early 1960s used in up to half of French maternity cases, doubtless contributed mightily to the diversification of practice and to its reconciliation with conventional obstetrics.

Although French firebrands insisted that "we must shout from the rooftops, there is no psychoprophylaxis with anesthesia," they fought a losing battle.[73] The widespread integration of psychoprophylaxis into the practice of active management of labor led Vellay, pictured at work in fig. 5.4, and others, by the mid-1960s, to see a need to clarify their position with regard to the relationship between drugs and psychoprophylactic practice. Concern arose over the quality of psychoprophylactic instruction and what psychoprophylaxis even meant in cases when obstetricians turned to drugs too freely. Vellay was unequivocal in his support for the use of drugs that sped labor's progress and eased pain, but he cautioned the need for conservatism and recommended the minimal dose necessary to achieve efficacy. He worried that inexperienced personnel were heavy-handed with dosages, robbing women of full and active participation in birth.[74] Hersilie, director of Les Bluets' maternity clinic, rejected the use of "aggressive 'cocktails'" that compromised women's consciousness, but viewed local or regional anesthetics as wholly compatible with psychoprophylaxis.[75]

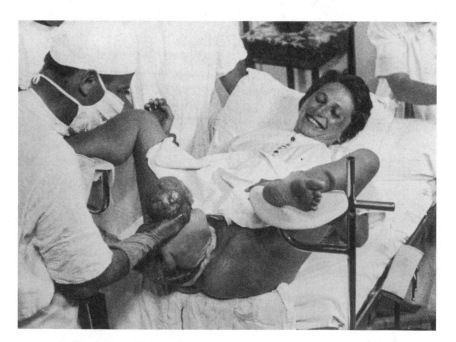

Figure 5.4: Vellay attending a birth in Paris, ca. early 1960s. Courtesy of the Schelsinger Library, Radcliffe Institute, Harvard University.

This increasingly accepting attitude toward the use of drugs to augment psychoprophylaxis was accomplished by a related shift in the understanding of the method's objective. A new emphasis on psychoprophylaxis as a tool to reduce and manage suffering replaced earlier, grandiose claims about its ability to eliminate pain. The benefits of psychoprophylaxis were many, including giving women a sense of pride and satisfaction, but it was no panacea for labor pain.[76] French discussions of the 1960s echoed those in Kiev in 1956, when the USSR retreated from its advocacy of psychoprophylaxis as a stand-alone practice and embraced instead its supplementation, when necessary, with pharmacological pain relief.

Freudian understandings of the mind-body connection came to play an increasingly prominent role in explanations of how the method worked and what it could accomplish. These theories did not supplant the Pavlovian neuropsychological foundation of the method, but supplemented it. Soviet de-Stalinization pushed French, leftist psychiatrists and obstetricians to question orthodox Pavlovism and move toward Freudian psychosomatics. A new level of engagement with their American colleagues, recent converts to the Lamaze method, may have reinforced these inclinations. Psychiatrist René Angelergues, once Lamaze's collaborator at Les Bluets and an ardent Pavlovian, did a sharp reversal in favor of "the wholesale rejection" of Pavlovian neuropsychology.[77] Freudian-inspired works on female psychology by Deutsch and, to a lesser degree, Marie Bonaparte found widespread integration into French discussion of pregnancy and childbirth, which were seen as a moment of both psychological crisis and therapeutic opportunity.[78]

This transition from a psychoneurological toward a psychosomatic understanding of psychoprophylaxis was not a pivot, but a process. The two perspectives coexisted in the 1960s, with Freudian ideas slowly becoming more central to French explanations of psychoprophylaxis. In the early 1960s, Vellay fretted about the dominance of psychoanalytical perspectives and their antimaterialist basis. He feared psychoanalysts' "total ignorance of obstetrical problems" that originated in the body, not the mind. Vellay expressed concern that Freudian thinking, particularly as propounded by American psychoanalysts, would distort psychoprophylaxis and lead to "confusion" and poor practice, undermining the Lamaze movement.[79] In later years, Vellay himself came to write about the therapeutic value of psychoprophylaxis to engage with and resolve questions connected with a list of psychological maladies that he understood through a Freudian lens: castration, masochism, narcissism, the oedipal complex, and penis envy.[80]

While Vellay moved, albeit with trepidation, toward Freudian psychosomatic medicine, others sought to stem the tide through social-psychological explanations that grounded the individual in society and elaborated on historical-cultural explanations put forth in earlier decades. Bernard Muldworf shared Vellay's concern with "the excessive value placed on psychology, which inevitably leads to speculative, abstract constructions, as is evident in certain works of psychoanalysis."[81] He argued that individual attitudes and behaviors needed to be understood both "from below," from the perspective of early childhood experiences inside the family and, more importantly, "from above," situated in a larger, social context.[82] While he saw individual and social forces working in tandem, he emphasized the latter, unlike his more psychoanalytically inclined colleagues. Muldworf drew on Simone de Beauvoir's feminist writings to explain supposed female passivity as socioculturally contingent, rejecting Freudian ideas that gave primacy to biologically determined male and female psychosexual development.[83] Hersilie similarly resisted what he characterized as an "anatomical determinism" in Freudianism, with its focus on the sex drive as the defining trait in psychological development.[84] Emphasizing the use of biology as mere "pretext" for, not the source of, gender roles, Hersilie's thinking, too, seems influenced by de Beauvoir. He asserted that the sociocultural, historical underpinning to human behavior, not the individual psyche, needed understanding to best enable women to take on an active and empowered role during childbirth.[85] These social-psychological elements were not alien to Vellay's thinking, but Hersilie and Muldworf deployed them in resistance to the growing incursion of psychoanalytic theorizing about psychoprophylaxis.

***

Esoteric professional debates that pitted Freud against Pavlov were distant from women's concerns for their personal birth experiences. But like arguments over the complementarity of psychoprophylaxis and drugs to ease pain and stimulate uterine contractions, these conflicts shaped the care women received at the clinical level. Reigning beliefs about female psychology, the mind-body relationship, and what, in fact, the objective of psychoprophylaxis was—behavior modification or pain alleviation—all fed into decisions made by women and their caregivers about how to proceed during labor and birth.

European and American debates over patient care and management framed popular discussions about what constituted a desirable birth experience. In the United States, ASPO leaders focused public attention on what they believed, apart from a healthy baby, women wanted most from their childbirth experience: dignity and satisfaction. Grassroots consumer enthusiasm was critical to the method's popularization.[86]

As new mother and US television personality Betsy Palmer reflected in 1962, "childbirth with dignity was something I'd begun to think about. You see, being married to an obstetrician, I knew some women carry on a lot. . . . I didn't like the idea. . . . Why should I suffer indignities if I could help it?"[87] According to one study, the majority of French women using psychoprophylaxis, too, appreciated the sense of dignity and the feeling of accomplishment for a job well done that this method imparted.[88] What did dignity in childbirth mean to these women? Above all else, it meant not crying or screaming, not grunting or groaning, remaining instead calm, quiet, and wide awake, ready to receive their babies with open arms.

As the 1960s gave way to the 1970s, these culturally determined value judgments about what constituted a desirable birth experience changed markedly. Society was in a process of transformation, as antiwar, countercultural, and social revolutionary values came more into the mainstream, at least among young, urban women and men. France's Generation of '68 rocked Paris, Nanterre, and beyond with antiwar demonstrations and calls for the democratization of the educational system. American hippies and Yippies poured out of classrooms and onto campus greens to air their grievances. Even those who led perfectly conventional, middle-class lives, quietly and without protest graduating from college and getting jobs, did so in a world where sensibilities in virtually every realm were changing. Questions of race relations, gender roles, and social justice filled newspapers, airwaves, and dinner-table conversations. In this environment, dignity in birth became disentangled from quiet, calm compliance and a satisfying, desirable birth experience started to look and sound very different. Rather than believing that the body should be conquered by the mind, women interested in a less medicated, more "natural" childbirth experience came to value the mind yielding to the body, and psychoprophylaxis changed with the times.

CHAPTER 6

✛

American Gains and Global Decline, 1968–80

In a 1970 newsletter for the Los Angeles chapter of ASPO, writer Theodore Sturgeon depicted natural childbirth as a path to an authentic and powerful embodied experience. Describing his partner's birth, he observed that

> within the borders of Lamaze control she was a she-wolf, fighting with all her soul and heart—and deeply enjoying it....In delivery she tapped some mysterious source of power and unleashed a force unlike anything else I have ever seen....She was Woman and by that I don't mean don't-muss-my-hair woman, or eek-a-mouse woman; I mean Woman of the earth and sky and origins, the creator, the living source of love and caring and strength. And in that wet-faced, vein-stretching baretoothed effort, she was truly beautiful.[1]

Sturgeon's words linked the natural childbirth movement to the American counterculture, with its affinity for antimaterialist, anticonsumerist spirituality. One reluctant Lamaze father conveyed disdain for this same synergy, writing that "the Lamaze idea, I associate with half-baked stimulus-response psychology, longhairs, loveins and other things of no account."[2] Whether celebrated or ridiculed, this vision of the Lamaze method as connected to mysterious, even mystical forces was a far cry from anything that the Soviet developers or their French students of psychoprophylaxis ever imagined. Sturgeon's phrase "Lamaze control" might have sounded familiar to the Soviet, French, and American obstetricians who valued psychoprophylaxis's ability to "discipline" the laboring woman, but the Lamaze method as path to New Age self-realization belongs uniquely to the United States in the 1970s.

In the late 1960s and early 1970s, readily apparent, tectonic social shifts shook the United States and Western Europe. Young people active in the counterculture and the emergent women's movement sought the transformation of economic structures and interpersonal relations. It was arguably in family relations and gender dynamics that the most fundamental and pervasive changes were wrought. The range of roles available to men and women in both the public and private sphere underwent a sea change. As society roiled, it appeared to many people at the time that the challenges to the status quo would end with nothing short of a total revolution in how we organize ourselves economically, socially, and politically. The reality has fallen short of the most grandiose objectives, but the United States and Western Europe were unquestionably transformed by the countercultural and feminist movements of the era, with ramifications for birth practices. In a clear shift from an earlier generation, expectant American mothers in the 1970s turned to psychoprophylaxis not primarily to suppress pain, but to weather it. They certainly wanted to avoid suffering, but pain's valorization among middle-class, educated, white women in the United States elevated the rejection of pharmacological relief to a rite of passage.

Despite psychoprophylaxis's roots in the world of medicalized and hospitalized birth, the faith of its advocates in a less interventionist practice of obstetrics caught the attention of those active in and sympathetic to the counterculture. Countercultural values seeped into middle-class, white America, finding expression in a desire to "get loose," to attain a more relaxed, natural, and authentic existence.[3] Young people sought "experiential abandon,...the desire to transcend mundane experiences through intense personal and interpersonal sensual experiences, such as drugs, sexuality, yoga, meditation, concern with the occult and the like."[4] When wedded to a new, countercultural ethos of natural, authentic living, Lamaze and other natural childbirth practices took on fresh meanings and forms. For many couples in the 1970s, natural childbirth offered a path to experiential abandon. This new aspiration came to color women's expectations about birth and to inform how we today commonly understand what defines natural childbirth.

How women described what they wanted out of a Lamaze birth points to the prevalence of countercultural sensibilities. Women sought a birth experience that was not just manageable, but "near ecstasy," as California Lamaze mother Wendy Johnston described it in 1971.[5] Bearing witness to a home birth in terms that captured the spiritual, New Age aesthetic, feminist Jeanne Hirsch felt the "powerful life energy vibrations from a room filled with holy madonnas. Transition [at the end of the first stage of labor] comes and her breathing turns to a pant,...the room is filled with panting. Earth Mother mounts her holy throne—she is queen of the birthing throne."[6] Hirsch references Lamaze breathing, but its use in a home birth, attended by a midwife and imbued with mysticism, marks a new turn.

In the changed atmosphere of the late 1960s and early 1970s, the Lamaze method appeared to some childbearing women and birth activists staid and regimented, better suited to the conventional hospital setting in which it had emerged. Those active in the counterculture sought an alternative way of childbirth well beyond the innovations ASPO advocated. The Tennessee commune The Farm offers a particularly vivid and prominent example. The community's co-founder and midwife Ina May Gaskin strove to promote a way of birth inspired by the counterculture and illustrative of just how conservative conventional Lamaze practice now looked by comparison. Rejecting modern hospital birth, Gaskin sought the restoration of what historians Richard Wertz and Dorothy Wertz term "social childbirth," an event located in the home and shared by the expectant mother's community of friends and family.[7] Unlike the quiet, composed demeanor Lamaze advocates encouraged, Gaskin emphasized a sensuous, primal engagement with the act of labor, supported by what she called "spiritual midwifery."[8] Women on The Farm and like-minded birth activists elsewhere embraced birth as an embodied experience in a way antithetical to the teachings of Lamaze and his American followers, for whom the mind's conquest of the body defined success.

For the most part, ASPO's core constituency remained pretty square—white, middle-class, well-educated, heterosexual, urban and suburban couples. Even as they took on new overtones, the aspirations of these childbearing women in the 1970s were not a decisive break with those women who had been drawn to natural childbirth a decade earlier. Johnston, the California mother who found childbirth to be an ecstatic experience, also felt "in total control, able to help every step of the way by responding to [the doctor's] directions."[9] With these words she expresses her connection to an earlier cohort of Lamaze mothers, even if other aspects of her motives differed markedly. Like her predecessors, Johnston appreciated the sense of self-mastery that the method imparted. She also quite clearly saw her physician as an authority figure. Johnston shared with members of the counterculture the view that an unmedicated birth offered a more authentic experience, but she pursued this goal in the confines of a conventional medical setting. It was not for ASPO but for Gaskin and those who shared her vision of social childbirth to posit a radical alternative.

Like those in the counterculture, women in the feminist movement iden-tified something useful in psychoprophylaxis and, in doing so, brought new meaning to the method. In 1973 American health activist Lolly Hirsch and psychologist Dorothy Tennov organized the First International Childbirth Conference, held at a Stamford, Connecticut, middle school. The confer-ence grew out of Tennov's work gathering women's birth stories, which captured the misogynistic, disempowering, degrading obstetric practices that American feminists had begun to critique. In advance of the Stamford conference, a New York City radio station aired some of these interviews, prompting one listener to write to Tennov of the anger these women's sto-ries stirred up in her. While listening,

> all of a sudden I started to cry and cry and cry…because I have repressed (in order to survive) the sense of loss in my life—how all the experiences that should be good and natural have been pure shit. I realize that I have *oceans* of rage in me and do not want to deal with it.…I have been in doubt about going to the confer-ence because of these feelings.…I'm enclosing all I have in my checking account for use for whatever you see fit to best overthrow the fucking male world.[10]

Like the women who shared their birth stories with Tennov, this listener was finding her voice in a rapidly changing environment. The burgeoning feminist movement provided women with a conceptual framework for articulating their frustrations with the status quo in obstetrics.

Two slim, forcefully written, foundational feminist histories of women and medicine appeared in 1973, the same year as the Stamford conference, and informed the feminist critique of contemporary childbirth practices. Barbara Ehrenreich and Deirdre English sketched the marginalization of female healers and the takeover of medical care by men in Europe and the United States in *Witches, Midwives, and Nurses*. With bold strokes, their book *Complaints and Disorders* described modern medicine's pathologiza-tion of the female body. Acting in their own economic interests, medical men had in centuries past denounced lay midwives and other women heal-ers as dangerous and ignorant. Eventually they created a male monopoly over the care of female bodies, including in childbirth. Ehrenreich and English identify class as central to the understanding and treatment of female bodies at the hands of this newly founded medical establishment. Wealthy women were seen as too frail to bear the rigors of modern life. Medical arguments legitimated the privileged woman's preservation in the gilded cage of the Victorian home. Ehrenreich and English observe that by the mid-twentieth century, the justification for women's exclusion from the public sphere had shifted. Middle- and upper-class women's bodies were no longer imagined as too weak to function outside the home, but their constant domestic presence was still required. Freudian theories about the mother's indispensable, non-transferable role in the child's formative years shifted the justification, but preserved the bourgeois gender order. Ehrenreich and English's writings offer historical background to explain in part what Betty Friedan had identified in 1963's *The Feminine Mystique* as "the problem that has no name"—the unhappiness and disappointment evident among middle-class housewives despite their material comfort. Told that she would find contentment in selfless devotion to husband and children, the American housewife felt a nagging dissatisfaction with life. Like Friedan, Ehrenreich and English critique Freudian ideas about female psychology, deepening that analysis by situating Freudianism in a long line of medical constructs oppressive to women.[11]

Ehrenreich and English were two of about 150 women from twelve states and four countries to participate in the Stamford conference. It was a gathering of unprecedented scale for the discussion of maternity and motherhood through the lens of feminism.[12] Speakers addressed the potential expansion of midwifery and home birth, the erotic pleasures of childbearing and breastfeeding, and the misogynistic foundations of conventional maternity care. A sense of potential for revolutionizing American birth filled the air. Feminism and the counterculture came together in the shared belief that childbirth was most empowering when experienced as naturally as possible. It was not only about the return to a purer, more authentic way of life, or fear of the harmful effects of powerful drugs; feminist childbirth activists attacked the power relations through which conventional obstetric practices were enacted. Drugs that desensitized women's bodies and clouded their minds subjugated them to male authority and control during what could otherwise be an empowering, gratifying lifecycle event. As lay midwife Cheryl Anderson said during the conference's open mike session, "the way we are born is ripped off from us. The authority is given over first of all to the AMA [American Medical Association]."[13] Feminist birth meant wresting control from male physicians and putting it back in the hands of birthing women and female caregivers, as had been the practice in the era of social childbirth. Moreover, as one Stamford conference speaker asserted, "eight centimeters is not the time to fight."[14] Women needed to make their demands and establish their authority well before they were in the throes of labor.

The renunciation of obstetric anesthesia was central to the feminist vision of an empowered birth and psychoprophylaxis offered a tool for pain management without dependence on what feminists characterized as a patriarchal medical establishment. As Deirdre English stated succinctly at the Stamford conference, "by removing the active participation—and even the consciousness—of the mother herself. . . . childbirth is no longer a healthy and powerful female act, but a ritual of female dependence on the male doctor."[15] Another speaker similarly observed that "the more drugs a woman takes the more she is forced to depend on the doctor and the less she is able to depend on herself."[16] Feminists asserted that psychoprophylaxis "affords the woman self-dignity during the birth process rather than uncontrolled, submissive emotions and unnecessary pain."[17] A turn away from pain medication opened up the possibility of home birth with a midwife in attendance, though legal hurdles posed a challenge in almost all states to lay and professional midwifery practice outside the hospital setting. For women who continued to prefer an obstetrician's care in a hospital, or who lived where midwifery services were unavailable, the rejection of drugs, feminists argued, enabled laboring women to maintain greater control over their bodies and faculties. From this feminist perspective, there was little room for distinguishing reliance on drugs from dependence on them, or for seeing the embrace of drugs as an expression of active participation, rather than passive submission.

Feminist enthusiasm was a welcome boon for those active in the Lamaze movement, but the question of home birth illustrates the uneasiness of this alliance. Endorsed by both feminists and those active in and inspired by the counterculture, home birth met a chilly reception from ASPO. Arguably the most influential voice in American childbirth education, ASPO founder Elisabeth Bing came out firmly against home birth. In 1976 she wrote that younger women "are justly opposed to the present mechanization of the obstetrical [wards]. But . . . they go to the opposite extreme by having their children at home attended only by lay-midwives. I do not believe that it is possible in this or any other field to turn back the clock. The price is too high."[18] Many rank and file ASPO members and Lamaze-trained mothers concurred with Bing. In a 1978 letter to *Ms. Magazine*, for example, one new Lamaze mother excoriated advocates of home birth for taking what she believed to be serious risks with a baby's health and safety. She was "sick and tired of laments about the Terror of Technology vs. The Joy of the Natural Earth Mother Way. I would rather lie on a metal table attended by doctors and machines than deliver a dead or defective baby in a cozy four poster at home."[19] Though she had turned to the Lamaze method as an alternative to pharmacological pain relief, this mother saw home birth as beyond the pale and clearly resented what she perceived to be the feminist position—that her decision to have an otherwise conventional birth somehow diminished her experience.

A 1974 incident in Buffalo, New York, illuminates the tensions between pro- and anti–home birth factions within the natural childbirth movement.

Newly arrived in the area, a young woman was expecting her second child. She had had a home birth for her first child and sought to do the same again. In preparation, she contacted the local ASPO chapter to find a Lamaze instructor and happened to mention that she was planning a home birth. Much to her surprise, she was informed that "she would not be permitted in an ASPO class, but would have to go to the Red Cross or look around for a non-ASPO hospital-sponsored class."[20] Stunned by the chapter's policy on home birth, she complained to ASPO's national office. Fearing possible legal repercussions, ASPO's director Vivian Mills upbraided the local Lamaze instructor for a rigid stance that had "public relations implications for ASPO."[21] Mills was no enthusiast for home birth, but believed Lamaze instruction had to be available to all expectant mothers. However, local chapters also had to be careful not to alienate physicians, whose livelihoods were threatened by home birth and whose backing was critical to the validation and promotion of psychoprophylaxis. Advocacy for home birth would have imperiled ASPO's positive working relationship with the physicians and the hospital administrators on whom ASPO depended for access to clients. With aid from physicians who promoted psychoprophylaxis and family-centered maternity care, Mills believed that in-hospital maternity care "would be every bit as humane, comfortable, geared to the individual and homelike as home itself."[22] ASPO dedicated itself to humanizing hospital birth, undermining momentum for home birth, and preserving the role of Lamaze instructors within the medical establishment.

Despite tensions, ASPO built common cause with those in the feminist and countercultural communities, and the early 1970s saw a "Lamaze explosion," as one ASPO activist described it at the time.[23] The Lamaze method became the most widely recognized approach to prenatal education and the most popular method of natural childbirth in the United States. From 1971 to 1973, the number of hospitals offering prenatal education courses grew five-fold, to encompass 25 percent of the seven thousand hospitals in the United States. By the close of the decade, childbirth preparation classes, like the one pictured in fig. 6.1, were nearly universally taught in American hospitals. Most of these courses offered either psychoprophylactic training or some variant inspired by or derived from it.[24]

An emergent social movement coalesced around the drive for psychoprophylaxis, which pushed beyond the northeastern American metropolises where it had made its initial impact. The Los Angeles ASPO chapter saw exponential growth, while in the South, no hotbed of Lamaze activism in the early days, interest in the method boomed. In Charlotte, North Carolina, for example, in 1966 the first Lamaze classes were taught to less than a dozen couples; in 1974, seven hundred Charlotte couples

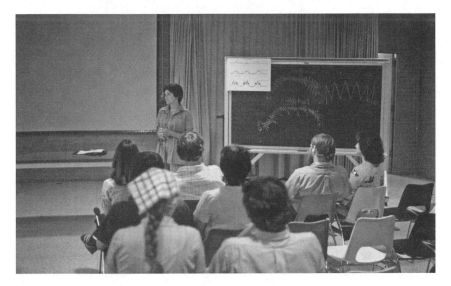

Figure 6.1: Lamaze class lecture, ca. 1970s. Courtesy of the Schlesinger Library, Radcliffe Institute, Harvard University.

enrolled in Lamaze courses. The Lamaze method also extended its reach in the Midwest, where in the 1960s there had been only isolated pockets of support. In 1968 no childbirth preparation courses were offered in Lincoln, Nebraska, but by 1974, fifty-five couples received training in each six-week course cycle. With chapters peppering the country, one hundred inquiries per month poured in to ASPO national headquarters regarding teacher training. Moved by their own positive, profound birth experiences, women—and even a few men—wanted to dedicate themselves to helping others to achieve the same thing. Certified Lamaze teacher rolls swelled to 1,200 by the mid-1970s.[25]

As psychoprophylaxis became an integral part of American birth, confusion grew over what, exactly, the method was. A common belief that the Lamaze method meant labor and birth without the use of any drugs whatsoever oversimplified ASPO's more complicated official position on pharmacological pain relief.[26] ASPO had fought unsuccessfully against the phrase "natural childbirth," which was in the 1970s popularly used as a synonym for psychoprophylaxis. With the intention of correcting the conflation with the Read method and of tamping down women's high expectation for a birth free of all medical intervention, ASPO promoted the term "prepared childbirth," which conveyed a more flexible stance toward anesthetics and analgesics. This effort met with mixed results. There seemed to be no way to dislodge natural childbirth from the American lexicon, and some thought it not worth the fight to try. They advocated instead a terminological reconciliation. In 1972 ASPO activist Sunnye Strickland wrote, "I, for one, am sick of hearing Dick-Read pitted against Lamaze."[27] Whatever the method's name or content, of preeminent importance was the shared goal of a safe, satisfying, empowered birth experience.

As the bright line between the Read and Lamaze methods lost its utility, methodological orthodoxy yielded to ecumenicism, and the ASPO leadership worried about what, exactly, their instructors were teaching in ASPO-endorsed classes. So diversified had the method's practice become that, writing to the national headquarters in 1975, the Central Jersey Chapter underscored the "desperate need to define that body of knowledge unique to [psychoprophylaxis]. Either there is a method called psychoprophylaxis (Lamaze) or there is not."[28] A proliferation of breathing patterns over the course of the 1960s and early 1970s compounded the confusion. British birth activist Sheila Kitzinger noted in 1977 that, when she lectured on either side of the Atlantic, students often asked if she advocated "'huff and puff,' 'slump and blow,' 'choo-choo breathing,' 'the sigh,' 'levels A, B, C and D,' 'H out, H out, Hoo-hoo,' 'sss-sss,' 'tune-tapping,' or whatever. I do not know if the mothers were as confused as I was. Certainly it all tended to be very noisy."[29] What had once been just a few breathing patterns had multiplied into a complex array of subtly varied forms that were hard to remember, let alone to master. Intended to give women more options, this diversification rendered psychoprophylaxis daunting and overly complicated.

With the Lamaze method's popularization also came organizational growing pains within ASPO. Local chapters sought support from the national office, but wanted to preserve their autonomy. At the national headquarters, originally in New York City and, beginning in 1974, in Washington, DC, ASPO leaders worked to reign in local chapters. The national office wanted to move ASPO away from its original model of loosely affiliated local groups and toward a centralized, cohesive, professional organization supported by a network of local offices. These conflicts came to a head in 1971, when the Los Angeles ASPO chapter received an anonymous donation to make a new childbirth education film. The national office demanded that the LA chapter remit the donation to headquarters, while the LA chapter, which had already begun the film's production, believed it had the authority and autonomy to dispense the funds locally. A debate over the relationship between the national organization and local chapters crystalized around this fight and precipitated a struggle for control of ASPO's Board of Directors in 1972.[30] In the short term, the local chapters came out on top. Opponents of centralization won control of the board, which began to better represent chapters outside the northeast, where control of ASPO had been concentrated since its inception. The LA chapter produced an award-winning film, *The Story of Eric* (1971), which became the center-piece of Lamaze courses for a decade. In the long run, though, the national office consolidated control. By the close of the 1970s, ASPO was beginning to take on the contours of a new breed of corporatized nonprofit organization. ASPO's national leadership focused its effort on the profession-alization of childbirth education through teacher certification. Standard teacher-training materials appeared, courses sprang up around the country, and ASPO accreditation of childbirth educators began to carry weight. ASPO sought to monopolize teacher certification, but it faced competition from organizations like the Council of Childbirth Education Specialists (CCES), itself led by a group formerly active in ASPO and on the losing side of the fight for Board control.[31] Despite such challenges, the 1970s was something of a golden age, as ASPO's ranks swelled and the Lamaze method's popularity and name recognition outstripped that of any other approach to childbirth preparation.

FEMINIST BACKLASH

As psychoprophylaxis boomed in the United States, its trajectory was in steep decline in France. The method had been losing support among women due to two mutually reinforcing trends: bad press and low quality instruction. Following great interest and press exposure in the 1950s, psychoprophylaxis suffered from what its advocates described as a campaign of "counter-propaganda" to discredit it. Stories began to circulate about the considerable number of women who had had negative experiences with psychoprophylaxis. The method's proponents, however, argued that some physicians, who merely wanted to cash in on the popularity of psychopro-phylaxis, were giving the method a bad name by promoting "counterfeit painless childbirth."[32] Irrespective of the truth of these charges, psychopro-phylaxis lost the luster it initially enjoyed in France with the circulation of these negative stories in the press and by word of mouth.

Inspired by leftist student unrest in May 1968, French feminism also posed a challenge to psychoprophylaxis. Pursuing many of the same objectives, such as reproductive freedom, as second-wave feminists in the United States, the *Mouvement de Libération des Femmes* (Women's Liberation Movement, or MLF) encompassed diverse political groups. With the legal-ization of contraception and abortion, the MLF pushed the questions of accessibility and costs, pressing for full coverage under *Sécurité sociale*.

Hampering its efficacy, the MLF was fragmented and conflict-ridden, fall-ing apart by 1980. While it was relatively short-lived as a political move-ment, the MLF nonetheless had a long-lasting impact on women's position in French society. French women in the 1970s spoke with a new frank-ness about their lives and their bodies, including their experiences of maternity.[33]

Although psychoprophylaxis continued to have its devotees, criticism surfaced with far greater frequency than in the previous two decades. Nearly three-quarters of respondents to a 1979 survey of women who used the maternity services at Les Bluets made negative comments about their stay. The bulk of complaints concerned material conditions, such as the quality of the meals and the coarseness of the toilet paper, but they also registered dissatisfaction with everything from poor organization to cranky personnel.[34] Letters of complaint regularly crossed the desks of Les Bluets' administrators, and several intensely critical books and articles appeared over the course of the 1970s and early 1980s, arguing that "far too many women still give birth in deplorable conditions."[35] Reliance on psychoprophylaxis as the primary, usually sole approach to pain manage-ment bore the brunt of women's ire and was seen as emblematic of indiffer-ent, inhumane maternity care. Women wrote of searing pain during labor that went untreated by a patronizing staff resistant to fulfilling patient requests for anesthetics or analgesics. In response to an exit survey in the late 1970s, Madame A. shared her traumatic experience at Les Bluets. She recognized that "objectively" all had gone well. She and her baby were doing fine physically, but "in my head, things aren't going so well sometimes." She asked herself, "how do you forget such an intense pain?... The night of my birth was torture." Madame A. recounted her experience of the psychopro-phylactic method: "I wanted to throw myself out the window....I didn't say [to the staff] what I really meant, that is—ease my pain, do something, meaning something effective." Her caregivers stood by, telling her to "be brave" and watching her suffer.[36]

Women complained about rude treatment and the inaccessibility of care-givers, who seemed to be overtaxed by their patient load both in prena-tal education classrooms and in the maternity ward. Despite the fact that Lamaze and his team had emphasized the need for constant support at the laboring woman's side, they sometimes found themselves abandoned by the medical staff for hours at a time.[37] At a maternity ward in Clamart, not far from Paris, Madame G. B. labored alone for nearly twelve hours after her admission to the maternity ward. Nurses came in, took her tem-perature, and promptly left.[38] Laboring without any professional support appears to have been common. According to a 1975 textbook for childbirth educators, such treatment was routine as, due to staff shortages, "one cannot expect midwives to stay the whole time with the laboring woman, because they often have to attend to other pressing matters. In that case, the laboring woman stays by herself and should cope as best she can."[39] Of women who participated in a qualitative study of French maternity care published in 1980, a negligible number were well-attended throughout the first stage of labor.[40]

French women denounced proponents of psychoprophylaxis for misleading expectant mothers with fairy tales about the method's efficacy and benefits, all touted as scientifically proven. A thirty-year-old mother of three, Veronique described psychoprophylactic training as "a catastrophe." In her estimation, filling women's heads with stories of how easy, beautiful, and painless labor is did little to ready women for birth. "That is why I felt cheated during my birth. With or without [psychoprophylaxis], there is a moment when suffering is unbearable and I was enraged. Telling women such nonsense seems monstrous to me."[41] Rather than risk being refused access to anesthesia if she desired it, Madame F. transferred her maternity care from Les Bluets late in her pregnancy because "I would be terrified by the idea of giving birth in your clinic, thinking that no one would really help me, but instead test my training or judge if I had prepared well or poorly."[42] The remarks of Madame P. show just how much Madame F. had to fear. In 1976 Madame P. wrote that "after 6 centimeters dilation, the pain was intense. Despite the encouragement of the midwife about my 'good cooperation' and 'good preparation,'. . . I would have preferred an epidural, because I have not chosen to be a masochist."[43] Not only does Madame P.'s testimony imply that the staff dismissed the severity of women's pain by denying access to pharmacological pain relief, but her reference to the midwife's compliment that she had shown "good cooperation" reveals how medical staff sought to ease their own burden by encouraging compliant behavior with praise. Maria-José Jaubert, the most prolific and outspoken French critic of psychoprophylaxis, went so far as to assert that women did not find relief using the method because it was not really about treating pain, but about training women to submit to medical control.[44]

Feminist critiques challenged clinicians' psychologizing of women's pain. A patient at Les Bluets, Madame M., had an episiotomy that required a couple of stitches. Four months after she gave birth, however, she continued to have perineal discomfort and sought help. The gynecologist at Les Bluets "saw nothing there but told me that it was 'psychological.'" She returned several times complaining of pain and was repeatedly informed that the problem was in her mind. She began to fret about her mental state in light of what the doctors said, even telling herself "I should see a psychiatrist if this continues." [45] After six months, she went to a gynecologist at another clinic. He found an infection where the thread from the stitches had neither been absorbed into the tissue nor removed. The quick resort to psychological explanations for women's pain was far from the unique experience of this woman. Recent studies indicate that women continue to receive less treatment for pain than men and are more frequently than men prescribed sedatives rather than pain relievers in response to complaints of pain.[46] French feminists understood such incidents in gendered terms, as an expression of male domination and control. They argued that, resentful of women's capacity to bring life into the world, male obstetric authorities (and the female midwives and nurses enmeshed in the medical system) work to "humiliate you, treat you with contempt, they try to put you back in your place."[47]

Though in the United States most feminists linked psychoprophylaxis to the notion of empowerment, reservations about the method were evident there as well. Like their French counterparts, some American feminists raged about having been bamboozled by the method's proponents, who sold them "an enchanted fairytale version of birth" that turned out to be "just another shuck."[48] As one disappointed new mother wrote in 1971, in their enthusiasm for psychoprophylaxis, "the radical sisters...left unchallenged the total power of doctors over their patients and deceived women into believing that natural birth somehow liberates them from the traditional female straightjacket."[49] In a letter written to the organizers of the Stamford conference, one woman expressed fear that the Lamaze method was

> used as one more demand for some women to be Super Mom....I'm talking about the women who have genuinely hard and long labors and are regarded as coward[s], scorned for 'carrying on' while the successful Lamaze [mother] (and her husband 'coach') breeze through a relatively short endeavor....I have seen and heard women who have never fully recovered [from] the shame and humiliation of their failure at Lamaze. How about women who have to, or decide to, receive 'help.' Weak. Hysterical. They are subject to...self-righteous, snickering judgment.[50]

Unlike earlier, psychoanalytic critiques from medical professionals who claimed that natural childbirth taxed nervous, emotionally fragile women, this woman took aim at the method's detrimental effect on sisterhood. For women who had had positive natural childbirth experiences, it could be challenging to sympathize with those who had not. Some of them blamed women who accepted forceps, cesarean sections, and other interventions as having yielded out of weakness, not necessity, to male obstetric authority.[51]

In *Immaculate Deception* (1975), a groundbreaking feminist analysis of American birth practices, Suzanne Arms offers the most sustained critique of psychoprophylaxis and other methods of natural childbirth, a term she denounces as a "gross misnomer."[52] Arms examines the limitations of natural childbirth as pursued in a hospital setting. The hospital staff's "expectation of failure" and "patronizing, negative attitude" undermined women's efforts and rendered "natural childbirth a deception in the modern hospital."[53] A supposedly "successful" Lamaze birth was, in Arms's estimate, "not to be confused with a natural birth, which can only take place in an atmosphere of calm and quiet faith within a natural environment."[54] In-hospital Lamaze birth stood outside her understanding of natural childbirth because of its high degree of medicalization. As a 1979 New York newspaper pointed out, "'natural childbirth' mother[s] use some form of anesthesia up to 75 percent of the time. In some hospitals, they are hooked up to fetal monitors and a variety of intravenous fluids and drugs 100 percent of the time."[55] Arms rightly observes that what ASPO advocated was a revision of, rather than a revolution in, standard, medicalized birth.

THE RISING TIDE OF TECHNOLOGY

Whether they advocated for access to pharmacological pain relief on demand, as many did in France, or pressed to express their authority through resistance to those same drugs, as they did in the United States, women in both national contexts faced a trend toward greater obstetric intervention fueled by the integration of new technologies and drugs. The use of technology expanded in maternity wards beginning in the 1970s and continuing in the 1980s. The presence of machines to monitor fetal heart rates increasingly became routine. Available in earlier decades, the application of drugs used to induce labor and strengthen contractions gained popularity. The obstetric application of epidural anesthesia grew by leaps and bounds. Among other factors, this reliance on technology to monitor and guide labor and birth contributed to skyrocketing rates of cesarean section. From 1970 to 1978 the US cesarean section rate nearly tripled, from 5.5 percent to 15.2 percent.[56] With American cesarean section rates in the early twenty-first century exceeding 30 percent, such figures seem modest by comparison, but the sharp uptick was unmistakable at the time and triggered growing concern.

Reliance on technology and a readiness to intervene stemmed from both financial pressures and the desire to reduce adverse outcomes. A 1979 magazine article captured this trend, observing that many physicians turned to technology "'just in case' it's indicated—which means all the time."[57] They feared malpractice suits if babies were stillborn or born with brain damage from a lack of oxygen. Slick salesmen and ad campaigns also encouraged physicians' and hospital administrators' faith in this technology, while the cost needed to be recouped through high usage, with the resulting expenses passed on to the consumer.[58]

Lamaze instructors attempted to prepare their students for the increased likelihood of technological intervention in hospital birth, while at the same time they resisted this trend. Bing believed that by the mid-1970s ASPO's task had become far more complicated due to the rising use of fetal monitors, epidurals, and other interventions. She asked, "how far can we support this machine age without losing our own humanity? I think this is a very real question, especially for all of us, who fought so hard for the participation of the parents in giving birth to their child. The main part of the fight was only against over-dosages of medication, almost an easy fight in retrospect.... The lines of battle are far more intricate today."[59] ASPO leaders insisted that interventions had to be medically indicated, not routine. In practice, however, determining medical necessity was often a subjective process that left a lot of women asking questions of themselves and their physicians in the wake of obstetric intervention.

The rise of epidural anesthesia posed the most direct challenge to Lamaze advocates. With precursors dating from the early twentieth century, modern epidural anesthesia has roots in the work of a California physician in the mid-1940s. Only in the 1970s and, especially, the 1980s did access to epidural anesthesia grow, as hospitals began to have on staff more anesthesiologists, whose routine work in obstetrics promised a lucrative revenue stream. There are, of course, drawbacks and dangers to epidural anesthesia, including the fact that the laboring woman is confined to the hospital bed. Epidurals earn blame for slowed or stalled labors, and sometimes do not wear off in time for a woman to push effectively during birth. With the anesthesia crossing the placenta, some babies are born too groggy to breastfeed properly in the hours just after birth. New mothers sometimes experience severe headaches after the anesthesia wears off, or soreness at the site of the drug's administration. But despite these negatives, epidural anesthesia won praise from obstetricians and their patients. It seemed to promise the very objective that psychoprophylaxis sought—to allow the laboring woman to be "awake and aware"—but with considerably less effort and, for almost all women, much greater physical comfort. In comparison to older, powerful drug cocktails and general anesthesia, epidural anesthesia was a safer alternative that allowed women to maintain consciousness and clarity of mind. Hospitals, which stood to profit from the increased use of epidural anesthesia, helped to persuade consumers by both subtle and direct means that the advantages outweighed the risks.[60]

ASPO had to change with the times, revising its curriculum in light of new demands and desires from both patients and hospitals. For childbirth educators, that meant devoting time to teaching about epidural anesthesia. In classes taught at hospitals, administrators sometimes required instructors to grant anesthesiologists the opportunity to speak to prospective parents and to distribute literature lauding the benefits and safety of epidural anesthesia. It is impossible to say how much this marketing swayed consumers and how much hospitals responded to consumer pressure to provide access to epidural anesthesia. The end result was that, from the mid-1970s through the 1980s, childbirth education courses became less about training women to use tools intended to minimize their reliance on pharmacological pain relief. Those childbirth educators who remained committed to the avoidance of drugs in childbirth used their contact hours with expectant parents to offer a more balanced view of epidural anesthesia than that offered by anesthesiologists and to encourage them to question the necessity of interventions done as a matter of routine, rather than medical necessity. With the goal of empowering their clients, childbirth educators emphasized to couples their right "to use assertive techniques to acquire the birth experience they want."[61]

When students asked why psychoprophylaxis was worth the bother when they could have an epidural, Lamaze instructors were ready with a litany of reasons that closely resembled those offered up against the debilitating drug cocktails widely used in previous decades.[62] To those women who rejected epidural anesthesia, they promised quicker recuperation after birth and "(usually) more satisfaction."[63] Indeed, for some mothers, epidural anesthesia proved so effective at suppressing pain that it left them feeling detached from the experience of birth. As one Boston mother wrote in 1972, "I found that watching the baby being born in the mirror [while under epidural anesthesia] was like watching a movie in class. I was too removed."[64] To childbearing couples, the benefit for the baby of avoiding exposure to anesthesia was perhaps the most compelling argument. Following her drug-free birth, one Lamaze mother commented that, when the nurse brought her baby to her in her hospital room, she "saw the benefits of the Lamaze method. Because she was so alert, so active and obviously so free of any drowsiness or grogginess from drugs. We realized then that the method was just as much for her sake as it was for ours and that it was the least we could give her as a good start in the world."[65] What parents would not want to give their baby the best possible start? But it was becoming difficult to accomplish in a hospital setting, where fetal monitors proclaimed risks, and doctors, anxious to avoid prolonged, potentially complicated labors, rushed women along with uterine stimulants that brought on powerful contractions and taxed their abilities to cope without the use of pharmacological pain relief.

French medical practitioners and childbearing women had their eyes on the popularization in the United States of epidural anesthesia in obstetrics. In the 1970s the French epidural rate was negligible; as of 1981, it stood at only 4 percent, compared to 22 percent that year in the United States. But interest was on the rise, and discussion of epidural anesthesia's pros and cons made its way into the medical and popular press. In 1972, for example, leading French practitioners of psychoprophylaxis gathered to debate, among other questions, the place of epidural anesthesia. Some came out forcefully against it as carrying unjustifiable risk. Others denounced it as a crutch that undermined women's and physicians' commitment to and faith in psychoprophylaxis. Several obstetricians spoke in favor of epidural anesthesia as perfectly compatible with psychoprophylactic practice and a useful tool for women who, for whatever reason, did not find adequate pain relief in non-pharmacological measures.[66] Strausbourg's Dr. Muller endorsed epidural anesthesia as a complement to psychoprophylaxis. After nearly two decades of obstetric practice using psychoprophylaxis, Muller had first-hand experience with the method's limitations and he welcomed the advent of what, in his judgment, was a safe and effective path to a satisfying birth. Muller took a pragmatic stance. Epidural anesthesia was no panacea; it carried certain (to him, minor) risks, but it could be valuable in circumstances when psychoprophylaxis was not enough. Like many of his colleagues who opposed epidural anesthesia, he feared that it encouraged passivity on the woman's part. Muller was also explicit that a woman's demand for pharmacological pain relief was a "questionable" and insufficient reason to administer it.[67] It was for the physician to judge whether it was truly necessary. Vellay described as "seductive" the capacity of the epidural to ease a woman's pain without dulling her mind. He cautioned that it should "neither be systematically rejected, not systematically applied," but used judiciously when the physician deemed it necessary.[68]

A number of obstacles blocked the more rapid integration of epidural anesthesia into French obstetrics. Dogmatic proponents of psychoprophylaxis challenged its safety, but material conditions no doubt played a decisive role in hampering its rise. Midwives delivered 85 percent of French babies in the 1970s and they were not authorized to administer epidurals. Only certified anesthesiologists, specialists who were in severe shortage in France, could do the procedure. It was also expensive and, under the terms of the socialized medical system, anesthesiologists were paid by *Sécurité sociale* solely in cases that were deemed medically necessary, such as cesarean sections. Epidurals strictly for pain management were not covered by *Sécurité sociale* and only patients who carried some types of supplementary private health insurance could expect reimbursement. In the context of French health care in the 1970s, epidural anesthesia was considered a luxury.[69]

French feminists argued that beneath the personnel shortages and financial impediments lay an intractable, insideous indifference to women's suffering, but they were also wary of physicians who pushed women to submit to epidural anesthesia. They emphasized the safety of most anesthetics and analgesics, and underscored that the intensity of labor pain justified at least the same level of care and consideration as dental work.[70] In striking contrast to most of their American counterparts, French feminists argued that "women who freely choose epidurals are less dependent" on their medical caregivers.[71] Women liberated from oppressive physical suffering during labor could sit in clear-headed judgment of the medical staff, rather than submit meekly to authoritarian abuse and manipulation. At the same time, feminists pointed to the potential for anesthesia to be used in ways, in their judgment, as coercive and disempowering as psychoprophylaxis. One Parisian maternity ward had an epidural rate that exceeded 65 percent in 1980, roughly sixteen times the national average. At a Normandy facility, eight out of ten women received epidural anesthesia.[72] Did all these women choose pharmacological pain relief, or were they pressed to use it? A woman named Marion attested that at the maternity ward where she gave birth, "we had no choice. Here there is complete opposition to all methods other than epidurals." The head of the facility told her that "'the epidural has become the usual practice and the medical staff do not support traditional births'" that used any other form of pain relief, including psychoprophylaxis.[73] Jaubert argued that "it is for the woman, she alone, to choose her own way of giving birth. [The physician] should give her the choice."[74] She accused medical professionals of preying on women's fear of pain to coerce them into using epidural anesthesia, just as they had earlier been, in her view, frightened into rejecting anesthesia for fear of harming their baby. As one mother expressed it, "maybe I would have so much pain that I'd choose an epidural. But it is for me to judge" whether it is needed or not. It took until 1994 for standard French perinatal care practices and benefits under *Sécurité sociale* to conform to this view that patient request was an adequate reason to administer or to eschew pharmacological pain relief.[75]

Two trends, evident in France but more pronounced in the United States in the 1970s, pulled maternity care in opposite directions. On the one hand, the integration of technology proceeded apace. On the other hand, influenced by feminist and countercultural values, consumers pushed for gentler, more humane care. Hospital administrators, physicians, and Lamaze activists in the United States tried to address consumer dissatisfaction and to head off any threat from the home birth movement to hospitals' monopoly on maternity care through a number of strategies. Topping out at 1 percent, American home birth in the 1970s never really posed a serious concern, but the medical establishment feared rising interest and sought to preempt any challenge to its market share.[76] To exude a homier feel, the physical space of the obstetric ward underwent renovation to make it more inviting and to reflect a purportedly new, depathologized view of hospital-based maternity care. Rocking chairs, abundant pillows, and large tubs offered to women the amenities of home in exchange for their business. According to a 1978 survey, 90 percent of hospitals in New York State either offered or planned to provide within a few months such comforts to their obstetric clients. Certainly New York was ahead of the rest of the nation, but changes there indicated which way the wind was blowing.[77]

New maternity ward layouts purportedly furthered care that emphasized less intervention in normal birth. To woo women who might otherwise consider home birth, hospitals also compromised on procedures that were not medically necessary. Enemas and genital shaving, which had been routine, began to fall out of fashion. There was some pressure to move away from the policy of "nothing by mouth," which banned laboring women from food or drink taken orally for fear that, should anesthesia become necessary, they might aspirate vomit and choke. To stave off dehydration, it had become standard practice to administer fluids via an intravenous line (IV). This unpleasant and usually unnecessary practice came under fire in the face of consumer pressure. As Yale University pediatrics professor Morris A. Wessel stated, "You have women who are sitting up to ask for a cup of tea and they get an IV. So women are having babies at home."[78] By liberating women from a mandatory IV, US hospitals positioned themselves to retain customers who wanted the perceived safety and security of the hospital, but sought minimal intervention in labor.

Sometimes referred to as freestanding birth centers or childbearing centers, alternative birth centers (ABCs) emerged as another tactic to counter the trend toward technology in obstetrics and the allure of home birth. These facilities were typically staffed by nurse-midwives and maintained affiliation with a nearby hospital. MCA founded the first American ABC in New York City in 1975; in the late 1970s ABCs popped up around the county. Some ABCs, like MCA's, were independent, while others were owned and operated by hospitals that hoped to stem what they feared was an imminent exodus from conventional maternity wards. In 1979 San Francisco's Mount Zion Hospital found that 30 percent of the women who availed themselves of its ABC said that, had the ABC not been available, they would have opted for a home birth. Women drawn to ABCs wanted midwifery care, but also the comfort of knowing that emergency equipment was on hand and a hospital transfer could be accomplished rapidly if necessary.[79] The less medicalized, home-like environment of the ABC seemed to avert a disaster for hospitals' bottom line and, perhaps, "helped to wear down some of the time-encrusted attitudes of diehard nurses [and] doctors" who had resisted change.[80]

There were efforts to imbue patient care in ABCs and hospital-based maternity wards with more humane interpersonal dynamics, in keeping with the demands of those women who sought a more natural birth. French obstetrician Frédérick Leboyer's philosophy of "childbirth without violence" spoke to this aspiration. His work gained notoriety in France beginning in 1974 and he quickly found an American audience.[81] Leboyer focused new attention on the baby's welcome into the world. He advocated the transformation of the delivery room into a serene environment with low lights, hushed voices, and gentle music. Leboyer supported the immediate immersion of the newborn into a warm bath intended to mimic the soothing atmosphere of the womb. Some Leboyer enthusiasts sought to extend that atmosphere into prenatal training, encouraging women to listen to music for fifteen minutes each day as a soothing addition to their psychoprophylactic preparation.[82]

Leboyer's method inspired mixed reactions in France and the United States. With greater emphasis on communication with and reception of the baby, and less focus on women's comportment during labor, Leboyer's ideas "certainly created a new climate" for childbirth.[83] But Jean-Marie Cheynier, who in the mid-1970s headed the maternity clinic at Les Bluets, believed that Leboyer's ideas were at odds with the objectives of psychoprophylaxis. Cheynier argued that "for Leboyer the mother is a completely passive object," little more than a vessel for the newborn, who alone occupies center stage.[84] Jaubert concurred, denouncing Leboyer as "a misogynistic guru" who promoted an "ersatz mystic religion."[85] In her estimation, Leboyer advocated the erasure of the mother from her role in childbirth, dismissing her as "pathetic, stupid" and a "prison of flesh" for the baby.[86] ASPO leaders, too, remained unconvinced. Bing expressed skepticism, saying that dim lights might sound pleasant, but she would "rather see what the baby looks like."[87] As for the immediate transfer to a warm bath, Bing cautioned that "water is a chill factor and we're very concerned to keep the baby warm."[88]

With views closer to those of Gaskin than Bing, Leboyer's compatriot and colleague Michel Odent worked to redress the criticism that Leboyer had forgotten the woman and her needs in childbirth. He endorsed a vision of birth as a primal, embodied experience. Toward the close of the 1970s, Odent began to practice water birth. Rather than transfer the newborn to a warm bath, as Leboyer preached, Odent advocated birthing in a tub. The aqueous environment eased the pain of labor, promoted relaxation, and provided the baby with a gentle transition from womb to world. Beginning in the 1960s, Soviet male midwife Igor Charkovsky had pioneered water birth.[89] Charkovsky's work came to Odent's attention and, following Odent's efforts in France, water birth began to gain adherents in the United States in the early 1980s. But Odent was not without his detractors. For all his talk about a gentle, humane childbirth experience for both mother and baby, in Jaubert's view Odent demonstrated a disdain for women's pain in labor and a refusal to take its treatment seriously when non-pharmacological methods of relief proved inadequate.[90]

Taking inspiration from the French yet again, American Lamaze enthusiasts made a unique contribution to the effort to humanize and demedicalize birth through their promotion of the "monitrice," whose role was akin to that of today's doula. As part of his drive to maximize the success of psychoprophylaxis, Lamaze early on added the monitrice to the labor support team in his private practice. Typically a nurse or physical therapist, the monitrice encouraged and guided the mother-to-be during the whole of her journey through labor and birth. A few American hospitals tried to adopt the monitrice model, but it never took root. In 1970 the Detroit-based Childbirth without Pain Education Association began to offer monitrice certification. The organization's founder, Flora Hommel, had trained as a monitrice under Lamaze and Vellay at Les Bluets. Monitrice programs were launched in Los Angeles and Connecticut in the mid-1970s. Finances proved to be the primary obstacle to success. It was too costly to provide constant, professional companionship in the context of privatized American maternity care. Confident that they knew what they wanted and how to get it, couples saw no need to pay out-of-pocket for additional professional support.[91] As hospital staff became more familiar with and sympathetic to what women were trying to accomplish through their rejection of pain medication, there was less perceived need for a monitrice to serve as the couple's advocate. In 1972 a Boston-area childbirth educator observed that just a few years earlier Lamaze instructors "monitriced nearly every couple.... As hospitals have opened delivery rooms and come to better understand that a positive, healthy experience and not just doing the Lamaze method is a couple's main goal, the need for us monitricing is now practically non-existent," because at least some members of the staff worked to support the couples' efforts.[92]

A REVOLUTION IN AMERICAN FATHERHOOD

One reason why the monitrice failed to take hold in the United States was because the American father shouldered her duties. Linked to the drive for the Read method, the movement to integrate the father into childbirth germinated in the 1940s and 1950s, took root in the 1960s, and blossomed into a national phenomenon in the 1970s, when the father's presence during labor and birth went from being uncommon to the norm. This was a fight that consumers had to take on hospital by hospital against sometimes unwilling, arbitrary caregivers and administrators. By the time of psychoprophylaxis's arrival in the United States around 1960, strides had already been made to bring the father into the childbirth experience, but physicians, psychologists, and hospital administrators still argued that husbands would be in the way and, if an emergency arose, they might be traumatized by what they witnessed.[93] In 1961 one chief of a New York City hospital's obstetrics department said, "We've got a real battle on our hands. Half our staff want the fathers in the labor and delivery rooms; the other half want to keep the men out."[94] Health regulations, like one in California barring "visitors" from the delivery room, stood in the way of couples who sought to be together for the birth of their child. In the face of arguments that "the prepared husband had an important function to perform," and of statistics that demonstrated no adverse physical complications or increased hospital liability from his presence, the California law was struck down in 1964, paving the way in that state for fathers to witness the births of their children.[95] Hospitals did not quietly or quickly yield to pressure, and momentum on this issue should not be overstated. As of 1965, only sixty hospitals in eighteen states and the District of Columbia allowed fathers into the delivery room, though significantly more permitted men to stay with their wives during labor.[96] After years of struggle, the mid-1970s saw a decisive turn in favor of the father's presence.

Several important shifts occurred in the 1970s regarding the father's role in childbirth. The man's presence at the laboring woman's side—a role for which he trained, as seen in fig. 6.2—became a far more familiar sight. Once the threshold to the labor room had been breached, it was somewhat less of a hurdle to get into the delivery room. More and more hospitals,

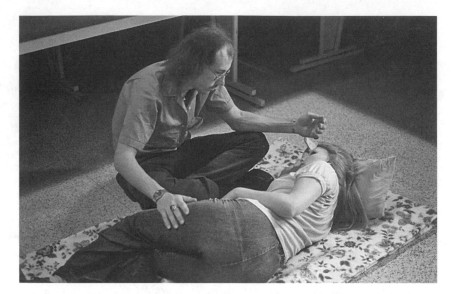

Figure 6.2: A couple practicing Lamaze techniques during a childbirth preparation class, ca. 1970s. Courtesy of the Schlesinger Library, Radcliffe Institute, Harvard University.

especially in the country's largest urban areas, were integrating labor and delivery into a single room, doing away with transferring the woman in the midst of transition. With a woman laboring and birthing in the same room, the husband's presence throughout was seamless. Moreover, pharmacological innovation meant that even in cases when anesthesia was used, the man's presence was still of value. Epidural anesthesia left the woman awake, clear-headed, and able to benefit from her husband's company in a way that had not been the case when labor ended in unconsciousness.

Economic pressures contributed to the integration of the father into American childbirth. It is no coincidence that one father described his role during labor's early stage as "mainly that of a nurse: comforting, puffing pillows, etc."[97] As noted above, some childbirth educators had initially monitriced their Lamaze students. Hospitals were often hostile to their presence in the labor room, there were not enough teachers to meet demand, and this was, in any case, an expensive option for the couple. According to Bing, "a new idea, therefore, presented itself to us: we had to make the husband his wife's coach."[98] Though she mistakes the origin of this practice, erasing the history of Dick-Read's and Lamaze's prior efforts to encourage the husband's participation, Bing points to a crucial difference in the role American fathers played in childbirth as compared to their British and French counterparts. Dick-Read and Lamaze had involved the father in childbirth as a source of emotional support for the laboring woman, but in the costly climate of privatized, hospitalized birth for the American middle-class, the father usually had to assume responsibility for being the laboring woman's sole constant companion. His presence supposedly freed up the nurses to attend to other obligations. Had American maternity wards welcomed the monitrice into hospital-based childbirth and had private insurance companies covered their services, there might have been a valuable, but less demanding role for American men at their wives' side.

Middle-class, white men—the typical Lamaze fathers—met their new responsibilities amid changing notions of American masculinity. With respect to men's role in childbirth, one again sees the twin impact of feminism and the counterculture. The women's movement redefined men's role in the domestic sphere, where they came to bear a greater, though still unequal, share of the burden for childrearing. Emerging out of both men's response to the women's movement and a counterculturally informed quest for authenticity, a more expressive, emotive, and empathic masculine ideal took shape. This is not to say that there were no other, competing, even more dominant models of American masculinity, but for many middle-class, well-educated, white American men, being a husband and father came to be more transparently invested with emotion. The 1950s' ideal of the strong, silent breadwinner gave way to new, more multidimensional models of manhood.[99]

The implication of these changes for men's presence during labor and birth was subtle, but clear. In earlier decades the man had often served as an extension of the physician's masculine authority and his job was to help control his wife. As natural childbirth advocate and ASPO member Robert Bradley wrote in 1965, the husband was the "'pregnancy policeman,' seeing that his wife practices her exercises."[100] And "should he catch her" bending at the waist instead of squatting to lift a heavy object, "a good-humored swat applied lightly to her posterior serves as a reminder that said posterior belongs down next to her heels—and further serves as a reminder that he loves her, he cares."[101] Setting aside the question of whether or not anything says "I love you" like a gentle spanking, Bradley clearly saw natural childbirth preparation as an opportunity to reinforce the husband's paternalistic, patriarchal authority in the home. By the mid-1970s, this sensibility was shifting, and the husband's role was less that of an authority figure than a gentle, emotionally present partner. The open and unselfconscious articulation of childbirth's emotional power and the intimacy this shared experience cultivated in the couple went beyond what was evident in earlier decades of the Lamaze movement's history both in the United States and in France. Husbands wrote and spoke about the closeness they felt to their wives, and how "it made the whole experience so much more meaningful because we were sharing [it] together," sentiments more commonly spoken by women than men in earlier decades.[102]

For men, these new demands for their physical and emotional presence were not always easy to meet. Some were squeamish. One new father, who had a positive experience at his wife's side, said in 1970 that initially he "couldn't think of anything less appealing than to watch my wife—the woman I love—in the middle of a messy business like childbirth."[103] Others experienced anxieties that went beyond mere unease. A father captured his sense of the tension between expectations for men and their experiences, writing that "while there's a great deal said about what a tremendous emotional experience is in store for parents who succeed in the Lamaze method, it seems to me that the emphasis has a drawback: if the father doesn't feel some overwhelming emotional wave of some sort he may suspect that he is cold or indifferent or freakish. I felt no great wave of anything on seeing [my son] born.... Actually, I had some moments of doubt and fear."[104] This father felt psychoprophylaxis was of value, especially in terms of his wife's ability to manage pain, but he worried that he had not measured up to society's new expectations for men.

To provide men with a safe environment to speak about their hopes and fears, "fathers only" childbirth education classes sprang up. A San Francisco physician found that "sometimes these groups get turned on in a beautiful way.... I listen to fathers rapping away with each other, sharing their common understandings and misunderstandings and anxiety."[105] Playing to conventional ideas about male camaraderie, the Nashville ASPO chapter tried to lighten things up with "Fathers' Beer Parties," from which "women were barred." Seasoned Lamaze dads brought in slides and photos of their children's births to share with first-timers who "would begin to open up (usually after the second beer)."[106] These courses included such topics as sex during and after pregnancy, aid to the woman during labor and birth, support of breastfeeding, and the adjustment to new parenthood.[107]

STAGNATION IN SOVIET PSYCHOPROPHYLAXIS

Discussion in the West over technology, humanization, feminist empowerment, and the father's role in childbirth were far removed from professional debates and clinical experiences in the USSR during the 1970s. Benjamin Segal visited Moscow's Maternity Ward No. 20 in 1970 and observed that, in contrast to the United States, "what impressed us most negatively was the absence of the husband from the scene."[108] Down to the USSR's demise, husbands had no place in Soviet birth practices. Soviet obstetricians remained adamant in their opposition to the father's presence inside the maternity ward, not to mention at his wife's side during labor and delivery. As Moscow's Dr. Golodnyi told Segal, Soviet obstetricians "saw no need for the husband's participation."[109] After birth, while mother and baby rested inside the maternity ward, "all the new fathers wandered about under the [ward] windows and shouted to their wives," as one former Soviet citizen later recalled.[110] There were small, isolated steps toward the integration of fathers into prenatal preparation courses, even as men remained banished from maternity wards. About 150 miles north of Kharkov, in the Russian region of Kursk, public health officials reported in 1974 that local pediatricians and gynecologists offered "Husband Seminars" for fathers-to-be. Like US Lamaze courses, expectant fathers saw birth films that demonstrated the use of psychoprophylaxis and reassured them that their wives would find labor and birth a comfortable experience. They learned about gestation, as well as infant care and safety, but as they would not be accompanying their wives through labor and birth, they did not need to learn about patterned breathing or comfort measures in any detail. The different curricular needs and perhaps the perception that mixed classes might prove uncomfortable led to segregated prenatal classes for men and women. It is unclear how widely available Husband Seminars were and how many men availed themselves of this opportunity, but every indication suggests that they were uncommon.[111]

The Soviet husband's absence from labor and birth highlights just one of many differences with Western psychoprophylactic practice. By the 1970s, there were few meaningful points of convergence, and professional contact between Soviet and Western researchers was limited. No grassroots support ever took shape inside the USSR. Neither the economic nor the political conditions that in the West had triggered challenges to the status quo in maternity care were in place in the Soviet Union. The lack of private market relations (outside of a black market for some goods and services) kept at bay the rise of a consumer movement. The population had no effective legal means to demand improvements, including in health care. Similarly, the authoritarian Soviet political system kept the countercultural and feminist movements from becoming mass phenomena. De jure equality between the sexes preempted the rise of an influential feminist movement. Official, state-sanctioned women's organizations promoted equity in the public sphere, while gender norms in the home remained inviolable.

A lack of alternatives, rather than faith in the method as the best course of action, inspired nominal state support for psychoprophylaxis. Research on psychoprophylaxis slowed to a trickle in the 1960s and the last Soviet investigation into its obstetric application was published in 1974.[112] A 1977 article in celebration of advances in obstetrics in the six decades since the October Revolution failed to even mention psychoprophylaxis.[113] Soviet obstetricians and the small but growing ranks of anesthesiologists continued their search for a more effective, equally safe approach to pain relief. Nitrous oxide remained a popular choice among obstetricians, but supply shortages persisted. Epidural anesthesia piqued some interest in the USSR, but saw virtually no clinical use.[114] As American physician and educator John Marlow observed, "if you gave [women in] the USSR the choice of whether to deliver without medication or with medication, assuming it was available, I feel certain that they would choose medication."[115] Of course, in the USSR no one asked women about their preferences because, in fact, they had no choices.

Archival records claim that psychoprophylactic training persisted through the last decades of the Soviet era. Official rates of psychoprophylactic preparation in the 1960s in urban areas typically ranged from 50 to 75 percent. Rural areas often reported figures considerably lower, in some regions dwindling to as little as 20 percent. Kharkov authorities claimed that in the 1960s and 1970s nearly 100 percent of women received training in the method. However, one must question not only the veracity of these figures but the content of the training. Anecdotal evidence suggests that these statistics were, if not outright fabricated, then greatly inflated. Dr. Ol'ga Valentinovna Grishchenko, a third-generation physician, observed that in the waning years of the USSR women were not compelled to attend childbirth preparation courses and the double burden of working full time both inside and outside the home often kept them away.[116] For those who did attend the course, lectures reportedly offered advice that was "superficial, consisting mainly of homilies about the importance of walks and the dangers of sweets. Such crucial subjects as breathing and massaging the stomach during labor [were] rarely mentioned more than once."[117] With minimal prenatal preparation and close to no access to pharmacological pain relief, Soviet women faced a grim reality at labor's onset.

Horror stories abound about the squalor and inhumanity of Soviet maternity wards in the 1960s, 1970s, and 1980s. Women typically labored without support, often in the company of three or four other women also in the throes of labor. In well-equipped, urban hospitals, a woman screaming in pain might receive some medication if her fuss began to irritate the physicians, but otherwise women's suffering met with indifference. In response to any requests or complaints, laboring women were frequently subjected to harsh reprimands from medical personnel.[118] As one Liudmila reflected, obstetric caregivers "take us for pigs. They don't give a damn. I mean, they treat us like cattle."[119]

Describing her experience giving birth in 1984 in Leningrad, one mother recalled that the staff treated patients "horribly, they all spoke haughtily; they had no time for us. It was very cold, -25 degrees [Celsius; -13 Fahrenheit] outside. There was no hot water...., no bathtub. The toilet was filthy. It's horrible to recall."[120] Another Soviet woman, who gave birth in Yaroslavl in 1989, attested that when a woman in her ward vomited during labor, the orderly "shoved a rag in her face and yelled, 'clean up after yourself!'"[121] After witnessing the gentle medical attention her daughter received at an Israeli maternity ward, one Soviet émigré reflected on her own experience decades earlier. "I pity the women of my generation," she wrote, "the poor girls of the 1970s, who could not even imagine that such [maternity care] happens."[122] Despite the important contribution the USSR had made to Western obstetrics through its development of psychoprophylaxis, Soviet women's lives went effectively untouched by the debates over how to humanize modern birth.

***

As psychoprophylactic practice peaked in the United States in the 1970s, signs of its decline as a global phenomenon were in evidence. Americans seemed to be taking their own path, with ASPO members participating less at international conferences and in the pages of international journals. Interest waned in France, Italy, and other countries that were once in the vanguard of the movement. By the end of the 1970s, the international journal and professional organizations dedicated to the promotion of psychoprophylaxis had folded, though the French journal hung on until 1994. In both France and the United States psychoprophylaxis faced technological and philosophical challenges. Some American women and their caregivers were beginning to turn increasingly to epidural anesthesia, while others, inspired by feminism and the counterculture rather than Pavlovian neuropsychology, embraced unmedicated childbirth. In the Soviet Union, Vel'vovskii retired without an heir apparent. Younger researchers pursued other avenues in their study of obstetric pain, and inquiry into psychoprophylaxis ceased. Instruction and practice continued in the USSR only in the most nominal ways. Ongoing shortages of anesthetics and analgesics kept women from receiving pharmacological pain relief, and they had neither the economic or political leverage to spur any of the changes wrought in the West.

CHAPTER 7

ᕯᕲ

Revolution or Cooptation?

By the early 1980s, a revolution had been wrought in American child-birth practices, with some parallels emerging in France and on the horizon for the Soviet successor states. How and with whom American women birthed differed strikingly from the status quo two decades earlier. Women were awake and aware, and free to enjoy and to benefit from the support of a loving companion at their sides. Nearly all American hospital administrators responding to a 1983 survey stated that their facilities allowed the father to be at the mother's side throughout labor and birth. Eighty-nine percent allowed someone other than the biological father to serve as a support person. Obstetricians nearly universally recommended childbirth preparation classes. More than 70 percent of responding hospitals reported that in excess of half their maternity cases underwent Lamaze preparation, though only 37 percent of hospitals offered Lamaze classes on site. Most surprisingly (and perhaps dubiously), researchers claimed to find no meaningful differences in rates of Lamaze use based on socioeconomic or ethnic background.[1] In other words, the Lamaze method—or at least elements of it—had become an integral part of the American way of birth.

The revolution in American maternity care was not a radical one. The broad changes to women's health care envisioned in the early editions of *Our Bodies, Ourselves*, which foretold a movement toward community-based, women-centered clinics, never materialized.[2] By the early 1980s, alternative clinical facilities, for either maternity services or women's health care more generally, remained the exception rather than the rule. How and with whom women birthed had changed, but where and under whose watchful eye had not. Hospitals succeeded in averting a large-scale shift toward home birth or independent ABCs staffed by midwives. They lured couples who might have chosen home birth back into the hospital by marrying some aspects of home birth—the companionship of a loved one and a homier, non-clinical atmosphere—with the reassuring promise of ready access to state-of-the-art medical care if it should prove necessary. Couples appreciated the opportunity to give birth in an environment that felt more appropriate to a normal, natural life cycle event, rather than a medical crisis. Rooming-in, too, became more readily available to those who preferred it to the use of the hospital nursery.

These concessions to the American consumer allowed hospitals and physicians to blunt the impact of challenges to their monopoly of control over birth. In the 1980s, the revival of midwifery gained momentum in the United States, but this movement never really threatened to unseat the hold obstetricians had over American birth. Lay midwives who entered the field in the 1970s sought state certification of their credentials and not infrequently came to see the benefits of qualifying as nurse-midwives. In the course of this turn toward professionalization, their practice in the 1980s moved increasingly into institutionalized, medicalized environments. The majority of midwives have in recent decades worked in hospitals, and it has been a hard-fought and incomplete struggle for them to carve out an autonomous practice, without the interference and oversight of obstetricians whose livelihoods midwifery seems to threaten. Obstetricians, hospitals, and insurance companies were so obstructionist in their efforts to deny midwives hospital privileges that the Federal Trade Commission had to intervene in the mid-1980s to force open hospital doors and break obstetricians' monopoly. From 1984 to 2010, the percentage of American midwives practicing in hospitals went from 78 to over 97 percent, a figure that speaks not only to the growing professionalization and integration of midwifery into conventional American maternity care, but to the home birth movement's failure to gain momentum.[3]

With the challenges posed by home birth and midwifery neutralized, within the walls of the hospital the medicalization and pathologization of childbirth continued apace. As noted previously, beginning in the 1970s the American cesarean section rate began a dramatic climb for complex and hotly contested reasons. A popular misconception attributes this marked upswing, discernible in both the United States and in Western Europe, to consumer demand, but studies suggest this factor plays far less a role than the medical community and the popular media make it seem. Among other considerations, labor induction—the artificial stimulation of labor through pharmacological and physical means—has nearly doubled in the United States since 1990 and likely factors as the first step down a slippery slope of interventions that culminate in cesarean section for about one in three American women by the early twenty-first century. The US figures are high when viewed in a global context, but European rates are also on the rise and exceed the World Health Organization's recommendation of optimal national rates in the range of 5 to 15 percent. Asia and Latin America appear to be following a similar course in recent years, with a rise in cesarean section rates that is nothing short of explosive.[4]

Of most direct relevance to the practice of psychoprophylaxis and, likely also contributing to the rise in cesarean section numbers, epidural anesthesia has taken firm hold in the US and much of Western Europe. In 1981 22 percent of American women in labor received epidural anesthesia. This figure climbed to nearly two-thirds by 1997. As of 2009 the number hovered around 75 percent.[5] Trends in France lag slightly behind chronologically, but parallel those in the United States. Over the course of the 1980s, the epidural rate more than quintupled from 4 to 21 percent, then jumped to 49 percent by 1995.[6] There remained in France uneven and inequitable access to anesthesia until 1994, when *Sécurité sociale* began to cover epidural anesthesia on patient demand. The 1994 plan stressed that in the maternity ward, "the principle to uphold is to seek to develop a policy that favors the greatest autonomy for laboring women."[7] Trained professionals, of course, continued to limit access in uncommon cases of contraindication, but French women's ability to avail themselves of pharmacological pain relief in childbirth ostensibly became a right and the norm. After two decades of advocacy, French feminists' demands for greater access to obstetric anesthesia finally met with satisfaction. Today, as in the United States, approximately three-quarters of French women receive epidural anesthesia during labor.[8]

In both France and the United States, what women sought from birth as a personal experience had changed, and advocates for unanesthetized childbirth found themselves with a dwindling audience. In a 2001 interview, Elisabeth Bing lamented that "women are not on our side anymore. They are too reliant on machines and want to get childbirth over quickly. They no longer care about achieving anything with their bodies."[9] Bing's judgment of contemporary women is clear, as is her appreciation that her own views have fallen out of favor. It "isn't just the epidural—it's the attitude toward childbirth.... Even with regard to pain—there is no satisfaction achieved because the woman does not have to work for anything. We've minimized the sense of achievement one obtains when mastering a difficult experience."[10] One could certainly challenge Bing's claim that a birth with epidural anesthesia is an unsatisfying experience, but she is correct that natural childbirth had fallen from favor. As of 2005, only 14 percent of US women gave birth without the use of any form of pharmacological pain relief.[11]

Mounting evidence against the grandiose claims made about psychoprophylaxis's efficacy reinforced the consumer's movement toward pharmacological pain relief. Informing professional medical opinion, new studies in psychology, obstetrics, and nursing challenged a quarter-century of psychoprophylactic research as methodologically unsound. Investigators demonstrated that relaxation, not the method's hallmark breathing techniques, was the most effective aspect of Lamaze preparation. The complicated breathing patterns did not really do much and only about 25 percent of women experienced significant mitigation of pain thanks to psychoprophylaxis. Ronald Melzack, a towering figure in the field of pain studies, found that with prepared childbirth, including Lamaze and other methods, "pain is diminished but remains severe."[12] Childbirth preparation classes were helpful in lowering women's perception of pain, but they were not predictive of resort to obstetric anesthesia or analgesia. Nor did psychoprophylaxis significantly shorten labor or improve outcomes, claims made frequently by its promoters.[13] Melzack acknowledged the medical advantages of birth without the use of anesthetics and analgesics, but emphasized that both prepared childbirth and epidural anesthesia are "aimed at assisting women in childbirth to suffer less fear, anxiety and pain."[14] Rather than seeing epidural anesthesia as rendering childbirth preparation obsolete or the Lamaze method as an obstacle to the more widespread use of epidurals, Melzack envisioned these approaches at work in tandem to achieve a common goal: a safe, satisfying birth experience. In this way his words echoed those of Konstantinov, Nikolaev, Vellay, Muller, and others who had come to see psychoprophylaxis as not a substitute for pharmacological pain relief, but a complement to it.

From 1975 to 1985, ASPO's growth continued, but a changing consumer and obstetric climate redefined the organization's mission. In 1975 there were 3.1 million live births in the United States and 200,000 couples attended Lamaze classes. Many more couples took advantage of courses with content that was not strictly defined as psychoprophylaxis, but was influenced by the teachings of Lamaze and his American followers. By the mid-1980s, when about 3.7 million American babies were born annually, Lamaze was unchallenged as a brand, dominating the field of childbirth education, with more than one million American women a year trained in Lamaze courses.[15] Despite ASPO's strong market position, the content of these courses had moved decisively away from the patterned breathing and other techniques that had comprised psychoprophylactic practice.

To survive the myriad and interlocking consumer pressures and technological challenges of the 1980s, ASPO essentially abandoned psychoprophylaxis as anything resembling what Vel'vovskii, Lamaze, Bing, and others
had taught in the 1950s and 1960s. Throughout the 1970s the method had
undergone repeated revision in its approach to patterned breathing and in
its claims about the potential for painlessness in childbirth. The increasingly complex breathing patterns of the 1970s were pared down considerably in the early 1980s. In the mid-1980s ASPO broke definitively with its
past and, as one advocate puts it, "Lamaze changed from a method to a
philosophy."[16] Rather than promote a particular approach to natural childbirth, with its historic emphasis on patterned breathing, relaxation, and
conditioning, ASPO committed itself to advocacy for minimal interventions in cases of normal birth, the presence of the father or other support
person of the woman's choosing, and other measures in keeping with its
long-standing orientation to a less medicalized birth experience. The picture of the panting woman who refused pharmacological pain relief—for
lack of either need or desire—remains salient in the collective American
imagining of a Lamaze birth, but in practice it ostensibly ceased to exist
by 1990. Lamaze International, as ASPO is now known, today rejects completely the breathing techniques that were at psychoprophylaxis's core. Talk
of Pavlovian conditioning is nowhere to be found in contemporary literature, which instead likens the benefits of focus on the breath in childbirth
to that in yoga and meditation practice. Today's official literature in fact
notes that "'breathing' is no longer the hallmark of Lamaze."[17] Expectant
parents are warned to "be wary of 'Lamaze' classes that spend a lot of time
practicing relaxation and breathing and little or no time building your confidence or discussing how to keep things simple and how to have the safe,
healthy birth you want in the birth setting you have chosen."[18] With these
statements, the organization that had been founded to promote psychoprophylaxis makes its break with the past complete.

In an effort to secure its dominant standing in the field of childbirth
preparation, ASPO took a decisive turn toward a more corporatist nonprofit organizational structure in the mid-1980s. Recognizing the need
to find new streams of revenue if the organization was to remain financially viable in the more competitive environment of the day, ASPO began
to encourage its teacher members to peddle ASPO-endorsed products in
their classes. To supplement their meager incomes, teachers earned a cut
of the profits. Some Lamaze-certified instructors were already selling products to their clients, including breastfeeding aids, their own relaxation and
labor-support audio cassette tapes, and the like. In 1986 ASPO surveyed
its members to gauge their interest in selling prenatal, childbirth, and

postpartum supplies and found misgivings about this commercialization. Some respondents were positive about the profit for themselves and the convenience for their clients of selling relevant supplies, but others replied that it was a "hassle," in "poor taste," or "not appropriate." Reflecting a widely shared sentiment, one stated that "I am an educator, not a sales-man."[19] When solicited to sell a home video in her childbirth education class, an Illinois childbirth educator wrote to ASPO to express her distaste for the video's content, which she claimed promoted exercises "that actually hurt." She resented the crass, "commercial turn that my organization ASPO/Lamaze is taking."[20]

ASPO also began to pursue an unprecedented level of collaboration with hospitals across the country. ASPO's 1986 business plan called for the development of an accreditation program in family-centered maternity care (FCMC) for 4,200 American hospitals. It sought to parlay its standing in the field into a profitable, mutually beneficial arrangement with these facilities. ASPO set itself up as a credible assessor of FCMC services. Hospitals earned ASPO's imprimatur and in exchange ASPO benefited from increased brand name recognition and a foot in the door with institutions that would offer childbirth preparation courses in-house. While not necessarily the primary motive, the potential for "a degree of financial benefit from the process" of FCMC accreditation certainly had appeal.[21]

The plan to move into FCMC accreditation was just one step that ASPO took in a new direction, a shift enshrined in a new mission statement and structural reorganization in the late 1980s. ASPO diversified its mission, expanding its "focus beyond the last trimester of pregnancy." The parent division, part of the organization since its inception, would no longer require dues for membership. Instead, baby product manufacturers were to support an advertisement-rich quarterly magazine for distribution to expectant parents and aimed at the promotion of products for infants 0 to 6 months of age. ASPO asked parents for permission to pass their names on to companies for mailings and questionnaires. Like the FCMC accreditation program that put ASPO in bed with the hospitals, this scheme to serve as middlemen in the relationship between businesses and expectant parents moved ASPO quite decisively away from its advocacy roots and toward a business model of operation. ASPO's leadership saw this as "the most exciting and innovative thinking ever undertaken in this organization's history."[22] In effect, it codified a change that was already apparent: the demise of Lamaze as a grassroots movement and its rise as a business, replete with a brand of plush infant toys.

Today, Lamaze International advocates six key childbirth practices: the avoidance of medically unnecessary interventions; the spontaneous start to labor; mobility during labor; the continuous support of a companion; the avoidance of giving birth on one's back; and rooming-in. It objects to epidural anesthesia—along with restrictions on eating and drinking during labor, the routine use of IV fluids, continuous electronic fetal monitoring, the artificial rupture of membranes, and the use of uterine stimulants—as medically unnecessary interventions. Lamaze International asserts that in instances of normal labor and birth, "if you are free to move and encouraged to find comfort in a variety of ways, you are less likely to need an epidural, to need one early in labor, or to need as much medicine." [23] There is some acknowledgment that in the case of a long, exhausting labor, epidural anesthesia can provide welcome relief, even if it is not strictly a medical necessity. This is a nuanced and moderate position toward pharmacological pain relief, in line with decades of ASPO advocacy for the restrained, judicious use of drugs. To some degree the contemporary position is more explicitly against the use of pain relief medications because it sets medical necessity, rather than physician judgment or patient desire, as the standard for decision-making.[24]

CONCLUSION

At the heart of the rise and fall of natural childbirth's popularity and, along with it, the global Lamaze movement, lay shifting technologies, economies, politics, and social values. With his 1933 book, Grantly Dick-Read proposed Natural Childbirth as a way to achieve what he believed to be a social and political good: greater fecundity, resulting from women's increased satisfaction in birth and securing Britain's demographic vitality and economic stability. Women took pride in participating fully in birth, which had been precluded by the incapacitating anesthetics available for obstetric use at the time. By the 1940s, amid a baby boom, a rising sense of consumer empowerment, and a desire for togetherness, couples on both sides of the Atlantic turned to the Read method to give them what they wanted out of their childbirth experience. They sought the healthiest, safest birth for their babies and a profound, shared emotional experience for themselves. The Read method and, later, psychoprophylaxis, also promised women the ability to bear their children with dignity, which in the 1950s and for most of the 1960s meant the maintenance of a quiet, calm demeanor that belied the extraordinary physical challenges of labor and birth.

In the USSR, maternal dignity and satisfaction played no role in the rise of psychoprophylaxis. Absent a consumer-driven medical marketplace, other motives led Vel'vovskii and his Soviet colleagues to craft their psychological approach to pain relief in childbirth. When psychoprophylaxis came on the scene in the USSR in the last years of the Stalin era, the Soviet government was unable to meet the demands for analgesics and anesthetics. Psychoprophylaxis offered a low-cost, low-tech alternative, feasible on a national scale. Ideological motives incentivized the regime's embrace of psychoprophylaxis over other alternatives, both psychological and pharmacological, while fiscal and personnel shortages made it the best option at the time. Instituted from the top down by government fiat, results on the ground proved disappointing. Stalin's death and the resultant shift in political climate undermined the push for psychoprophylaxis. Records state that the method continued to be taught down to the USSR's 1991 demise, but one is hard pressed to find anyone to attest to anything beyond the most cursory prenatal preparation. For those who can afford high quality, private care, childbirth in the post-Soviet period has begun to resemble more closely the experience of most American and Western European women. Epidural use is on the rise and, though it remains far from a universal choice, the father is increasingly at the laboring woman's side.[25] Ironically, materials for childbirth preparation courses like those promoted by Lamaze International are being translated into Russian, Ukrainian, and other languages of the former USSR, with no awareness of the Soviet Union's place in the history of the prepared childbirth movement.

In France, as in the United States, there was no shortage of drugs, but there were other reasons why psychoprophylaxis earned a following. While American women in the 1950s were turning in increasing numbers to Dick-Read's Natural Childbirth, French women expressed their dissatisfaction with the mid-century status quo in maternity care through their embrace of psychoprophylaxis. Among other factors, ideology played a role in the promotion of the Soviet method over Dick-Read's, with the UFF, the PCF, and other leftist organization favoring it as representative of the progressive, benevolent, and uplifting quality of Soviet power for working-class women. But ideology alone does not explain psychoprophylaxis's French success. It surfaced at the right moment, when urban French women sought something more satisfying from their childbirth experiences. Like their British and American sisters drawn to the Read method, they wanted a tool to maintain an even keel during labor and birth, and psychoprophylaxis fit the bill.

In France and in the United States in the late 1960s and early 1970s, the quest for dignity yielded to a desire for authenticity, experiential abandon, and empowerment. Women continued to seek control, over themselves and the situation around them, but they and their partners attempted to utilize that control to weather a visceral, embodied experience of birth.

Psychoprophylaxis offered a way to mitigate, rather than obliterate, sensation. The method's promoters no longer held out the possibility of "painless childbirth," as had been touted in the 1950s and early 1960s. Over the course of the 1970s, they backed well away from earlier, grandiose promises and emphasized instead the method's role as a coping tool. At the same time, a rising tide of both French and American voices critiqued psychoprophylaxis as a sham, just another tool for the exertion of medical authority over women and their bodies.

The feminist health movement of the 1970s bequeathed to American women an understanding of the need to educate themselves about their bodies and their options. When it came to maternity care, many middle class, white women of that era equated this agenda with the rejection of anesthetics or analgesics, marking a break with the past. In general, American women in the 1950s and 1960s had not viewed their natural childbirth experiences as marred or compromised by resort to a moderate use of anesthetics, analgesics, or sedatives. In fact, throughout the 1950s and 1960s Demerol and similar drugs were routinely used in what Americans nonetheless defined as natural childbirth. By the late 1960s, natural childbirth had not just become more popular; the very definition had changed to proscribe the use of drugs. ASPO literature was unequivocal, as it had been all along, that pain medication had a place in obstetrics when used judiciously. Nonetheless, expectant mothers got the message, through the popular media, in their childbirth preparation classes, and from peers, that anesthetics and analgesics were dangerous, unnatural, disempowering, and to be avoided at all costs.

By the mid-1980s, the technological, economic, and social context in which American women gave birth had changed in important ways. The rise of epidural anesthesia led to further revision of the Lamaze method and ASPO's mission. Epidural anesthesia became more widely available and what women wanted in birth began to shift. Unlike the women of the 1950s and 1960s, who did not have good options for drugs that were safe, effective, and preserved their clarity of mind, or the women of the 1970s, who valued an authentic, embodied experience of childbirth even if it meant enduring pain, women in the 1980s and beyond have by and large not seen any particular value to foregoing anesthetics and analgesics in childbirth. The marketing of anesthesiologists' services to patients played an important role, but there was a cultural shift at work as well.

The counterculturally inflected values of the 1970s lost their pull on a younger generation of childbearing women and their partners, who saw no added medical or personal payoff in a low-tech childbirth experience. Instead, these women valued the ease and relief made possible by epidural anesthesia and they believed the benefits more than outweighed the risks. Today's proponents of natural childbirth argue that these women are not making fully informed decisions and do not know the whole truth about the drawbacks of epidural anesthesia for themselves and their babies. It is indisputable that the playing field is not level, as hospital-based childbirth preparation classes have a captive audience for the promotion of the services of anesthesiologists. However, to dismiss the vast majority of today's childbearing women as dupes is to do them a disservice. Many of them make a clear, conscious, and fully informed decision that reflects a different set of values and priorities than those held by natural childbirth advocates; their choice to turn to epidural anesthesia in and of itself is no less feminist or empowered. Their preferences arguably harken back to the values and priorities propounded by first-wave feminists, who lauded the benefits of twilight sleep. And, like enthusiasts for natural childbirth in the 1950s and early 1960s, they value the ability to comport themselves calmly throughout labor and birth.[26]

In the last quarter-century in the United States, France, and, more recently, the Soviet successor states, "choice" in medicine, including in maternity care, has become a mantra and with it have come a number of problems.[27] Enmeshed in the Western heritage of the Enlightenment, the linkage between choice and freedom is a central tenant of capitalism. In a market economy, the consumer supposedly has "freedom of choice...to cast 'dollar votes' for goods and services that best satisfy their needs."[28] Of course, those choices in medical care are limited from the start and not only with respect to affordability. As Fredric Jameson observes, the "market as a concept rarely has anything to do with choice or freedom, since those are all determined for us in advance, whether we are talking about new model cars, toys, or television programs," or, in the case at hand, maternity care. "[W]e select among those, no doubt, but we can scarcely be said to have a say in actually choosing any of them."[29] In rural areas, choice in the medical market is curtailed by the number of available practitioners and facilities. For those living in or near poverty, options are also curtailed. They may be priced out of certain choices and, if they rely on governmental assistance, certain caregivers, types of care, or care settings may be beyond what the state is willing to pay. And what of alternatives that are nowhere on offer? Freedom of choice is touted as the order of the day, but consumer options are everywhere circumscribed.

To degrees that vary by national context, medical practitioners must compete in the marketplace, responding, or at least seeming to respond, to consumer demand. The rising tide of the consumer rights movement very much informed the groundswell of American support for the Lamaze method, as well as the backlash against psychoprophylaxis in France in the 1970s. But despite rhetoric that asserts that women can now write their "birth plans" and tailor their experience to their desires—have an epidural, or don't have one; choose a midwife, or an obstetrician; give birth in a homey hospital-based "birthing suite," or in an independent ABC—there is persistent dissatisfaction among obstetric customers. Nowhere is this more the case than in the United States, where, although survey data indicates high levels of satisfaction among obstetric patients, one finds mommy groups and the blogosphere perennially abuzz with chatter of disappointing childbirth experiences.[30]

Choice has become a substitute for empowerment.[31] In their responses to the patriarchal obstetric establishment, American and French feminism offered women in the 1970s two markedly different visions of what constituted empowerment in childbirth. For American women, a feminist, empowered birth meant the avoidance of drugs and other interventions that kept them from a fully active, conscious, embodied experience. This ideal of a feminist birth emerged in the context of the world's most medicalized, pathologized approach to obstetric care. Empowerment meant reclaiming birth from patriarchal physicians, who had wrested control of the natural, normal process of childbirth from women. Responding to a very different obstetric environment, French feminists fought against "the myth of painless childbirth." They channeled their energy into demanding greater access to the kinds of analgesics and anesthetics that American women battled to resist. Underneath these two divergent visions of empowerment lay common ground, as both French and American feminist health advocates saw education about one's body and one's options as key. Only through education about choices and their relative benefits and risks could women make truly informed and empowered decisions about what was best for them and their babies. It is worth noting that, down to the USSR's 1991 collapse, questions of choice, self-education, and empowerment had virtually no place in the maternity care of Soviet women. Economic crisis through the 1990s, and persistent regional and class inequities, make empowerment as medical consumers a pipe dream for most women in the former Soviet republics.

The contemporary fixation on choice leads to a false consciousness, an ersatz sense of freedom in place of genuine empowerment, which I understand as an active stance toward and meaningful ability to exert influence over one's own health care. Bioethicist and ethnographer Annemarie Mol offers an instructive critique of the limitations of what she calls "the logic of choice," juxtaposing it to "the logic of care." Following the logic of choice, the patient is empowered to choose among options "delineated as the product on offer and... you may choose it or not." By contrast, "care is a process: it does not have clear boundaries. It is open-ended.... Care is not a (small or large) product that changes hands, but a matter of various hands working together (over time) towards a result. Care is not a transaction in which something is exchanged (a product against a price); but an interaction in which the action goes back and forth (in an ongoing process)."[32] It is not that choice means a cold, impersonal market relationship and care is a warm and fuzzy return to the paternalistic medicine of yore, but rather that the logic of care roots medical practice not in the act of buying and selling clearly defined and bounded goods and services, but in an interpersonal dynamic.

What would it mean for maternity services to be governed by the logic of care, rather than choice? Could a reorientation toward care rather than choice open up an opportunity to more meaningfully infuse hospital-based childbirth with any of the elements of social birth for which American feminists in the 1970s fought? Crafting a clearer picture of what we mean by distinct but interconnected concepts such as control and empowerment in childbirth may be a decisive step toward developing maternity care that seeks to yield not satisfied customers, but satisfied recipients of care. An empowered birth might, for example, require continuity of care not just throughout the course of labor and birth, but for the duration of prenatal and perinatal care. Rather than be attended by whomever happens to be on call from an obstetric or midwifery practice when she went into labor, the expectant mother might be better served by someone with whom she has developed a rapport during her pregnancy and who understands her priorities and preferences.

Recent studies show that constant companionship and support exerts a powerful influence on a woman's ability to manage the pain in labor without the use of drugs.[33] For maternity services oriented around care, rather than choice, labor support might not be left primarily in the valuable but inexpert hands of a partner, friend, or relative. The American medical practitioner's responsibility for the woman's physical comfort and for her ability to work with and through her pain at present seems to end with her choice to accept or refuse epidural anesthesia. The logic of care would suggest that, rather than abandon the women who choose to forego anesthesia, an alternative path to pain management would follow. The ongoing, knowledgeable support of a trained professional, be she a doula, a midwife, or a nurse, could supplement the presence of a loved one. Doulas are at present gaining in popularity, as women seek to enhance the support of a partner or friend with someone who has not just patience and compassion, but expert knowledge. Lamaze International today encourages expectant mothers to consider the services of a doula, but this option is accessible only to those who live in the select communities where they are available, and who can afford to hire them privately.[34] In a maternity service ordered by the logic of care, what is today an uncommon luxury would be transformed into a routine, integral part of labor and birth.

Birth without anesthesia, however, is not intrinsically a more feminist, empowered, or care-driven practice. The belief that an unanesthetized labor is the gold standard of feminist empowerment in childbirth is a legacy of the 1970s. Feminist health activists opposed patronizing, patriarchal obstetricians who struggled to sustain a status quo in which women had little say in their own course of care. Physician authority and patient dependence certainly persist, but the caregiver-patient dynamic today is much changed from what it was when unanesthetized birth came to define an American feminist ideal. Moreover, drug options have changed as well and, though questions of safety remain, the dangers posed by today's anesthetics are not as clear and grave as they were in the mid-twentieth century. Of no less importance has been a shift away from the valorization of labor pain. Can the use of epidural anesthesia be part of a feminist, empowered birth? It hinges only on the meaning with which we imbue this practice and, as this study demonstrates, those meanings are mutable and context-sensitive.

The international history of psychoprophylaxis speaks to how we arrived at today's status quo, but perhaps more significantly it also reminds us that the values and meanings that we attribute to certain obstetric interventions, like the use of anesthesia, are not constant, but provisional. Practices are historical products of specific technological, economic, social, and political conditions. What constituted a desirable birth experience changed with the times, as issues of safety, dignity, control, and power each came to be reconfigured under both national and international influences. Contributing to revisions of the psychoprophylactic method as practiced on the clinical level and as justified to medical professionals and the general public alike, shifts in beliefs about female psychology and the mind-body relationship reverberated in maternity wards. By excavating the story of psychoprophylaxis, this book demonstrates the rootedness of maternity care in big, broad, and fundamental social, political, and economic considerations.

Situating the American experience of the Lamaze method in a transnational perspective offers an important corrective to a history typically understood as framed by the nation-state's boundaries. Restoring the USSR's role in the story of psychoprophylaxis's rise, spread, and decline renders vivid the contingent and constructed meanings that Americans reflexively link to natural childbirth. The Soviet case, even more so than the French one, demonstrates how a clinical practice could take hold thanks to sharply divergent political, social, and material conditions and come to convey very different meanings. With its failure to meet the demands of medical caregivers—and, presumably, patients, though their desires are muted in the sources—the Soviet effort to ease the pain of labor highlights, by way of contrast, the power and responsiveness of a consumer-driven economy. Soviet physicians and public health leaders had knowledge of all the medications available in the West to ease the pain of labor, but the centralized, planned economy combined with the regime's priorities to keep women from availing themselves of these drugs. Unlike Soviet women, French and American women had the power to leverage their position as consumers in democratic societies to effect positive, if incomplete, changes in maternity care.

With the Lamaze movement as a case in point, this book shows that how, where, and with whom we birth says a lot about who we are. A more empowered birth, one that moves us past the dead-end, polarized, and limited logic of choice, will require vision and effort to forge, but holds the potential, as one longtime American childbirth educator put it recently, to help "people find meaning in the most basic experiences: of becoming pregnant, of becoming parents, of raising children....When these most basic things are...trivialized or sanitized or produced by somebody else, I think we're [left] hungry. I think there's a void and not only are our individual lives less for that, but we seek things out that...aren't so good for the whole culture."[35] Maternity care for women and their children, for our sisters and our friends, for us, is a matter of personal responsibility and of self-education, as feminist health activists preached in the 1970s. But there is another dimension to their message of empowerment that has fallen into the shadows: that medicine and health reflect and are structured within economic, social, and political systems marked by the unequal exertion of power and by inequitable access. Careful examination of the historical record reminds us of the potential for change, and offers an instructive starting point from which to launch consideration of how best to redress these imbalances and to offer more humane, empowering, safer care for all women.

NOTES

INTRODUCTION

1. On earlier models of mental ailments and the place of gender in their construction, see Janet Oppenheim, *"Shattered Nerves": Doctors, Patients, and Depression in Victorian England* (New York: Oxford University Press, 1991), esp. 181–232; Mathew Thomson, "Neurasthenia in Britain: An Overview," in *Cultures of Neurasthenia: From Beard to the First World War*, ed. Marijke Gijswijt-Hofstra and Roy Porter (Amsterdam: Rodopi, 2001), 77–96; Hilary Marland, "'Uterine Mischief': W. S. Playfair and His Neurasthenic Patients," in *Cultures of Neurasthenia*, 117–40.
2. Helene Deutsch, *The Psychology of Women* (New York: Grune and Stratton, 1945), 2: 234.
3. Ibid., 235.
4. Ziv Eisenberg, "Clear and Pregnant Danger: The Making of Prenatal Psychology in Mid-Twentieth-Century America," *Journal of Women's History* 22 (Fall 2010): 112–35.
5. Deutsch, *Psychology of Women*, 2: 138.
6. Ibid., 227. For a clear, concise analysis of the place of Deutsch's writings in thinking about psychological approaches to obstetric pain, particularly with respect to psychoprophylaxis in France, see Marilène Vuille, *Accouchement et douleur: Une étude sociologique* (Lausanne: Éditions Antipodes, 1998), 58–60.
7. Rebecca L. Davis, "'Not Marriage At All, but Simple Harlotry': The Companionate Marriage Controversy," *Journal of American History* 94 (Mar. 2008): 1137–63.
8. Stephanie Coontz, *The Way We Never Were: American Families and the Nostalgia Trap* (New York: Basic Books, 1992).
9. Elaine Tyler May, *Homeward Bound: American Families in the Cold War Era*, rev. ed. (New York: Basic Books, 2008), 109–28; Jessica Weiss, *To Have and To Hold: Marriage, the Baby Boom, and Social Change* (Chicago: The University of Chicago Press, 2000), 83–139; Peter G. Filene, *Him/Her/Self: Sex Roles in Modern America*, 2nd ed. (Baltimore: Johns Hopkins University Press, 1986), 172. See also Christopher Lasch, *Haven in a Heartless World: The Family Besieged* (New York: Basic Books, 1977); Robert Moeller, *Protecting Motherhood: Women and the Family in the Politics of Postwar West Germany* (Berkeley: University of California Press, 1993).
10. See Rebecca Jo Plant, *Mom: The Transformation of Motherhood in Modern America* (Chicago: University of Chicago Press, 2010).

11. Oral histories would have been impractical on any large, systematic scale given the amount of time that has passed since psychoprophylaxis was practiced in the USSR and, especially, given the limited degree to which it ever made inroads at the clinical level. Inquiries in Kharkiv, the birthplace of psychoprophylaxis, failed to yield even a single interlocutor who had experienced or witnessed a birth using the method. An article in a local newspaper in the Russian city of Yekaterinburg soliciting birth stories produced not one response.

CHAPTER 1

1. Brigitte Jordan, *Birth in Four Cultures: A Crosscultural Investigation of Childbirth in Yucatan, Holland, Sweden, and the United States*, 4th rev. ed. (Long Grove, IL: Waveland, 1992). See also Brigitte Jordan, "Childbirth and Authoritative Knowledge," in *Childbirth and Authoritative Knowledge: Cross-Cultural Perspectives*, ed. Robbie E. Davis-Floyd and Carolyn F. Sargent (Berkeley: University of California Press, 1997), 55–79.

2. The standard studies of the history of American birth practices include Judith Walzer Leavitt, *Brought to Bed: Childbearing in America, 1750–1950* (New York: Oxford University Press, 1986); Judith Pence Rooks, *Midwifery and Childbirth in America* (Philadelphia: Temple University Press, 1997); Richard W. Wertz and Dorothy C. Wertz, *Lying-In: A History of Childbirth in America*, rev. ed. (New Haven, CT: Yale University Press, 1989).

3. Timothy B. Smith, "The Social Transformation of Hospitals and the Rise of Medical Insurance in France, 1914–1943," *The Historical Journal* 41 (Dec. 1998): 1060; Yvonne Knibiehler, *Accoucher: Femmes, sages-femmes et médecins depuis le milieu du XXe siècle* (Rennes: Éditions de l'École Nationale de la Santé Publique, 2007), 21, 25, 31.

4. Tania McIntosh, "Profession, Skill, or Domestic Duty? Midwifery in Sheffield, 1881–1936," *Social History of Medicine* 11 (Jan. 1998), 414; Brooke Victoria Heagerty, "Class, Gender and Professionalization: The Struggle for British Midwifery, 1900–1936" (PhD diss., Michigan State University, 1990); Brooke V. Heagerty, "Reassessing the Guilty: The Midwives Act and the Control of English Midwives in the Early 20th Century," in *Supervision of Midwives*, ed. Mavis Kirkham (Hale, Cheshire, England: Books for Midwives, 1996), 13–27. See also Julia Allison and Mavis Kirkham, "Supervision of Midwives in Nottingham, 1948–1972," in *Supervision of Midwives*, 28–37; Jean Towler and Joan Bramall, *Midwives in History and Society* (London: Croom Helm, 1986), 177–246; Jean Donnison, *Midwives and Medical Men: A History of the Struggle for the Control of Childbirth*, 2nd ed. (New Barnet, Herts, UK: Historical Publications, 1988); A. Susan Williams, *Women and Childbirth in the Twentieth Century: A History of the National Birthday Trust Fund, 1928–1993* (Phoenix Mill, Gloucestershire, UK: Sutton Publishing, 1997), 141.

5. During World War II, the Soviet state still battled lay midwifery, a phenomenon already ostensibly extinguished for decades by that point in Britain and the United States. Mie Nakachi, "Replacing the Dead: The Politics of Reproduction in the Postwar Soviet Union, 1945–1955" (PhD diss., University of Chicago, 2008), 253. On midwifery in the postwar Soviet periphery, see Paula A. Michaels, *Curative Powers: Medicine and Empire in Stalin's Central Asia* (Pittsburgh: University of Pittsburgh Press, 2003), 149.

6. Sherwin B. Nuland, *The Doctor's Plague: Germs, Childbed Fever, and the Strange Story of Ignác Semmelweis* (New York: Norton, 2003); Irvine Loudin, *Death in*

Childbirth: An International Study of Maternal Care and Maternal Mortality, 1800–1950 (London: Clarendon Press, 1992); Irvine Loudin, *The Tragedy of Childbed Fever* (New York: Oxford University Press, 2000); Richard A. Meckel, *Save the Babies: American Public Health Reform and the Prevention of Infant Mortality, 1850–1929* (Baltimore: Johns Hopkins University Press, 1990). Dramatic declines in maternal mortality in the United States well illustrate the scale of these shifts. For example, between 1939 and 1943 the rates of maternal mortality among African American women declined 33 percent and among European American women 40 percent thanks to the availability of new drugs and stricter attention to sanitary condition for both hospital and home deliveries. Edwin P. Jordan, "Maternal Death Rate Lowered," *Evening Independent* (St. Petersburg, FL), Sept. 28, 1950.

7. Adrian E. Feldhusen, "The History of Midwifery and Childbirth in America: A Timeline," *Midwifery Today*, 2000, http://www.midwiferytoday.com/articles/timeline.asp; Jane Lewis, "Mothers and Maternity Politics in the Twentieth Century," in *The Politics of Maternity Care: Services for Childbearing Women in Twentieth-Century Britain*, ed. Jo Garcia, Robert Kilpatrick, and Martin Richards (Oxford: Clarendon, 1990), 21; Angus McLaren, *Twentieth-Century Sexuality: A History* (Malden, MA: Blackwell Publishing, 1999), 80; Angela Davis, *Modern Motherhood: Women and Family in England, c.1945–2000* (Manchester and New York: Manchester University Press, 2012), 84.

8. Smith, "The Social Transformation of Hospitals," 1074; Knibiehler, *Accoucher*, 32.

9. William A. Knaus, *Inside Russian Medicine: An American Doctor's First-Hand Report* (New York: Everest House, 1981), 203.

10. Jacqueline H. Wolf, *Deliver Me from Pain: Anesthesia and Birth in America* (Baltimore: Johns Hopkins University Press, 2009). See also Donald Caton, *What a Blessing She Had Chloroform: The Medical and Social Response to the Pain of Childbirth from 1800 to the Present* (New Haven, CT: Yale University Press, 1999); Margarete Sandelowski, *Pain, Pleasure, and American Childbirth: From the Twilight Sleep to the Read Method, 1914–1960* (Westport, CT: Greenwood Press, 1984); Cynthia De Haven Pitcock and Richard B. Clark, "From Fanny to Fernand: The Development of Consumerism in Pain Control during the Birth Process," *American Journal of Obstetrics and Gynecology* 167 (Sept. 1992): 581–87; A. P. Nikolaev, "K probleme obezbolivaniia rodov," *Akusherstvo i ginekologiia* 25 (Nov.–Dec. 1949): 7; W. Richards, G. D. Parbrook, and J. Wilson, "Stanislav Klikovich (1853–1910). Pioneer of Nitrous Oxide and Oxygen Analgesia," *Anesthesia* 31 (Sept. 1976): 933–40; G. F. Marx and T. Katsnelson, "The Introduction of Nitrous Oxide Analgesia into Obstetrics," *Obstetrics and Gynecology* 80 (Oct. 1992): 715–18. Familiarity in Russia with twilight sleep is demonstrated by the publication of Ganna Raion, *Obezboleznennye rody v "sumerechnom sne": Skopolamin-morfinovyi metod po dokladam vrachei i lichnym perezhivaniiam materei*, trans. M. Bedelar (Moscow: Moskovskoe izdatel'stvo, 1917), which had originally appeared in English in 1915 and met with considerable success in both the United States and Great Britain. Hanna Rion, *The Truth about Twilight Sleep* (New York: McBride, Nast, 1915) and *Painless Childbirth in Twilight Sleep* (London: T. Werner Laurie, 1915). On the use of ether and chloroform, see also F. V. Bukoemskii, *Obezbolivanie normal'nykh rodov vdykhaniiami efira i khloroforma* (Saint Petersburg: V. A. Vatslika, 1895).

11. Marguerite Tracy and Mary Boyd, *Painless Childbirth: A General Survey of All Painless Methods with Special Stress on "Twilight Sleep" and Its Extension to America* (New York: Frederick A. Stokes, 1915), 41.

12. Wolf, *Deliver Me from Pain*, 87.

13. Williams, *Women and Childbirth in the Twentieth Century*, 124–40.

14. Jennifer Beinart, "Obstetric Analgesia and the Control of Childbirth in Twentieth-Century Britain," in *The Politics of Maternity Care*, 121. See also Sarah Robinson, "Maintaining the Independence of the Midwifery Profession: A Continuing Struggle," in *The Politics of Maternity Care*, 61–91.

15. Nicky Leap and Billie Hunter, *The Midwife's Tale: An Oral History from Handywoman to Professional Midwife* (London: Scarlet Press, 1993), 143, 168.

16. On the benefits of this type of obstetric anesthesia and the obstacles to its popularization in the United States, see Jill [Arnold], "Call It a Comeback? The Many Faces of Nitrous Oxide for Labor Pain Relief," *RH Reality Check*, Dec. 16, 2010, http://www.rhrealitycheck.org/blog/2010/12/14/callcomeback-m any-faces-nitrous-oxide-labor-pain-relief; Sherry Boschert, "Nitrous Oxide Returns for Labor Pain Management," *Ob.Gyn. News*, June 18, 2013, http://www.obgynnews.com/specialty-focus/obstetrics/single-article-page/nitrous-o xide-returns-for-labor-pain-management.html; Williams, *Women and Childbirth in the Twentieth Century*, 144–45; Janet A. Pickett, "History of Obstetric Analgesia and Anaesthesia," in *Textbook of Obstetric Anesthesia*, ed. Rachel E. Collis, Felicity Plaat, and John Urquhart (London: Greenwich Medical Media, 2002), 6–7.

17. Wolf, *Deliver Me from Pain*, 126–30. For a long list of available choices in the United States at midcentury, see Clifford B. Lull and Robert A. Hingson, *Control of Pain in Childbirth: Anesthesia, Analgesia, Amnesia* (Philadelphia: J. B. Lippincott, 1944), 38–39.

18. See, for example, Judith Walzer Leavitt, *Brought to Bed*; Wertz and Wertz, *Lying-In*; Ann Oakley, *The Captured Womb: A History of the Medical Care of Pregnant Women* (New York: Basil Blackwell, 1984); Judith Pence Rooks, *Midwifery and Childbirth*. Lying beyond the relatively narrow range of the debate among most histories of childbirth in Great Britain and the United States is the work of Donald Caton, a physician and medical historian. He denies the coercive tactics of modern medical practices, the subtle and transparent ways that doctors and nurses coax compliance from patients. Caton, *What A Blessing She Had Chloroform*. More persuasive is the work of Jacqueline Wolf, who acknowledges women's initial enthusiasm for obstetric anesthesia without denying the ways that resort to anesthesia increased women's dependence on the authoritative knowledge of medical personnel, especially obstetricians. Wolf, *Deliver Me from Pain*.

19. Leavitt, *Brought to Bed*, 196.

20. Registered Nurse, "Sadism in Delivery Rooms?" *Ladies' Home Journal*, Nov. 1957, 4.

21. Gladys Denny Shultz, "Journal Mothers Testify to Cruelty in Maternity Wards," *Ladies' Home Journal*, Dec. 1958, 58–59, 135, 137–39. See also Gladys Denny Shultz, "Journal Mothers Testify on Cruelty in Maternity Wards," *Ladies' Home Journal*, May 1958, 44–45, 152–55.

22. Quoted in Shultz, "Journal Mothers Testify to Cruelty," 59.

23. Ibid., 137.

24. A. D. Farr cautions that nineteenth-century religious opposition to pharmacological pain relief never played a significant role and that most reluctance to use ether in childbirth stemmed from fears within the medical community over the drug's safety. A. D. Farr, "Religious Opposition to Obstetric Analgesia: A Myth?" *Annals of Science* 20 (1983): 159–77. See also Judith Walzer Leavitt, "Birthing and Anesthesia: The Debate over Twilight Sleep," *Signs* 6 (Autumn 1980): 147–64.

25. He primarily blamed anxious relatives who pushed for interference when patience was warranted. Irrespective of the validity of this accusation, he saw the hospital setting itself, with its routine inductions, use of sedatives and anesthesia, and consequent reliance on forceps as conducive to spiraling, unnecessary interventions. Chester D. Bradley, "The Urge to Interfere in Obstetrics," *North Carolina Medical Journal* 10 (July 1949): 343, 348.

26. For a brief overview of the interconnected threads of Mesmer, Coué, Charcot, et al., see Anne Harrington, *The Cure Within: A History of Mind-Body Medicine* (New York: Norton, 2008), 39–66, 103–22. Nineteenth-century French interest in the mind-body connection, particularly with respect to women, is also evident in the fact that more than 20 percent of psychiatric dissertations explored the question of "hysteria." See Mark S. Micale, "On the 'Disappearance' of Hysteria: A Study in the Clinical Deconstruction of a Diagnosis," *Isis* 84 (Sept. 1993), 497. See also Edward Shorter, *From Paralysis to Fatigue: A History of Psychosomatic Illness in the Modern Era* (New York: Free Press, 1992), esp. 69–128; Georges Didi-Huberman, *Invention of Hysteria: Charcot and the Photographic Iconography of the Salpêtrière*, trans. Alisa Hartz (Cambridge, MA: MIT Press, 2003). For background on the precursors to hypnosis in France, see also John Warne Monroe, *Laboratories of Faith: Mesmerism, Spiritualism, and Occultism in Modern France* (Ithaca, NY: Cornell University Press, 2008).

27. Emile Coué, *Self Mastery through Conscious Autosuggestion* (New York: Malkan, 1922), 118.

28. James Braid, *The Discovery of Hypnosis: The Complete Writings of James Braid, "The Father of Hypnotherapy,"* ed. Donald Robertson (London: National Council for Hypnotherapy, 2008), 108; John Milne Bramwell, *Hypnotism: Its History, Theory, and Practice*, 2nd ed. (London: Alexander Moring, 1906), 171–72.

29. I. Velvovsky, K. Platonov, V. Ploticher, and E. Shugom, *Painless Childbirth through Psychoprophylaxis* (1960; repr., Honolulu: University Press of the Pacific, 2003), 85–86, 88. Originally published as I. Z. Vel'vovskii, K. I. Platonov, V. A. Ploticher, and E. A. Shugom, *Psikhoprofilaktika boleĭ v rodakh: Lektsii dlia vrachei-akusherov* (Leningrad: Medgiz, 1954). Subsequent citations refer to the English-language edition. F. Schultze-Rhonhof, "Der hypnotische Geburtsdämmerschlaf," *Zentralblatt für Gynäkologie* 46 (1922): 247, cited in A. M. Michael, "Hypnosis in Childbirth," *British Medical Journal*, Apr. 5, 1952, 734.

30. Grantly Dick-Read, *Natural Childbirth* (London: William Heinemann, 1933). On Dick-Read and his life's work, see A. Noyes Thomas, *Dr. Courageous: The Story of Dr. Grantly Dick-Read* (New York: Harper, 1957); Valerie Allen, *The Legacy of Grantly Dick-Read* (London: National Childbirth Trust, 1991); Mary Thomas, ed. *Post-War Mothers: Childbirth Letters to Grantly Dick-Read, 1946–1956* (Rochester, NY: University of Rochester Press, 1997).

31. First published in the United Kingdom as *Revelation of Childbirth: The Principles and Practice of Natural Childbirth* (London: Heinemann, 1942), the book was reprinted with minor changes for the US market as *Childbirth without Fear* (New York: Harper & Brothers, 1944). Unless otherwise noted, all subsequent

citations refer to Grantly Dick-Read, *Childbirth without Fear: The Principles and Practice of Natural Childbirth*, 2nd rev. ed. (New York: Harper & Brothers, 1959), the last edition that Dick-Read oversaw. In all of his writing, the core ideas remain constant, but over the years he explicates them more fully, offers more illustrative examples, and expands his advice into realms such as prenatal nutrition and breastfeeding. See also Grantly Dick-Read, *Introduction to Motherhood* (London: William Heinemann Medical Books, 1950).

32. Dick-Read, *Natural Childbirth*, 101.
33. Ibid., 101.
34. Ibid., 50.
35. Dick-Read, *Childbirth without Fear*, 143.
36. Ibid., 201.
37. Dick-Read, *Natural Childbirth*, 100.
38. Ibid., 112.
39. Barbara Gelb, *The ABC of Natural Childbirth* (New York: Norton, 1954), 113; Marjorie F. Chappell, *Childbirth: Theory and Practical Training* (Edinburgh: E. & S. Livingstone, 1954), 119–20; Justine Kelliher, "Natural Childbirth in Boston," typescript, n.d., Boston Association for Childbirth Education Records, box 1, folder (hereafter cited as fol.) 1 (hereafter cited as MC515/BACE/1.1) Schlesinger Library, Radcliffe Institute for Advanced Study, Harvard University, Cambridge, MA (hereafter cited as SL). See also Judith Walzer Leavitt, *Make Room for Daddy: The Journey from Waiting Room to Birthing Room* (Chapel Hill: University of North Carolina Press, 2009).
40. Dick-Read, *Childbirth without Fear*, 185.
41. Ibid., 169.
42. Ibid., 176
43. Ibid., 189.
44. While advocating for the Read method, one UK textbook on midwifery promoted the use of drugs to stop women from pushing too soon: "the mother's urge is to bear down, while those in charge of her delivery want her to refrain.... The simplest method of controlling the situation is to muffle the urge to push by the use of an analgesic drug." Chappell, *Childbirth*, 77. The sedative Demerol was marketed in the United Kingdom as pethidine. Favored by some caregivers over nitrous oxide, the inhalant trilene was a widely used, self-administered anesthetic abandoned in the 1980s due to safety concerns. G. Chamberlain, "The History of Pain Relief in Labour," in *Pain and Its Relief in Childbirth: The Results of a National Survey Conducted by the National Birthday Trust*, ed. Geoffrey Chamberlain, Ann Wraight, and Philip Steer (London: Longman, 1993), 6–7.
45. E.g., Dale Clark, "A Man's Crusade for Easy Childbirth," *Esquire*, Oct. 1949, 51; Gelb, *The ABC of Natural Childbirth*, 39, 100, 114.
46. H. Lloyd Miller, "Prenatal Training in Private Practice: Report on 2140 Consecutive Deliveries," *Obstetrics and Gynecology* 8 (Oct. 1956): 477.
47. Herbert Thoms, *Understanding Natural Childbirth: A Book for the Expectant Mother* (New York: McGraw Hill, 1950), 81; Frederick W. Goodrich, Jr., *Natural Childbirth: A Manual for Expectant Parents* (New York: Prentice Hall, 1950), 11, 19; H. Lloyd Miller, "Education for Childbirth," *Obstetrics and Gynecology* 17 (Jan.–June 1961): 120–23; Cathleen Schurr, *Naturally Yours: A Personal Experience with Natural Childbirth* (New York: Rinehart & Company, 1953), 178.
48. Goodrich, *Natural Childbirth*, 150.
49. Redacted letter to Justine Kelliher, Nov. 20, 1954, MC515/BACE/6.17, SL.

50. For explicit references to Deutsch, see the writings of New Zealand–based Dick-Read enthusiasts Enid Cook and M. Bevan-Brown, *Psychological Preparation for Childbirth* (Christchurch: Christchurch Psychological Society, 1948), 3, 4, 7. On the history of the Read method and childbirth education in New Zealand, see Marie Bell, "The Pioneers of Parents' Centre: Movers and Shakers for Change in the Philosophies and Practice of Childbirth and Parent Education in New Zealand" (PhD diss., Victoria University of Wellington, 2004).

51. Dick-Read to J. Arthur Rank, [1954], Personal Papers of Grantly Dick-Read, section C.18, box 20 (hereafter cited as PP/GDR/C.18/20), Wellcome Library, London (hereafter cited as WL).

52. Schurr, *Naturally Yours*, 182. See also, for example, Chappell, *Childbirth*, vii.

53. *Childbirth without Fear* (dir. Grantly Dick-Read, 1956).

54. Grantly Dick-Read, *Motherhood in the Post-War World* (London: Wm. Heinemann Medical Books, 1944), 9, 19. See also O. Moscucci, "Holistic Obstetrics: The Origins of 'Natural Childbirth' in Britain," *Postgraduate Medical Journal* 79 (2003): 169; Sheryl Nestel, "'Other' Mothers: Race and Representation in Natural Childbirth Discourse," *Resources for Feminist Research* 23 (Winter 1994/1995): 5–19.

55. Dick-Read, *Natural Childbirth*, 42. For similar ideas from earlier writers, see Filip Sylvan, *Natural Painless Childbirth and the Determination of Sex* (London: Kigan Paul, Trench, Trubner, 1916), 29; John H. Dye, *Painless Childbirth, or Healthy Mothers and Healthy Children: A Book for All Women* (Buffalo, NY: Baker, Jones, 1889), 53, 60; Rion, *The Truth about Twilight Sleep*, 8. For insight into the hardships of maternity for impoverished British women in this era, see Ellen Ross, *Love and Toil: Motherhood in Outcast London, 1870–1918* (New York: Oxford University Press, 1993), esp. 91–127.

56. Dick-Read, *Motherhood in the Post-War World*, 18. For a broader perspective on British demographic anxieties, see Richard Soloway, *Demography and Degeneration: Eugenics and the Declining Birthrate in Britain* (Chapel Hill: University of North Carolina Press, 1990).

57. Dick-Read, *Natural Childbirth*, 90. This is a point that Dick-Read stresses repeatedly. See, for example, Dick-Read, *Childbirth without Fear*, 73, 76, 91, 227, 281, 333, and 345–48.

58. Dick-Read, *Natural Childbirth*, 65.

59. Dick-Read, *Childbirth without Fear*, 346.

60. Hazel Corbin, "Changing Maternity Service in a Changing World," *Canadian Nurse* 46 (Dec. 1950): 949–56; "Childbirth Pains Are Laid to Fears," *New York Times*, Jan. 21, 1949; Blackwell Sawyer, "Experiences with Labor Procedure of Grantly Dick Read," *American Journal of Obstetrics and Gynecology* 51 (June 1946): 852–58; "Medicine: Should It Hurt?" *Time*, July 22, 1946, http://www.time.com/time/magazine/article/0,9171,888278,00.html.

61. "Relates Technique in Painless Births," *New York Times*, Jan. 18, 1947; Thoms to Dick-Read, Feb. 10, 1948; Dick-Read to Thoms, Nov. 9, 1948; both in PP/GDR/D.196, WL; Greta Palmer, "Having Your Baby the New Way," *Collier's*, Nov. 1948, 26–27, 61. Dick-Read praised *Collier's* coverage of Thoms's work. Dick-Read to Thoms, Nov. 17, 1948, PP/GDR/D.196, WL. On Dick-Read's recognition of and praise for the vanguard role played by MCA, see Dick-Read to Hazel Corbin and Anne Stevens, Feb. 14, 1947, box 3, fol. 13, Maternity Center Association Records (hereafter cited as MCA), Augustus C. Long Health Sciences Library Archives and Special Collections, Columbia University,

New York (hereafter cited as LHSL). Childbirth preparation courses like those offered by the MCA had existed in the United States since the turn of the century, but they had historically targeted immigrant communities in an effort to suppress maternal and infant mortality rates in overcrowded urban tenements. Following the publication of *Childbirth without Fear*, the MCA increasingly turned its attention to meeting the needs of white, middle-class, nonimmigrant women who sought Natural Childbirth preparation courses. Dick-Read to Corbin, June 12, 1950, box 3, fol. 13, MCA, LHSL; *Maternity Center Association* (New York: [The Maternity Center Association], 1943). Today MCA is known as Childbirth Connection.

62. When Dick-Read toured fifteen cities in North America in 1957–58, he gave talks at hospitals where his American advocates practiced obstetrics, but a number of his speaking engagements were at grassroots childbirth preparation and mothercraft organizations. "Dr. Grantly Dick-Read: Itinerary of Lecture Tour in the U.S.A. and Canada, 1957–1958," MC515/BACE/1.10, SL.

63. Corbin, "Changing Maternity Services in a Changing World," 949.

64. Ibid., 950. Maternity care was typically not covered by health insurance in the 1950s, but Corbin's argument here suggests that couples came to see medicine as a consumer good and that this perception extended to their attitude toward maternity care, even if insurance coverage did not. On the rise of the American consumer culture, see Lizabeth Cohen, *A Consumers' Republic: The Politics of Mass Consumption in Postwar America* (New York: Vintage, 2003).

65. Corbin, "Changing Maternity Service in a Changing World," 950. On the "hardened" linkage in the 1950s between employment and health insurance, increasingly seen as an earned extension of wages, see Colin Gordon, *Dead on Arrival: The Politics of Health Care in Twentieth-Century America* (Princeton, NJ: Princeton University Press, 2003), 124.

66. Writing to express support for public funding of prenatal education, one British physician wrote that "the consumer...appreciates the efforts made" to prepare her for childbirth. Anthony Ryle, "Wither Natural Childbirth?" *British Medical Journal*, Mar. 19, 1955, 725. On the changing meaning of medical consumerism, see Glen O'Hara, "The Complexities of 'Consumerism': Choice, Collectivism and Participation with Britain's National Health Service, c.1961–c. 1979," *Social History of Medicine* 26 (May 2013): 288–304.

67. Corbin, "Changing Maternity Service in a Changing World," 953.

68. Quoted in ibid., 955.

69. Kelliher, "Natural Childbirth in Boston;" American College of Obstetricians and Gynecologists, *Manual of Standards* (Chicago: ACOG, 1959), 17, 23.

70. Thomas, *Post-War Mothers*, 167.

71. Ibid., 173.

72. Palmer, "Having Your Baby the New Way," 61.

73. Mrs. K. to Miss [Carol] Janeway, Apr. 16, 1949, box 129, fol. 1, MCA, LHSL. The letter is a typed transcription of a handwritten letter that was not preserved in the MCA files. Here, as throughout the book, I have used a pseudonym to identify this source. The use of pseudonyms was a stipulation of access to certain archival records and I have extended their utilization to all references to maternity patients in archival documentation and oral interviews. The initials I use do not reflect the patients' real names. Where published sources refer to patients using initials, real names, or pseudonyms, I have retained the original. In correspondence between public figures or among professional colleagues (that is,

in documents not of a personal, private nature), I use real names of writers and recipients.

74. Ibid. For a similar characterization of a maternity ward room, see Clark, "A Man's Crusade for Easy Childbirth," 51.

75. Mrs. K. to Janeway, Apr. 16, 1949, box 129, fol. 1, MCA, LHSL.

CHAPTER 2

1. On the history of medicine and public health in the USSR, see Chris Burton, "Medical Welfare during Late Stalinism: A Study of Doctors and the Soviet Health System, 1945–53," (PhD diss., University of Chicago, 2000); Frances L. Bernstein, Christopher Burton, and Dan Healey, eds. *Soviet Medicine: Culture, Practice, and Science* (DeKalb: Northern Illinois University Press, 2010); Michaels, *Curative Powers*; Susan Gross Solomon, ed., *Doing Medicine Together: Germany and Russia between the Wars* (Toronto: University of Toronto Press, 2006).

2. See Janet Evans, "The Communist Party of the Soviet Union and the Women's Question: The Case of the 1936 Decree 'In Defense of Mother and Child,'" *Journal of Contemporary History* 16 (Oct. 1981): 757–75; Wendy Z. Goldman, *Women, the State and Revolution* (New York: Cambridge University Press, 1993), 254–95; Paula A. Michaels, "Ethnicity, Patriotism, and Womanhood: Kazakhstan and the 1936 Ban on Abortion," *Feminist Studies* 27 (2001): 307–33.

3. Quoted in I. I. Feigel', "Akusherstvo i ginekologiia za 30 let," *Akusherstov i ginekologiia* 23 (Sept.–Oct. 1947): 1. Unless otherwise noted, all translations into English are the author's.

4. Ibid., 16.

5. Prikaz no. 537, Ministerstvo zdravookhraneniia Soiuza Sovetskikh Sotsialisticheskikh Respublik (hereafter cited as MZ SSSR), "Ob obezbolivanii rodov," July 22, 1949, Gosudarstvennyi arkhiv Rossiiskoi Federatsii, Moscow (hereafter cited as GARF), fond (hereafter cited as f.) r-8009, opis (hereafter cited as op.) 1, delo (hereafter cited as d.) 813, list (hereafter cited as l.) 313; Nakachi, "Replacing the Dead," 211.

6. Sostoianie obezbolivaniia rodov po Khar'kovskoi oblasti, Jan. 1, 1950, Tsentral'nyi derzhavnyi arkhiv vyshchykh organiv vlady ta upravlinnia Ukrainy, Kyiv (hereafter cited as TsDAVO), f. 342, op. 14, spravka (hereafter cited as spr.) 4202, arkush (hereafter cited as ark.) 217.

7. M. F. Levi, *Istoriia rodovspomozheniia v SSSR* (Moscow: Izdatel'stvo akademii meditsinskikh nauk SSSR, 1950), 185. It is axiomatic that these statistics need to be used cautiously. By contrast with the above modest figures, which themselves may well be inflated, A. P. Nikolaev offers the ludicrous estimate that 60 to 70 percent of prewar births were accompanied by pain relief measures. No evidence supports this number, which can only be explained by either blatant inflation or by folding in commonplace comfort measures such as the use of warm or cold compresses into these statistics. Unfortunately, neither Nikolaev nor Levi specify what types of pain-relief measures their figures take into account or what evidence supports their claims. See A. P. Nikolaev, "K probleme obezbolivaniia rodov," *Akusherstvo i ginekologiia* 25 (Nov.–Dec. 1949): 3.

8. Sostoianie obezbolivaniia rodov po Khar'kovskoi oblasti, TsDAVO, f. 342, op. 14, spr. 4202, ark. 217.

9. Analiz raboty rodovspomogatel'noi seti v gorodakh i sel'skikh mestnostiakh U[krainskoi] SSR (hereafter cited as USSR), 1947, TsDAVO, f. 342, op. 14, spr. 4057, ark. 23.

10. Vechernee zasedanie soveshchaniia inspektorov Okhrany materinstva i detstva, Jan. 30, 1945, Derzhavnyi arkhiv Kharkivskoi oblasti, Kharkiv (hereafter cited as DAKhO) f. R-5125, op. 1, spr. 47, ark. 9.

11. Stenogramma zasedaniia kollegii MZ SSSR, June 17, 1949, GARF, f. r-8009, op. 1, d. 777, l. 24; Analiz raboty rodovspomogatel'noi seti, TsDAVO, f. 342, op. 14, spr. 4057, ark. 3; Stenogramma oblastnogo soveshchaniia inspektorov okhmatdeta po Khar'kovskoi oblasti, Jan. 29–30, 1945, DAKhO, f. R-5125, op. 1, spr. 47, ark. 1obverse (hereafter cited as ob.); Stenogramma konferentsii akusherok Khar'kovskoi oblasti, Jan. 17, 1955, DAKhO, f. R-5125, op. 2, spr. 546, ark. 51–52; Spravka o sostoianii rodovspomozheniia v USSR, 1948, TsDAVO, f. 342, op. 14, spr. 529, ark. 231.

12. The most compelling portrayals of Soviet maternity care come from literary sources published in the last decade of Soviet power. Though they attest to conditions in a later period, they capture well the gruff manner of medical professionals and the low quality of care that were also characteristic of earlier years. For a novel that well conveys the atmosphere of a Soviet maternity ward, see Julia Voznesenskaya, *The Women's Decameron*, trans. W. B. Linton (London: Quartet Books, 1986). See also Liudmila Petrushevskaia, "Bednoe serdtse Pani," in *Taina doma* (Moscow: Kvadrat, 1995), 420–24; Natalia Sukhanova, "Delos," in *Zal ozhidaniia* (Moscow: Sovremennik, 1990), 3–28. I thank Beth Holmgren for suggesting to me these and other literary works set in Soviet maternity wards.

13. Komissiia rodovspomozheniia pri upravleniia MZ USSR to V. N. Khmelevskii, June 21, 1947, TsDAVO, f. 342, op. 14, spr. 4053, ark. 7. On the 1944 legislation and postwar Soviet pronatalism, see Nakachi, "Replacing the Dead."

14. Instruktsiia po primeneniiu prosteishikh metodov obezbolivaniia normal'nykh rodov, Apr. 14, 1948, TsDAVO, f. 342, op. 14, spr. 4157, ark. 1–9. The Obstetrics Commission met on March 2, 1948, when the members debated the Khmelevskii Method, made minor recommendations about the dosages and intervals of application, and endorsed the method. See Protokol no. 3, zasedaniia komissii rodovspomozheniia pri MZ USSR, Mar. 2, 1948, TsDAVO, f. 342, op. 14, spr. 4103, ark. 12–13.

15. Instruktsiia po primeneniiu prosteishikh metodov obezbolivaniia, TsDAVO, f. 342, op. 14, spr. 4157, ark. 3–6. On the benefits of vitamin B_1, see R. L. Shub, *Primenenie vitamina V^1 v akusherstve i ginekologii: Sposob fiziologicheskogo obezbolivaniia i uskoreniia rodov* (Leningrad: Tsentral'nyi institut akusherstva i ginekologii ministerstva zdravookhraneniia SSSR, 1946), the findings of which supported the use of vitamin B_1 for analgesic effect in the Khmelevskii method. Patushinskaia and Filina argued that vitamin B_1, while useful for speeding labor, was only effective in pain management in combination with other drugs, as was recommended in the Khmelevskii method. See F. P. Patushinskaia and E. I. Filina, "Vitamin V^1 v obezbolivanii rodov," *Akusherstvo i ginekologiia* 24 (Sept.–Oct. 1948): 35–37. Nikolaev, too, concurred with Khmelevskii, endorsing Vitamin B_1 for use during dilation and effacement, in combination with lydol, a narcotic analgesic and synthetic opioid similar to pantopon, described below. See Nikolaev, "K probleme obezbolivaniia rodov," 7. Others disagreed, describing it as ineffective for relieving labor pain and its ability to speed labor as "insignificant." K. Figurnov, *Painless Childbirth: Latest Achievements of Soviet Medicine in Obstetric Analgesia and Anesthesia* (Moscow: Foreign Languages Publishing House, [1953]), 18–19. See also B. Triantafillopoulo, "L'accouchement rapide: L'action biologique

de la thiamine (vitamine B$_1$) sur la fibre musculaire de l'utérus gravide,"
Gynécologie et obstétrique 57 (Mar. 1958): 313–26; Drew Middleton, "Soviet
Doctor Uses Vitamin B-1 to Ease Pain and Speed Childbirth, Moscow Paper
Says," *New York Times*, Aug. 30, 1946. Khmelevskii's recommended sup-
positories combined belladonna, pantopon, and antipyrine. Belladonna was
a botanical source for the drug scopolamine, used in twilight sleep. It continues to be used as a homeopathic remedy in childbirth. As homeopathy
originated and remained popular in Germany, it is not surprising that the
Germans pursued an interest in the obstetric application of belladonna. They
found it to be productive in calming women and stimulating labor's progress.
Introduced by Roche in 1909 and still available today in select markets, pantopon is Roche's longest selling product. The 1948 Instruction recommended
use of the non-opioid analgesic antipyrine, also called phenozone. First syn-
thesized at the close of the nineteenth century, it was used widely for pain,
discomfort, and fever reduction, but fears of its toxicity have minimized its
application in recent decades. On belladonna, see Hans Rieger, "Gefahrlose
Geburtserleichterung durch Belladonna-Exclud-Zäpfchen," *Die Medizinische
Zeitschrift*, Aug. 20, 1955: 1145–47; on pantopon, see Alexander L. Bieri,
Traditionally, Ahead of Its Time (Basel: Roche Historical Archives, 2008),
10–11, 65; on antipyrine, see Kay Brune, "The Early History of Non-Opioid
Anesthetics," *Acute Pain* 1 (Dec. 1997): 33–40. Ether and novocaine were
prized during this period and had been for decades in the West and Russia.
See, for example, F. I. Rabinovich-Brodskaia, *Obezbolivanie normal'nykh rodov*
(Ivanogo: Gosudarstvennoe izdatel'stvo Ivanovskoi oblasti, 1936), 26.

16. Instruktsiia po primeneniiu prosteishikh metodov obezbolivaniia,
    TsDAVO. f. 342, op. 14, spr. 4157, ark. 7.
17. Ibid., ark. 8. The document attributes the phrase "sterility of the word" to
    Pavlov. Vel'vovskii credits Platonov in I. Z. Vel'vovskii, V. A. Ploticher, and E. A.
    Shugom, "Psikhoprofilakticheskoe obezbolivanie rodov," *Akusherstvo i ginekolo-
    giia* 26 (Nov.–Dec. 1950): 9. On Platonov's understanding and interpretation of
    Pavlovian neuropsychology, see K. I. Platonov, *The Word as a Physiological and
    Therapeutic Factor: The Theory and Practice of Psychotherapy according to I. P. Pavlov.*
    2nd ed. (Moscow: Foreign Languages Publishing House, 1959). On Platonov,
    see the memoir of his son, K. K. Platonov, *Moi lichnye vstrechi na velikoi doroge
    zhizni: Vospominaniia starogo psikhologa* (Moscow: Izdatel'svto "Institut psik-
    hologii RAN", 2005), 46–55.
18. Instruktsiia po primeneniiu prosteishikh metodov obezbolivaniia,
    TsDAVO. f. 342, op. 14, spr. 4157, ark. 7–8.
19. I. Struev to A. I. Shchukin, Sept. 8, 1949, TsDAVO, f. 342, op. 14, spr. 4202,
    ark. 82. For similar examples, see Prikaz no. 258, MZ USSR, "Ob osushchest-
    vlenii massovogo obezbolivaniia rodov v respublike," Oct. 19, 1949, TsDAVO,
    f. 342, op. 14, spr. 7002, ark. 115–16; Dokladnaia zapiska ob osushchestvlenii
    massovogo obezbolivaniia rodov Vinnitskoi oblasti, 1949, spr. 4202, ark. 63;
    Soobshchenie ot Dnepropetrovskogo oblzdravotdela, Nov. 24, 1949, spr. 4202,
    ark. 69–70; all in TsDAVO, f. 342, op. 14. Spravka 4202 contains similar reports
    from several oblasts on the progress of the obstetric pain relief effort in the last
    quarter of 1949, including from Voroshilovgrad region (ark. 50); Vinnitsa region
    (ark. 54–63); Odessa region (ark. 158–61); Stalino region (ark. 183–84); Sumi
    region (ark. 191–93); Kharkov region (ark. 210–11); and the city of Kharkov
    (ark. 212–15).

20. Struev and Fel'dman to Shchukin, Dec. 1, 1949, spr. 4202, ark. 83; Otchet po proverke vypolneniia prikaza no. 258, vypolnenie nastoiashchego prikaza po gor. Zhitomiru, Troianovskomu i Korostyshevskomu raionakh, Jan. 24, 1950, spr.4202, ark. 24; Soobshchenie ot sektora lechprofpomoshchi detiam Volynskogo oblzdravotdela o meropriiatiiakh provedennykh po vypolneniiu prikaza MZ "O provedenii obezbolivanii rodov," Nov. 22, 1949, spr. 4202, ark. 64; all in TsDAVO, f. 342, op. 14.
21. Piatagorskii to M. D. Burova, Dec. 10, 1949, spr. 4202, ark. 204; Makarov to Burova, Dec. 10, 1949, spr. 4202, ark. 206. See also Doklad, Roddom no. 3, Dnepropetrovsk, Nov. 28, 1949, spr. 4202, ark. 76; [signature illegible], MZ USSR to E. K. Isaeva, Dec. 31, 1949, spr. 4202, ark. 18; Listengurt to Shchukin, Dec. 6, 1949, spr. 4202, ark. 81; Mikulaninets to Khodorovsko, Oct. 13, 1949, spr. 4202, ark. 89; [B.] Stroganov to Shchukin, Aug. 13, 1949, spr. 4202, ark. 94; S. Mel'nikov to Shchukin, Dec. 10, 1949, spr. 4202, ark. 105; Dopolnenie k spravke o vypolnenii prikaza no. 537, MZ SSSR, "Ob obezbolivanii rodov," [1950], spr. 4245, ark. 39; G. F. Vraga to Shchukin, Jan. 28, 1950, spr. 4202, ark. 237; Svedeniia o sostoianii obezbolivanie po Drogobychskoi oblasti, Apr. 3, 1950, spr. 4243, ark. 42; Shchukin to A. E. Shebeleva, Dec. 6, 1949, spr. 4243, ark. 74; Garagash'ian to Shchukin, May 26, 1950, spr. 4244, ark. 16; Stroganov to Shchukin, [1950], spr. 4245, ark. 26; all in TsDAVO, f. 342, op. 14.
22. Proverka sostoianiia obezbolivaniia rodov v rodosvpomogatel'nykh uchrezhdeniiakh g. Odessy, 1949, TsDAVO, f. 342, op. 14, spr. 4202, ark. 159, 161. Quote from ark. 161.
23. Doklad ot g. Dnepropetrovska, Dec. 6, 1949, TsDAVO, f. 342, op. 14, spr. 4202, ark. 72ob.
24. Otchet po proverke vypolneniia prikaza no. 258, MZ USSR, "Ob osushchestvlenii massovogo obezbolivaniia rodov v respublike," Jan. 24, 1950, TsDAVO, f. 342, op. 14, spr. 4202, ark. 24–28.
25. A report comparing the first eight months of 1947 and 1948 pointed to a 22-percent drop in the number of births. Nakachi, "Replacing the Dead," 401.
26. Kratkoe soderzhanie doklada na zasedanii kollegii MZ SSSR, June 17, 1949, GARF, f. r-8009, op. 1, d. 777, l. 57. Physicians and administrators clamored for nitrous oxide in numerous regional Ukrainian reports from the late 1940s. See Soobshchenie Stalinskogo oblzdravotdela o vypolenii prikaza no. 258, MZ USSR, Nov. 24, 1949, spr. 4202, ark. 183ob; Struev and Fel'dman to Shchukin, Dec. 1, 1949, spr. 4202, ark. 83; Spravka L'vovskoi oblasti o sostoianii vypolneniia prikazov MZ USSR, Nov. 12, 1950, spr. 4221, ark. 24; all in TsDAVO, f. 342, op. 14.
27. Stenogramma zasedaniia kollegii, GARF, f. r-8009, op. 1, d. 777, listy (hereafter cited as ll.) 14–26, 31.
28. Some argued that nitrous oxide was too expensive and that analgesics on hand in most maternity wards, like those used in the Khmelevskii method, were adequate to the task. Others responded that aspirin, belladonna, and the like were not sufficiently effective, and they, too, were often hard to come by. Stenogramma zasedaniia kollegii, GARF, f. r-8009, op. 1, d. 777, ll. 28–29, 44. The pharmaceutical industry's struggles in this era reached well beyond the realm of obstetric anesthesia. See Mary Schaeffer Conroy, "The Soviet Pharmaceutical Industry and Dispensing, 1945–1953," *Europe-Asia Studies* 56 (Nov. 2004): 963–91.
29. Prikaz no. 537, MZ SSSR, GARF, f. r-8009, op. 1, d. 813, ll. 313–20; Vremennaia instruktsiia po obezbolivaniiu rodov, MZ SSSR, Jan. 4, 1950, TsDAVO, f. 342,

op. 14, spr. 4245, ark. 5–8. On preliminary steps toward the issuance of new drug protocols for pain in normal birth, see Spravka o sostoianii rodovspomozheniia, TsDAVO, spr. 529, ark. 239; Dopolnenie k spravke o vypolnenii prikaza no. 537, MZ SSSR, spr. 4245, ark. 39; Prikaz no. 258, MZ USSR, Oct. 19, 1949, spr. 7002, ark. 115–20; all in TsDAVO, f. 342, op. 14. See also Prikaz no. 537, MZ SSSR, July 22, 1949, GARF, f. r-8009, op. 1, d. 813, ll. 313–20.

30. On the failure to expand the availability of pharmacological pain relief in the wake of Moscow's mandate, see [signature illegible], MZ USSR to Isaeva, Dec. 31, 1949, TsDAVO, f. 342, op. 14, spr. 4202, ark. 18; Stenogramma zasedaniia kollegii, GARF, f. r-8009, op. 1, d. 777, ll. 17–18; Spravka o khode vypolneniia prikaza no. 142, "O vnedrenii v praktiku psikhoprofilaktiki bolei v rodakh" i no. 555, "O merakh po uluchsheniiu organizatsii i kachestva obezbolivaniia rodov," Apr. 19, 1952, GARF, f. r-8009, op. 22, d. 249, ll. 119–26; Stenogrammy soveshchaniia pri zam. ministra t. Kovriginoi glavnykh akusherov i ginekologov soiuznykh respublik, pt. 1, Moscow, Jan. 1950, GARF, f. r-8009, op. 22, d. 215, l. 375.

31. Maternity ward workers were taken to task, for example, for mishandling the application of silver nitrate to the eyes of newborns. The improper administration of this common treatment to prevent the transmission of gonorrhea from mother to baby led to burns on several newborns. Protokol no. 36, reshenie kollegii MZ USSR, TsDAVO, f. 342, op. 14, spr. 530, ark. 212.

32. For example, the 277-page 1948 edition of a popular obstetric and gynecologic nursing textbook offers only a half-page discussion on pain relief measures. A. L. Kaplan, *Uchebnik akusherstva i zhenskikh boleznei: Dlia shkol medsester*, 3rd ed. (Moscow-Leningrad: Medgiz, 1948), 127. Unless otherwise noted, subsequent references refer to this edition. A sixteen-page article commemorating thirty years of Soviet obstetrics and gynecology in the field's premier journal devoted one lone paragraph to anesthetics and analgesics and underscored the shortcomings to date. See Feigel', "Akusherstvo i ginekologiia," 6.

33. The archival record is clear that the fundamental problem was access, not safety, but to avoid open indictment of the Soviet pharmaceutical industry's inability to meet obstetric needs, proponents of psychoprophylaxis often made their case publicly in terms of the risk of drugs to mother and fetus. E.g., V. N. Shishkova, R. M. Bronshtein, E. I. Ivanova, and P. P. Nikulin,, "Psikhoprofilakticheskoe obezbolivanie v rodakh," in *Obezbolivanie v rodakh: Trudy konferentsii v g. Leningrade, 29–31 ianvaria 1951 g.*, ed. A. P. Nikolaev (Moscow: Izdatel'stvo akademii meditsinskikh nauk SSSR, 1952), 54; Stenogramma konferentsii akusherok Khar'kovskoi oblasti, DAKhO, f. R-5125, op. 2, spr. 546, ark. 27.

34. Soobshchenie po vypolneniiu prikaza no. 537, MZ SSSR, May 22, 1950, spr. 4245, ark. 80; Dokladnaia zapiska ob osushchestvlenii massovogo obezbolivaniia rodov, spr. 4202, ark. 55ob; both in TsDAVO, f. 342, op. 14. K. I. Platonov, "O znachenii slova v obezbolivanii rodov," typescript, n.d., DAKhO, f. R-5833, op. 1, spr. 176, ark. 8. Archivists marked the Platonov text as "no earlier than 1948," but it cannot predate 1950. Platonov uses the term psychoprophylaxis, which Nikolaev introduced into this context only in December 1949.

35. No public repository holds Vel'vovskii's personal papers, a resource that might have fleshed out his personality and private thoughts in a way comparable to Dick-Read's voluminous archive, and his daughter declined my request in 2006 for an interview. B. V. Mikhailov, one of his former students, remembers Vel'vovskii as a "vivid" figure whose lectures were well-attended "because he was

so interesting and dynamic." His engaged psychotherapeutic method was dictated "by temperament. It is not possible that someone so vibrant could be otherwise." Boris Volodimirovich Mikhailov (chair, Department of Psychotherapy, Kharkiv Academy of Postgraduate Medical Education), interview by the author, Apr. 4, 2006.

36. Platonov and Vel'vovskii published prodigiously, and their research on hypnosis was known abroad. C. Platonoff and G. Z. Velvosky, "Sur l'application de l'hypnose en chirurgie, accouchement et gynécologie," *Revue franco-russe de médecine et de biologie* 1 (June-Sept. 1925): 54–62. During his career, Vel'vovskii held affiliations with a number of institutions: the Southern Railway Psychoneurological Institute; Kharkov's Institute for Advanced Physician Training (today, KhMAPO); and the Neuropathology Department, Kharkov Sanitation-Hygiene Institute. In 1962 Vel'vovskii founded the Department of Psychotherapy, Psychoprophylaxis, and Psychohygiene at the Institute for Advanced Physician Training. Platonov's vision of the interrelationship of neurology and psychology and its therapeutic implications animated the department's organization and approach. "Terapevtychnyi fakul'tet," in *Kharkivs'kyi instytut udoskonalennia likariv: Iuvileine vydannia, 1923–1998* (Kharkiv: Kharkivs'kyi instytut udoskonalennia likariv, 1998), n. p.; "Biograficheskaia stat'ia: Vel'vovskii, Il'ia (Gilel') Zakharevich (Zel'manovich)," typescript, 2006, courtesy of KhMAPO, Kharkiv. On the broader context in which Platonov and Vel'vovskii worked, see B. V. Mikhailov, "Khar'kovskaia psikhoterapevticheskaia shkola." *Mezhdunarodnyi meditsinskii zhurnal* 10 (2004): 43–44; Anton Yasnitsky and Michel Ferrari, "Rethinking the Early History of Post-Vygotskian Psychology: The Case of the Kharkov School," *History of Psychology* 11 (May 2008): 101–21; Anton Yasnitsky and Michel Ferrari, "From Vygotsky to Vygotskian Psychology: Introduction to the History of the Kharkov School," *Journal of the History of Behavioral Sciences* 44 (Spring 2008): 119–45; S. G. Grinval'd, "Khar'kovskaia shkola psikhoterapii," 2010, http://grinvald.com/stati/harkovskaya-shkola-psihoterapii.html.
37. Vel'vovskii to Burova, [1950], TsDAVO, f. 342, op. 14, spr. 4246, ark. 22ob.
38. I. Velvovsky et al., *Painless Childbirth*, 167. Also Vel'vovskii, Ploticher, and Shugom, "Psikhoprofilakticheskoe obezbolivanie rodov."
39. Velvovsky et al., *Painless Childbirth*, 168.
40. Ibid., 168, 174; Vel'vovskii, Ploticher, and Shugom, "Psikhoprofilakticheskoe obezbolivanie rodov," 6. See also Sostoianie obezbolivaniia rodov po Khar'kovskoi oblasti, TsDAVO, f. 342, op. 14, spr. 4202, ark. 225; K. I. Platonov, "Kontseptsiia uslovno-reflektornogo proiskhozhdeniia rodovoi boli i ee profilaktika v svete ucheniia Pavlova," typescript, Jan. 30, 1950, DAKhO, f. R-5833, op. 1, spr. 157, ark 11.
41. In the USSR at this time, the majority of physicians were women, but most specialists, including obstetricians, were men.
42. Velvovsky et al., *Painless Childbirth*, 178, 218; Vel'vovskii, Ploticher and Shugom, "Psikhoprofilakticheskoe obezbolivanie rodov," 6.
43. Velvovsky et al., *Painless Childbirth*, 227.
44. Ibid., 233–44; quote from 240.
45. Ibid., 245.
46. Ibid., 245–59.
47. Ibid., 262; emphasis in original.
48. Ibid., 269–75; quotes from 274.
49. Ibid., 269.

50. Ibid., 170.
51. M. I. Donigevich, *Metod psikhoprofilaktiki bolei v rodakh* (Kiev: Gosudarstvennoe meditsinskoe izdatel'stvo, 1955), 16; John D. Bell, "Giving Birth to the New Soviet Man: Politics and Obstetrics in the USSR," *Slavic Review* 40 (Spring 1981): 9.
52. K. Platonov, "Zakliuchitel'noe slovo na konferentsii po psikhoterapevtiches-komu obezbolivaniiu rodov," stenographic transcript, Dec. 23, 1949, DAKhO, f. R-5833, op. 1, spr. 164, ark. 2; Spravka o khode vypolneniia prikaza no. 555 MZ SSSR, "O merakh po uluchsheniiu organizatsii i kachestva obezbolivaniia v rodakh," Apr. 6, 1951, MZ SSSR, GARF, f. r-8009, op. 22, d. 239, l. 83.
53. M. I. Koganov, "Obezbolivanie rodov vnusheniem bez predvaritel'noi gip-noticheskoi podgotovki," *Akusherstvo i ginekologiia* 27 (Mar.–Apr. 1951): 31–34.
54. V. P. Mikhailov to V. I. Pshenichnikov, Sept. 29, 1951, d. 1708, ll. 5–7; M. Koganov to Editor, *Akusherstvo i ginekologiia*, June 14, 1951, d. 1708, ll. 9–11; Protokol no. 38, zasedanie biuro prezidiuma UMS MZ SSSR, Oct. 11, 1951, d. 1641, ll. 1–4; all in GARF, f. r-8009, op. 2. I thank Benjamin Zajicek for putting me onto the scent of this controversy and for his generosity in providing the reference to and his notes on Protocol 38.
55. Vel'vovskii to Burova, TsDAVO, f. 342, op. 14, spr. 4246, ark. 21.
56. Quoted in Velvovsky et al., *Painless Childbirth*, 130.
57. On the negative suggestive influence of *War and Peace*, see V. N. Shishkova, *Obezbolivanie rodov* (Moscow: Medgiz, 1959), 7. For a case study that high-lights the influence of *Anna Karenina* on one young woman's expectations of childbirth, see Z. A. Kopil'-Levina, "Metodika obezbolivaniia rodov slovesnym vnusheniem," in *Voprosy psikhoterapii v akusherstve: Rodoobezbolivanie i neu-krotimaia rvota beremennykh*, ed. K. I. Platonov (Khar'kov: IKPS dorsanotdel IuZhD psikhonevrologicheskii institut, 1940), 44. Platonov and Vel'vovskii likely found inspiration for their understanding of collective reflex in the work of Bekhterev, but it was politically impossible for them to invoke his contribu-tion. Bekhterev developed the field of "reflexology," a term close to the notion of conditional response in the parlance of his more famous rival, Ivan Pavlov. Platonov and Vel'vovskii would have been familiar with his work on hypnosis and post-hypnotic suggestion but, even before Pavlovism's postwar hegemony, Bekhterev had fallen from grace. Shortly after his death in 1927, Bekhterev's Psychoneurological Institute in Leningrad closed. His writings were never banned outright, but they were not reprinted. Reference to Bekhterev's inves-tigations virtually disappeared from the scholarly literature, rendering his life's work invisible. Bekhterev died under suspicious circumstances and rumors per-sist that he had run afoul of Stalin, though a "smoking gun" to link Stalin to Bekhterev's sudden demise will likely never be found. In the 1930s, Bekhterev's children were arrested and sent to forced labor camps, where they perished. Only after Stalin's death in 1953 were his name and reputation restored, though the linkage of Platonov's and Vel'vovskii's work to Pavlov, rather than Bekhterev, persisted. Since the USSR's collapse Bekhterev's life and work has received renewed interest, but a biography has yet to be written. Vladimir Lerner, Jacob Margolin, and Eliezer Witztum, "Vladimir Bekhterev: His Life, His Work, and the Mystery of His Death," *History of Psychiatry* 16 (June 2005): 223–25. Bekhterev's work has recently enjoyed several new translations into English. See in particular V. M. Bekhterev, *Suggestion: Its Role in Social Life*, trans. Tzvetanka Dobreva-Martinova (New Brunswick, NJ: Transaction, 1998); V. M. Bekhterev,

Collective Reflexology: The Complete Edition, ed. Lloyd H. Strickland, trans. Eugenia Lockwood and Alisa Lockwood (New Brunswick, NJ: Transaction, 2001). My thanks to Anton Yasnitsky for directing me to Bekhterev's work and its likely connection to that of Platonov and Vel'vovskii.

58. Velvovsky et al., *Painless Childbirth*, 170.

59. Ibid., 177.

60. Dick-Read to Léon Chertok, Dec. 11, 1956, PP/GDR/D.216/55, WL.

61. The meeting was officially called the Scientific Session on the Physiological Teachings of Ivan P. Pavlov. See Ethan Pollock, *Stalin and the Soviet Science Wars* (Princeton, NJ: Princeton University Press, 2006), 136–67. On celebration of this occasion in Ukraine and around the USSR, see, for example, E. Babinskii, "Gordost' russkoi nauki: 100-letie so dnia rozhdeniia I. P. Pavlova," *Pravda Ukrainy*, Sept. 27, 1949; "Torzhestvennye zasedaniia, posviashchennye stoletiiu so dnia rozhdeniia I. P. Pavlova," *Pravda Ukrainy*, Sept 28, 1949; V. G. Butomo and V. A. Povzhitkov, "I. P. Pavlov i otrazhenie ego idei v akusherstve i ginekologii," *Akusherstvo i ginekologiia* 25 (Sept.–Oct. 1949): 3–7. Also Materialy iubileinoi sessii posviashchennoi 100-letiiu so dnia rozhdeniia akademika Pavlova: Tezisy doklady, vol. 1, July 5–Oct. 3, 1949, spr. 3347; Stenogramma sessii posviashchennoi 100 letiiu so dnia rozhdeniia akad. Pavlova, vol. 2, Sept. 30–Oct. 3, 1949, spr. 3348; Vypiska iz protokola no. 25 zasedaniia prezidiuma uchenogo meditsinskogo soveta MZ USSR, Sept. 11, 1950, spr. 4781, ark. 1; Studencheskaia nauchnaia konferentsiia posviashchennuiu fiziologicheskomu ucheniiu akademika I. P. Pavlova, Khar'kovskii meditsinskii institut, Dec. 9–10, 1950, spr. 4781, ark. 32–39; all in TsDAVO, f. 342, op. 14.

62. Vnedrenie ucheniia Pavlova v prepodavanie i nauchnoi rabote Khar'kovskogo medinstituta, 1949–50, TsDAVO, f. 342, op. 14, spr. 4751, ark. 77–109.

63. Martin A. Miller, *Freud and the Bolsheviks: Psychoanalysis in Imperial Russia and the Soviet Union* (New Haven, CT: Yale University Press, 1998); Alexander Etkind, *Eros of the Impossible: History of Psychoanalysis in Russia* (Boulder, CO: Westview Press, 1997); Pollock, *Stalin and the Soviet Science Wars*; Benjamin Zajicek, "Scientific Psychiatry in Stalin's Soviet Union: The Politics of Modern Medicine and the Struggle to Define 'Pavlovian' Psychiatry, 1939–1953" (PhD diss., University of Chicago, 2009); David Joravsky, *Russian Psychology: A Critical History* (Cambridge, MA.: Blackwell Press, 1989).

64. Platonov, "O znachenii slova v obezbolivanii rodov," DAKhO, f. R-5833, op. 1, spr. 176, ark. 3.

65. Platonov authored these two lectures. Velvovsky et al., *Painless Childbirth*, 9–69. See also A. P. Nikolaev, "Teoreticheskie osnovy i sovremennye metody obezbolivaniia rodov," *Vestnik akademii meditsinskikh nauk SSSR* 6 (July–Aug. 1951): 13–23; V. N. Shishkova, R. M. Bronshtein, and E. I. Ivanova, "Psikhoprofilakticheskoe obezbolivanie rodov," *Akusherstvo i ginekologiia* 27 (Mar.–Apr. 1951): 25, 26; B. K. Korabel'nik, D. Ia. Daron, O. G. Serdiukova, E. E. Melerovich, and N. I. Musatova, "Opyt obezbolivaniia rodov psikhoprofilakticheskim metodom," *Akusherstvo i ginekologiia* 27 (Mar.–Apr. 1951): 31.

66. Platonov, "Kontseptsiia uslovno-reflektornogo proiskhozhdeniia rodovoi boli," DAKhO, f. R-5833, op. 1, spr. 157, ark. 1. According to Bell, Vel'vovskii borrowed "the pretentious style of Lysenko and the Neo-Pavlovians" and "donned this Neo-Pavlovian armor." Bell, "Giving Birth to the New Soviet Man," 9. I agree that the excessive emphasis on Pavlov's theoretical contribution to psychoprophylaxis was a product of the times, as was the absence of reference to Bekhterev, but Bell

is too quick to dismiss Vel'vovskii's arguments about the relevance of Pavlovian neuropsychology to psychoprophylaxis as mere convenience. Vel'vovskii, Platonov, and others who were interested in hypnosuggestion for obstetric pain relief had long explained their approach with resort to Pavlov's theories. For early references to Pavlov in connection with hypnosis and post-hypnotic suggestion for pain relief in childbirth prior to both the cult of Pavlov and the turn to psychoprophylaxis, see, for example, Rabinovich-Brodskaia, *Obezbolivanie normal'nykh rodov*, 47. Among others, Rabinovich-Brodskaia makes reference to the work of Nikolaev in this area. See also K. Skrobanskii, *Kratkoe rukovodstvo po obezbolivaniiu normal'nykh rodov* (Moscow-Leningrad: Gosudarstvennoe izdatel'stvo biologicheskoi i meditsinskoi literatury, 1936), 40.

67. A. P. Nikolaev, "Teoreticheskie osnovy i sovremennye metody obezbolivaniia rodov," 13.

68. Platonov, "Zakliuchitel'noe slovo na konferentsii po psikhoterapevticheskomu obezbolivaniiu rodov," DAKhO, f. R-5833, op. 1, spr. 164, ark. 3.

69. Kaplan, *Uchebnik akusherstva i zhenskikh boleznei*, 127.

70. Babinskii, "Gordost' russkoi nauki."

71. Vel'vovskii, Ploticher, and Shugom, "Psikhoprofilakticheskoe obezbolivanie rodov," 10.

72. Ibid.

73. Velvovsky et al., *Painless Childbirth*, 311.

74. Ibid., 315–16.

75. For example, see ibid., 113, 179, 181, 230, 313–14, 316–17; Shishkova et al., "Psikhoprofilakticheskoe obezbolivanie rodov," 26.

76. Velvovsky et al., *Painless Chilldbirth*, 136, 149, 164, 179, 180, 313, 314, 317.

77. In Vel'vovskii, Ploticher, and Shugom, "Psikhoprofilakticheskoe obezbolivanie rodov," the authors refer to the women subjects of their study as "patients," substituting this word and an initial for the women's names. I have retained the initials used in the article, but choose not to label them "patients." Following the lead of Lamaze and Vellay, who identify the women in their studies by the word "Madame" and an initial, I have attempted to render an approximate Soviet equivalent here with the use of the word "Comrade" [*tovarishch*] and an initial. It would perhaps have been more precise to call these women "Citizens" [*grazhdanki*], which after the revolution became a substitute for titles such as "sir," "madam," "Mr.," and "Mrs." Though it was in the USSR often reserved for party members, "comrade" was used frequently as well. Here it suggests no party affiliation or loyalty.

78. Vel'vovskii, Ploticher, and Shugom, "Psikhoprofilakticheskoe obezbolivanie rodov," 11.

79. For example, see V. Bogoliubova, "Zdes' otdykhaiut budushchie materi," *Sovetskaia zhenshchina*, Dec. 1954, 28–31; "Na blago materinstva," *Sovetskaia zhenshchina*, July 1955, 40–41; M. D. Piradova and V. G. Khrenova, "Obezbolivanie rodov," *Zdorov'e*, Nov. 1955, 28–29.

80. Sostoianie obezbolivaniia rodov po Khar'kovskoi oblasti, TsDAVO, f. 342, op. 14, spr. 4202, ark. 223.

81. Prikaz no. 142 MZ SSSR, "O psikhoprofilaktike bolei v rodakh," Feb. 13, 1951, GARF, f. r-8009, op. 1, d. 988, ll. 199 205; also available in TsDAVO, f. 342, op. 15, spr. 14, ark. 167–78ob. The edict from Minzdrav confirmed the conclusions of a conference held a few weeks earlier in Leningrad on the question of obstetric anesthesia. Nikolaev, *Obezbolivanie v rodakh*. On the plan for training

medical cadres in psychoprophylaxis, see Vremennyi uchebnyi plan i programma kursov spetsializatsii vrachei-akusherov po metodu psikhoprofilaktiki bolei v rodakh, Apr. 4, 1951, GARF, f. r-8009, op. 22, d. 249, ll. 69–90.

82. Fernand Lamaze, "Vérités sur l'accouchement sans douleur," *L'Humanité diman-che*, Aug. 23, 1953. See also Marianne Caron-Leulliez and Jocelyne George, *L'accouchement sans douleur: Histoire d'une révolution oubliée* (Paris: Les Éditions de l'Atelier, 2004), 32; Christiane Chotard, "La belle histoire du docteur Lamaze," *La Revue des travailleuses* 1 (June–July 1953): 15. On the history of Les Bluets, see Michel Dreyfus, *Une belle santé: Hôpital des Métallurgistes Pierre Rouquès, 50ème anniversaire de la maternité* (Paris: Hôpital des Métallurgistes Pierre Rouquès, 1997). For Lamaze's biography, see Caroline Gutmann, *The Legacy of Dr. Lamaze: The Story of the Man who Changed Childbirth*, trans. Bruce Benderson (New York: St. Martin's, 2001).

83. Fernand Lamaze, "Experience of a French Doctor," typescript translation of an article in *Les Lettres francais* (July 9–16, 1953), GC/106, Special Collections, WL. On Lamaze's trip to the USSR, see also Lamaze, " Vérités sur l'accouchement sans douleur"; Fernand Lamaze and Pierre Vellay, "L'accouchement sans dou-leur," *La Semaine médicale* 28 (Jan. 2, 1952): 304; "Tu enfanteras dans la joie," *Radar*, Jan. 4, 1953, 10; Fernand Lamaze, typescript, Dec. 19, 1952, box G, Collection l'Accouchement sans Douleur, Archives de l'Union Fraternelle de la Métallurgie, L'Institut d'Histoire Sociale CGT de la Métallurgie, Paris (hereafter cited as UFM). A brief but detailed summary of Lamaze's trip can be found in Caron-Leulliez and George, *L'accouchement sans douleur*, 33–35.

84. Chotard, "La belle histoire," 16.

CHAPTER 3

1. On psychoprophylaxis in France, see Caron-Leulliez and George, *L'accouchement sans douleur*. Sociologist Marilène Vuille offers particularly balanced and judicious work on the French history of psychoprophylaxis. See Vuille, *Accouchement et douleur*; Marilène Vuille, "La naissance de l''accouchement sans douleur,'" *Revue médicale de la Suisse romande* 120 (2000): 991–98; Marilène Vuille, "Le militantisme en faveur de l'accouchement sans douleur," *Nouvelles questions féministes* 24 (2005): 50–67. See also Sandra Fayolle, "L'Union des Femmes Françaises: Une organisation féminine de masse du Parti communiste français (1945–1965)" (PhD diss., Université Paris-I-Panthéon-Sorbonne, 2005), esp. 333–40. For studies of the history of childbirth in France that con-textualize psychoprophylaxis, see Yvonne Knibiehler, *La révolution maternelle depuis 1945: Femmes, maternité, citoyenneté* (Paris: Perrin, 1997); Knibiehler, *Accoucher*; Françoise Thebaud, *Quand nos grand-mères donnaient la vie: La maternité en France dans l'entre-deux-guerres* (Lyon: Presses Universitaires de Lyon, 1986).

2. Léon Chertok, Isabelle Stengers, and Didier Gille, *Mémoires d'un hérétique* (Paris: Éditions La Découverte, 1990), 149.

3. See Jules Regnault, *Maternité sans douleur: Comment accoucher normalement sans douleur* (Paris: Éditions médicis, 1945), 171–224; Thebaud, *Quand nos grand-mères donnaient la vie*, 249–75. No cumulative interwar statistics quantify the extent of drug use for obstetric pain relief, but Thebaud implies its infre-quent application. Thebaud, *Quand nos grand-mères donnaient la vie*, 262. Though the idea of speeding labor, both to minimize women's suffering and to protect the fetus from possible danger, had been in circulation for decades, it was in the

1960s that Irish obstetricians first sought to make such interventions routine for the explicit purpose of decreasing the total time in labor to under twenty-four hours. They called their method active management of labor, a term I borrow to convey *accouchement dirigé*'s similar use of drugs to speed labor and ease pain, even if French obstetricians lacked the stated optimal time limit that their Irish colleagues later put on labor's duration. See Kieran O'Driscoll, Reginald J. A. Jackson, and John T. Gallagher, "Prevention of Prolonged Labor," *British Medical Journal*, May 24, 1969, 477–80. See also Ann Oakley, *The Captured Womb*, 204–05. I thank Anne Drapkin Lyerly for guidance on the genealogy of this practice.

4. Quoted in Alain Noirez, "L'accouchement sans douler: De la présence du conjoint à l'accouchement de son épouse. Le vécu de la paternité, le rôle du mari au cours de la gestation, la crise moderne de la paternité" (PhD diss., Université Pierre et Marie Curie, Paris-VI, 1976), 122.

5. Ibid.

6. Marc Rivière and Léo Chastrusse, "La douleur en obstétrique," *Revue française de gynécologie et d'obstétrique* 49 (Sept.–Oct. 1954): 267. For similar remarks by Pierre Vellay, see Corinne Poittevin, "P. P. O.: 'Une manière d'affirmer ma personnalité,'" *Heures claires*, May 1978, 9. As in the United States and Great Britain, the decline in French maternal mortality began well before the development of antibiotics, with greater attention to asepsis and the segregation of maternity patients from the general hospital population. Mary Lynn Stewart, *For Health and Beauty: Physical Culture for Frenchwomen, 1880s–1930s* (Baltimore: Johns Hopkins University Press, 2001), 128–29.

7. See Micale, "On the 'Disappearance' of Hysteria," 497; Harrington, *The Cure Within*, 53–62.

8. Gutmann asserts that Lamaze studied in Nancy under Charcot's contemporary and rival Hippolyte Bernheim, but the timing of Lamaze's studies, the disruption caused by World War I, and Bernheim's death in 1919 all raise questions about the plausibility of this claim. My thanks to Marilène Vuille for pointing out the absence of corroboration for Gutmann's claim and its unlikelihood. Gutmann, *The Legacy of Dr. Lamaze*, 29. On Bernheim and the Nancy School, see Leon Chertok and Raymond de Saussure, *The Therapeutic Revolution: From Mesmer to Freud*, trans. R. H. Ahrenfeldt (New York: Brunner/Mazel, 1979), 36–49.

9. For a useful discussion of Freudian and Pavlovian strains of psychosomatic medicine on both sides of the Iron Curtain, see L. Chertok, "Psychoprophylaxie ou psychothérapie obstétricale: Évolution des théories sur l'accouchement sans douleur," *Revue de médecine psychosomatique* 3 (1961): 5–15; Leon Chertok, "Psychosomatic Medicine in the West and in Eastern European Countries," *Psychosomatic Medicine* 31 (Nov.–Dec. 1969): 510–21. For a provocative attempt to square Freudianism with Marxism by a psychiatrist who, earlier in his career, was active in promoting psychoprophylaxis, see Bernard Muldworf, *Le divan et le prolétaire* (Paris: Messidor/Éditions sociales, 1986).

10. Sigmund Freud, "On the History of the Psycho-Analytic Movement," *The Standard Edition of the Complete Psychological Works of Sigmund Freud* (London: Hogarth Press, 1975), 14: 32, quoted in Marion Michel Oliner, *Cultivating Freud's Garden in France* (Northvale, NJ: Jason Aronson, 1988), 21. On the early history of French psychoanalysis, see also Chertok and de Saussure, *The Therapeutic Revolution*. For a concise history of French psychoanalysis, see Alain de Mijolla, "La psychoanalyse en France (1893–1965)," *Histoire de la psychanalyse*, ed. R. Jaccard (Paris: Hachette, 1982), 2: 9–105. Translated by Ruth Hoffman in an

abridged form as "France (1893–1965)," *Psychoanalysis International*, ed. Peter Kutter (Stuttgart: Friedrich Frommann Verlag, 1992), 1: 66–113.

11. France at the end of the twentieth century had more psychoanalysts per capita than any other country in the world. Elisabeth Roudinseco, "Psychoanalysis," *The Columbia History of Twentieth-Century French Thought*, ed. Lawrence D. Kritzman, Brian J. Reilly, and M. B. DeBevoise, trans. M. B. DeBevoise (New York: Columbia University Press, 2006), 100–01.

12. Chotard, "La belle histoire du docteur Lamaze," 16; Colette Jeanson, *Principes et pratique de l'accouchement sans douleur* (Paris: Édition du Seuil, 1954), 22; F. Lamaze, "L'accouchement sans douleur par la méthode psycho-prophylactique," typescript, Jan. 1955, box J-2, UFM.

13. For example, in the author's note to the 1953 French translation of *Childbirth without Fear*, Dick-Read romanticizes how "the calm strength and indomitable determination of the natural forces of reproduction" have the potential "to lead the human spirit toward fundamental truth and a greater understanding of the omnipotent, but invisible forces of the Universe." Grantly Dick-Read, *L'accouchement sans douleur: Les principes et la pratique de l'accouchement naturel*, trans. Jean-Marc Vaillant (Paris: Colbert, 1953), viii.

14. For a brief, excellent study that explains well the varied strains of thinking on the subject, see Karen Offen, "Depopulation, Nationalism, and Feminism in Fin-de-Siècle France," *The American Historical Review* 89 (June 1984): 648–76. See also William Schneider, *Quality and Quantity: The Quest for Biological Regeneration in Twentieth-Century France* (Cambridge: Cambridge University Press, 2002).

15. Karen Offen, "Body Politics: Women, Work and the Politics of Motherhood in France, 1920–1950," in *Maternity and Gender Policies: Women and the Rise of the European Welfare States, 1880s–1950s*, eds. Gisela Bock and Pat Thane (London: Routledge, 1991), 138–59; Antoine Prost, "L'évolution de la politique familiale en France de 1938 à 1981," *Le mouvement sociale* 129 (Oct.–Dec. 1984): 7–28; Mary Louise Roberts, *Civilization without Sexes: Reconstructing Gender in Postwar France, 1917–1927* (Chicago: University of Chicago Press, 1994), esp. 89–147; Cheryl A. Koos, "Gender, Anti-Individualism, and Nationalism: The Alliance Nationale and the Pronatalist Backlash against the Femme Moderne, 1933–1940," *French Historical Studies* 19 (Spring 1996): 699–723; Knibiehler, *La révolution maternelle*, 26–29.

16. H. P. Pétain, "Appel du 20 juin" (1940), in *Le Maréchal vous parle…: Recueil des discours et allocations prononcés par le Maréchal Pétain, chef de l'état du 16 juin au 31 décembre 1940* (Le Mans: Éditions CEP, 1941), unpaginated, cited in Offen, "Body Politics," 154, n. 6. During World War II, racialist and eugenicist ideas that had long circulated in France gained new prominence in debates over demographic revival, but Vichy's fall, Germany's defeat, and revelations of Nazi atrocities largely discredited such thinking. Miranda Pollard, *Reign of Virtue: Mobilizing Gender in Vichy France* (Chicago: University of Chicago Press, 1998); Francine Muel-Dreyfus, *Vichy and the Eternal Feminine: A Contribution to a Political Sociology of Gender*, trans. Kathleen A. Johnson (Durham, NC: Duke University Press, 2001).

17. Claire Duchen, *Women's Rights and Women's Lives in France, 1944–1968* (London: Routledge, 1994), 103; Prost, "L'évolution de la politique familiale." On more recent French incarnations of pronatalism, see Leslie King, "'France Needs

Children': Pronatalism, Nationalism and Women's Equality," *The Sociological Quarterly* 39 (Jan. 1998): 33–52.

18. A 1967 law gave women the right to contraception and in 1975 abortion became legal in France. See Marie-Françoise Lévy, "Le mouvement français pour le planning familial et les jeunes," *Vingtième Siècle. Revue d'histoire*. No. 75, Numéro special: Histoire des femmes, histoire des genres (July–Sept. 2002): 75–84; Claire Duchen, *Feminism in France: From May '68 to Mitterrand* (London: Routledge & Kegan Paul, 1986), 49–66.

19. See Richard F. Kuisel, *Seducing the French: The Dilemma of Americanization* (Berkeley: University of California Press, 1993), esp. 52–69.

20. The Left had a history of resistance to neo-Malthusianism in the interwar era. See Offen, "Body Politics."

21. Knibiehler, *La révolution maternelle*, 131; Prost, "L'évolution de la politique familiale," 10–15. Only a small number of vocal opponents on the Left, most notably through the organization Happy Motherhood (*Heureuse Maternité*), broke with the French consensus on pronatalism and familialism in the 1950s. Dr. Marie-Andrée Lagroua Weill-Hallé, who had been among the Communist doctors and sympathizers who, along with Dr. Lamaze, went to the USSR in 1951, led Happy Motherhood in its opposition to the PCF's position against birth control. According to Fayolle, the UFF remained silent in the 1950s on the question of birth control and abortion, perhaps in an effort to avoid a split within the organization between proponents and opponents. Fayolle, "L'Union des Femmes Françaises," 251–353; Sylvie Chaperon, *Les années Beauvoir, 1945–1970* (Paris: Librairie Arthème Fayard, 2000), 247–52; Duchen, *Women's Rights and Women's Lives*, 109–10, 119–27.

22. "Déclaration du Docteur Lamaze à son retour d'un voyage d'études médicales en URSS," 1951, box H, UFM.

23. Caron-Leulliez and George, *L'accouchement sans douleur*, 50–53. A kinesiologist specializes in the study of human anatomy and the mechanics of body movement.

24. Gutmann, *The Legacy of Dr. Lamaze*, 187. PCF colleagues at Les Bluets considered him "not only a man of rare honesty and dedication, but a Communist who lacks only the [membership] card." Dacour, Lefebvre, Bougon, and Devoret to unnamed PCF comrade, [Jan. 1953], box B, UFM. Caron-Leulliez and George emphasize Lamaze's links to and sympathy with the PCF. Caron-Leulliez and George, *L'accouchement sans douleur*, 28.

25. Le Guay went under the auspices of Le Mouvement de la Paix, a French pacifist organization founded in 1948 and allied with the PCF. On connections in Eastern Europe, see correspondence, box J-2, UFM.

26. F. Lamaze to Ho Dac Di, Apr. 26, 1955, box J-1, UFM.

27. Dominique Desanti, "Nous avons vu se forger l'avenir d'un enfant," *La revue des travailleuses* 1 (June–July 1953): 35.

28. "Grand Succès de la conférence des Professeurs Nicolaev et Khilov," *L'Humanité*, Oct. 31, 1953. For Nikolaev's Paris speech, see Professeur A. Nicolaev, "Les principaux problèmes d'obstétrique et de gynécologie à la lumière de la théorie de Pavlov," typescript, [1953], box H, UFM. On the France-USSR Association, see "La France devant les échanges et les relations avec l'URSS: Introduction à une grande consultation nationale," Paris, 1975, box 15, 88A5 Association France-URSS, Archives nationales de France, Paris (hereafter cited as ANF).

29. Largely suspended as the Cold War heated up at the close of World War II, American travel to the USSR resumed in small ways after Stalin's death in 1953. Soviet-American exchanges of medical workers occurred in 1955 and 1956, but only in 1958 did a bilateral agreement establish formal, regular exchanges in public health, science, education, and other fields. Until the 1980s, the number of exchangees traveling in both directions remained small. H. B. Shaffer, "Cultural Exchanges with Soviet Russia," *Editorial Research Reports 1959*, 11 (Washington, DC: CQ Press, 1959), http://library.cqpress.com/cqresearcher/document.php?id=cqresrre1959070300#.UmNC_VBkN8E; see also Yale Richmond, *Cultural Exchange and the Cold War: Raising the Iron Curtain* (University Park: Pennsylvania State University, 2003).

30. Nikolaev's trip also appears to have sparked interest in translating his writings into French. M[ichel] Sapir to unknown [F. Le Guay?], Nov. 14, 1953, box I, UFM. For a typescript of Lamaze's France-USSR Association–sponsored talk in the Parisian suburb of Argenteuil in April 1956, see box H, UFM. For evidence of continuing communication, see Nikolaev to Lamaze, July 11, 1954, box H, UFM.

31. Pierre Vellay and Aline Vellay-Dalsace, *Témoignages sur l'accouchement sans douleur par la méthode psycho-prophylactique* (Paris: Éditions du Seuil, 1956), 339–40. The archives are silent on whether Vel'vovskii was denied permission to travel abroad for scholarly conferences. He had no shortage of invitations and submitted papers but to the best of my knowledge he never traveled to the West.

32. "Editorial," *Cahiers de médecine soviétique* 2 (Nov. 1955): 227–28.

33. Fernand Lamaze, "Experience of a French Doctor," GC/106, Special Collections, WL. See also F. Lamaze, P. Vellay, J. Hersilie, R. Angelergues, [A.] Bourrel et les Sages-Femmes, "Expérience pratiquée à la maternité du Centre 'Pierre-Rouquès' sur la méthode d'accouchement sans douleur par psycho-prophylaxie," *Bulletin de l'Académie nationale de médecine* 138 (Jan. 26–Feb. 2, 1954): 54.

34. "Evelyne a (sans souffrance) donné le jour à Michèle," *Regards*, Jan. 1953, 5–6; "Observations," *Revue de la nouvelle médecine* 1 (May 1954): 105. For a description of the film, see Jeanson, *Principes et pratique de l'accouchement sans douleur*, 111. With rare exception, most notably to persuade government officials to support coverage of psychoprophylaxis under *Sécurité sociale* and to train medical and paramedical personnel, the film was used exclusively for prenatal classes and was not shown publically. Le Guay to Madame Paulette Auguet, Jan. 12, 1955, box M, UFM; Lamaze, "L'accouchement sans douleur par la méthode psycho-prophylactique," box J-2, UFM.

35. Jeanson, *Principes et pratique de l'accouchement sans douleur*, 90; André Bourrel, "Mettre tous les atouts dans son jeu…" *La revue des travailleuses* 1 (June–July 1953): 26–27; Fernand Lamaze, *Qu'est-ce que l'accouchement sans douleur* (Paris: La Farandole, 1956), 121–219.

36. Elisabeth Roudinesco, *Jacques Lacan & Co.: A History of Psychoanalysis in France, 1925–1985*, trans. Jeffrey Mehlman (Chicago: University of Chicago Press, 1990), 180.

37. René Angelergues, "Introduction à l'étude de Pavlov: L'activité nerveuse supérieure base de la pathologie cortico-viscérale," *Revue de la nouvelle médecine* 1 (June 1953): 36. As part of a broader push to promote the Left's progressive medical and public health agenda, a group of Communist doctors launched the journal *Revue de la nouvelle médecine*, which ran from 1953 to 1957. Much of the journal's first issue was devoted to the discussion of psychoprophylaxis, including

an article by Lamaze and Vellay. F. Lamaze and P. Vellay, "Considérations sur l'accouchement sans douleur par la méthode psycho-physique. Travail de la maternité de la Polyclinique des Métallurgistes," *Revue de la nouvelle médecine* 1 (June 1953): 71–77.

38. Angelergues, "Introduction à l'étude de Pavlov," 35, 36.
39. Ibid., 39.
40. "Une interview du Dr. Lamaze," *La Quinzaine*, Dec. 1, 1953, 12.
41. For an excellent analysis of thinking among activists for psychoprophylaxis on pain as a sociohistorical phenomenon, see Vuille, *Accouchement et douleur*, 53–63. The totality of this faith in the painless nature of normal birth is challenging to accept given our beliefs at present, but is well-articulated in the words of one journalist, who said, "all normal women from now on can give birth absolutely pain free, without the aid of any anesthetic or drugs, and without any risk to themselves or their babies." Louis Dalmas, "500 Femmes vous racontent leur accouchement sans douleur," *France dimanche*, Feb. 14, 1953.
42. Lamaze, "L'accouchement sans douleur par la méthode psycho-prophylactique," box J-2, UFM.
43. [Fernand] Lamaze and [Pierre] Vellay, "L'accouchement sans douleur par la méthode psychophysique," *Gazette médicale de France* 59 (Dec. 1952): 1459. See also F. Lamaze and P. Vellay, "Il faut rompre avec la tradition," *Revue de l'économe* 19 (Oct. 1953): 1197.
44. Typescript report from Ch. Lefeuvre, July 12, 1953, box C, UFM.
45. Caron-Leulliez and George characterize psychoprophylaxis as an expression of resistance to obstetric authority and a radical alternative to conventional birth practices. Caron-Leulliez and George, *L'accouchement sans douleur*, 231.
46. Molly Lobban, "N. M. Study Tour of the USSR," *Nursing Mirror*, Aug. 27, 1965, iv. Lobban had the opportunity to see several Soviet maternity wards in Moscow, Leningrad, and Kiev. Members of her group repeatedly raised the issue of the husband's presence and participation during labor and birth with their Soviet counterparts, only to find that "there was never any question of husbands visiting during labor, much less to be present at delivery.... [O]ur hostesses seemed reluctant even to consider the possibility.... We put forward various reasons as to why we encourage it but mostly they refused to discuss the matter further, dismissing it on the grounds that it would introduce infection."
47. Leavitt, *Make Room for Daddy*, esp. 86–119.
48. Annie Rolland and Paul Rolland, "L'accouchement sans douleur à domicile, à la campagne," *Revue de la nouvelle médecine* 1 (Dec. 1954): 57. See also, Vellay and Vellay-Dalsace, *Témoignages sur l'accouchement sans douleur*, 337.
49. Jeannette Coutant, "La première expérience d'accouchement sans douleur à domicile," *Femmes françaises*, June 5, 1954, 5; A. Rolland to Lamaze, [1954], box I, UFM; Annie Rolland, "Journal d'une médecine de campagne," *Heures claires*, Mar. 1955, 13; "20 Accouchées sans douleur vous parlent," *France dimanche*, Jan. 20, 1956; Caron-Leulliez and George, *L'accouchement sans douleur*, 61. As one American living in Paris attested following her baby's birth at Les Bluets, "the father participates in his child's birth. This is useful, even necessary and he can say, 'I saw my child born.' Leaving the labor room, he too has a wonderful memory. Certainly, he is already attached to his child and he appreciates appropriately the value of his wife's effort." Vellay and Vellay-Dalsace, *Témoignages sur l'accouchement sans douleur*, 271.

50. Lamaze strongly endorsed an enhanced role for the husband, who contributes to the positive " 'psychological climate' that his presence creates and that concretely and effectively aids in the woman's adaptability." Fernand Lamaze, *La suppression de la douleur liée à la contraction de l'utérus en travail: Méthode psycho-prophylactique* (n.p., [1955]), 20. This pamphlet was reprinted as Fernand Lamaze, "La suppression de la douleur liée à la contraction de l'utérus en travail," *Revue de la nouvelle médecine* 3 (June 1956): 61–91. Quote appears on p. 80. On the husband and doctor working as a team, see, for example, R. Demeusy, "L'accouchement psycho-prophylactique," *Formulaire dimanche*, July 24, 1955; Pierre Vellay, "Il faut lutter," *L'Humanité dimanche*, Aug. 23, 1953.

51. For example, see "20 Accouchées sans douleur vous parlent;" Vellay and Vellay-Dalsace, *Témoignages sur l'accouchement sans douleur*, 146.

52. Typescript report from Ch. Lefeuvre, box C, UFM.

53. Vellay and Vellay-Dalsace, *Témoignages sur l'accouchement sans douleur*, 306.

54. Ibid., 226. The husband's presence was not always a source of comfort. For example, Madame Dutilleul found her husband's movements and commands distracting. He had not participated in the preparatory courses nor tutored her in the relaxation and breathing techniques at home. Ibid., 231.

55. Ibid., 293.

56. Ibid., 297.

57. Ibid., 200.

58. "L'accouchement sans douleur fait son chemin," *Regards*, [April? 1955], 4, press clipping, box I, UFM.

59. "J'attends mon bébé d'un moment à l'autre," *Regards*, [April? 1955], 20, press clipping, box I, UFM.

60. Victor Lafitte, "La douleur c'est le passé!" *La revue des travailleuses* 1 (June–July 1953): 31.

61. Vellay and Vellay-Dalsace, *Témoignages sur l'accouchement sans douleur*, 41.

62. Dalmas, "500 Femmes vous racontent leur accouchement sans douleur."

63. Maurice Mayer and Jacques Bonhomme, "La méthode de l'accouchement naturel, son utilisation en pratique hospitalière," *La vie médicale*, Dec. 1953, 762; Réunion de l'équipe de la Maternité du Métallurgiste, meeting minutes, Nov. 14, 1954, box H, UFM.

64. Lamaze and Vellay, "L'accouchement sans douleur par la méthode psychophysique," 1450, 1454. Quote appears on p. 1454.

65. Lamaze, *La suppression de la douleur liée à la contraction de l'utérus en travail*, 17.

66. Lamaze and Vellay, "L'accouchement sans douleur par la méthode psychophysique," 1448.

67. Chaperon, *Les années Beauvoir*, 125.

68. Rolland, "Journal d'un médecin de campagne," 13.

69. Lamaze and Vellay, "L'accouchement sans douleur par la méthode psychophysique," 1448.

70. Quoted in Coutant, "La première expérience d'accouchement sans douleur à domicile," 4.

71. "Les enfants se portent-ils mieux?" *Heures claires*, Mar. 1955, 32.

72. "Observations," 98.

73. Geneviève Clairbois, "Oui, il est possible d'accoucher sans douleur," *La Quinzaine*, Dec. 1, 1953, 14.

74. Vuille, *Accouchement et douleur*, 58–60.

75. Lamaze and Vellay, "L'accouchement sans douleur par la méthode psychophysique," 1450. Emphasis in original.

76. Ibid., 1456. Emphasis in original.

77. Yvette Churlet, "Quatre Lyonnaises ont accouché sans peur, sans douleur," *La République—La Patriote*, Dec. 22, 1953.

78. Lamaze and Vellay, "L'accouchement sans douleur par la méthode psychophysique," 1450–51.

79. E.g., Jeanson, *Principes et pratique de l'accouchement sans douleur*. We know, for example, that American Marjorie Karmel read Colette Jeanson's book when she was a patient in Dr. Lamaze's private practice. Before the birth of her second child, she read Vellay and Vellay-Dalsace's collection of patient testimonials. Marjorie Karmel, *Thank You Dr. Lamaze* (1959; repr. London: Pinter & Martin, 2005), 58, 137. For other examples of the influence of the testimonials that appear in Jeanson's book, see Vellay and Vellay-Dalsace, *Témoignages sur l'accouchement sans douleur*, 96, 99, 196, 238, 285, 291, 295; Madame Fournier, "J'ai accouché sans douleur à domicile et à la campagne," *Femmes françaises*, Dec. 4, 1954, 19.

80. For example, see Isabelle Barontini, "Le journal d'une accouchée sans douleur," *Femmes françaises*, Nov. 27, 1954, 7; "Observations," 98; Vellay and Vellay-Dalsace, *Témoignages sur l'accouchement sans douleur*, 55, 67.

81. "Evelyne a (sans souffrance) donné le jour à Michèle," 8. See also, for example, Vellay and Vellay-Dalsace, *Témoignages sur l'accouchement sans douleur*, 48.

82. Quote from "Observations," 101. On the benefits of continuous labor support, see Jeanne Green, Debby Amis, and Barbara Hotelling, "Care Practice #3: Continuous Support," *Journal of Perinatal Education* 16 (Summer 2007): 25–28.

83. Lamaze and Vellay, "L'accouchement sans douleur par la méthode psychophysique," 1448. Emphasis mine.

84. F. Lamaze, "L'accouchement sans douleur par la méthode psycho-prophylactique," box J-2, UFM, F. Lamaze, P. Vellay, and H. Hersilie, "Essai d'interprétation des causes d'échec," *Revue de la nouvelle médecine* 1 (May 1954): 136; Vellay and Vellay-Dalsace, *Témoignages sur l'accouchement sans douleur*, 32, 146, 235, 260.

85. Vellay and Vellay-Dalsace, *Témoignages sur l'accouchement sans douleur*, 249–50.

86. Rolland and Rolland, "L'accouchement sans douleur à domicile, à la campagne," 59. Loosely based on Rolland's experience promoting psychoprophylaxis in the countryside, the film *Le cas du docteur Laurent* (1957) depicts vividly the powerful influence one woman's success with the method had in winning adherents for the method.

87. Ibid., 64.

88. Pierre Vellay, "Réalités et perspectives de l'accouchement sans douleur," *Heures claires*, March 1955, 4.

89. Jeannette Coutant, "J'ai vu une femme accoucher sans douleur," *Femmes françaises*, Oct. 13, 1951, 12–13; "Orientation de l'action des femmes pour la diffusion de l'accouchement sans douleur," memo to USTM Secretariat, [1953 or 1954], box B, UFM; Lamaze to Raymond Guyot, Oct. 23, 1954, box B, UFM.

90. "Accoucher sans douleur," *Femmes françaises*, May 27, 1954, 19; "Pour qu'ils naissent dans la soie...à travers nos départements," *Femmes françaises*, Nov. 20, 1954, 7; "Toutes les femmes veulent et peuvent accoucher sans douleur," *Femmes françaises*, Apr. 24, 1954, 9; Bilan de l'activité connue des départements et fonctionnement des Commissions, Commission nationale de l'enfance et des

activités sociale de l'UFF, Nov. 1954–Feb. 1955; Feb. 10–28, 1955; Mar. 1–31, 1955, box I, UFM.

91. "Il existe maintenant de nombreuses villes de France où des médecins pratiquent l'accouchement sans douleur," *Femmes françaises*, Oct. 16, 1954, 7; *Comment nous préparer à accoucher sans douleur par la méthode psycho-prophylactique* (Paris: Union des Femmes Françaises, 1955). See also "Demain sera dans toute la France la journée de l'accouchement sans douleur," *L'Humanité*, May 17, 1955; Bilan de l'activité connue des départements et fonctionnement des Commissions, Commission nationale de l'enfance et des activités sociales de l'UFF, Mar. 1–31, 1955; Apr. 1–May 31, 1955, box I, UFM; "Comment nous préparer à accoucher sans douleur," *Femmes françaises*, Apr. 9, 1955, 8; "Des victoires dont nous sommes fières," *Femmes françaises*, Mar. 3, 1956, 18.

92. François Le Guay, "Une réalisation dont nous sommes fiers," *La revue des travailleuses* 1 (June–July 1953): 32.

93. Not only his publications but lectures abroad, also, elevated his stature. He traveled to Cuba, Brazil, and elsewhere to promote psychoprophylaxis. On his trip to Brazil, see Lamaze to Edson Augusto de Almeida, May 3, 1956, box M, UFM. For the text of Lamaze's presentation in Cuba in December 1955, see Lamaze, "La suppression de la douleur liée à la contraction de l'utérus en travail."

94. Lamaze, "L'accouchement sans douleur par la méthode psycho-prophylactique," box J-2, UFM; Lamaze, *Qu'est-ce que l'accouchement sans douleur*, 92; Vellay and Vellay-Dalsace, *Témoignages sur l'accouchement sans douleur*, 329. A department is an administrative district in France.

95. On Lamaze's fame, see W. C. W. Nixon, presentation at "Problèmes médicaux et sanitaires dans les différentes sphères d'activité de l'*American Joint-Distribution Committee*" conference, UNESCO, Paris, June 28-July 1, 1954, typescript, box C, UFM. For representative letters from prospective students, see Asher Segall to Dr. Gasches, Nov. 9, 1954, box J-1, UFM; Edward B. Winheld to Lamaze, Aug. 25, 1955, box J-1, UFM.

96. Lamaze to Madeleine Jaegle, Nov. 9, 1954, box M, UFM; [signature illegible], UFF Departmental Committee, Angers to Lamaze, Sept. 20, 1954, box M, UFM; "Pour qu'ils naissent dans la joie," *Femmes françaises*, Dec. 25, 1954, 5; F. Lamaze, P. Vellay, and H. Hersilie, "Réponse à quelques questions," *Révue de la nouvelle médecine* 1 (May 1954): 125.

97. Réunion de l'équipe de la Maternité du Métallurgiste, box H, UFM; Paula A. Michaels, "Comrades in the Labor Room: The Lamaze Method of Childbirth Preparation and France's Cold War Home Front, 1951–1957," *The American Historical Review* 115 (Oct. 2010): 1045–47.

98. Pierre Muller, "Remarques sur l'accouchement sans douleur pratiqué à Mulhouse depuis février 1954," Nov. 1954, typescript, box C, UFM.

99. Two decades later, Muller found women and their obstetricians in the region to be early and enthusiastic adopters of epidural anesthesia. P. Muller, "Anesthésie péridurale et psycho-prophylaxie obstétricale," *Bulletin officiel de la Société française de psycho-prophylaxie obstétricale*, no. 69 (July–Sept. 1977): 6.

100. Vellay, "Réalités et perspectives de l'accouchement sans douleur," 4–5. Vellay makes similar comments in Vellay and Vellay-Dalsace, *Témoignages sur l'accouchement sans douleur*, 264.

101. Vellay and Vellay-Dalsace, *Témoignages sur l'accouchement sans douleur*, 21.

102. As one article in *Radar* asserted, "women of still uncivilized populations give birth with an ease that always boggles observers. They have maintained an

instinctive sense of the most favorable position. We should take a page from their book." "Mesdames accouchez sans douleur!" *Radar*, Feb. 7, 1954, 9. For similar views on non-European women, see Rivière and Chastrusse, "La douleur en obstétrique," 252. Lamaze took offense at the views articulated in the *Radar* article and personally wrote to the editors to clarify that the positions, exercises, and ideas expressed in this article had nothing to do with psychoprophylaxis. Lamaze to General Director, *Radar*, Feb. 9, 1954, box E, UFM. Even Lamaze's supporters expressed these views on so-called uncivilized peoples. See Pierre Joffroy, "Nathalie née sans douleur," *Paris Match*, Apr. 2, 1955, 80. Lamaze held similar views on the painlessness of childbirth for French peasant women. See Rose Vincent, "Catherine est née 'sans douleur,' grâce à l'accouchement naturel," *Elle*, Apr. 22, 1955, 29.

103. Jean Larribère to Lamaze, Dec. 11, 1954, box C, UFM.

CHAPTER 4

1. Dick-Read to Miguel Cioc, Feb. 9, 1959, PP/GDR/D.216/55, WL.
2. Meeting minutes, Natural Childbirth Trust of Great Britain (hereafter cited as NCT), May 7, 1959, PP/GDR/D.249/57, WL.
3. For an attempt to schematize the differences among Vel'vovskii, Lamaze, and Read, see L. Chertok, "L''accouchement naturel' et l''accouchement psychopro-phylactique,'" *Concours médical* 79 (Nov. 23, 1957): 5105–08. Chertok was in a unique position to transcend ideological, theoretical, and methodological divides. Born near Vilnius, Chertok's native language was Russian, enabling him to access directly the Soviet scholarship on psychoprophylaxis. Unlike many of the Soviet method's French supporters, he had no ideological incentive to support psychoprophylaxis, though neither was he anti-Soviet. See Chertok, Stengers, and Gille, *Mémoires d'un hérétique*.
4. Dick-Read, *Childbirth without Fear*, 148–49.
5. *Natural Childbirth: A Documentary Record of the Birth of a Baby Supervised by Dr. Grantly Dick-Read* (n.p.: Westminster Recording, 1957); *L'accouchement sans douleur: Reportage de Francis Crémieux* ([Paris]: Voix de son maitre, 1955).
6. One British woman active in the promotion of the Read method suggested that "natural childbirth might suit the British mother better than the psy-choprophylactic method breathing, which might be better suited to the more emotional Continental women." Meeting minutes, NCT, May 7, 1959, PP/GDR/D.249/57, WL.
7. Jenny Kitzinger, "Strategies of the Early Childbirth Movement: A Case-Study of the National Childbirth Trust," in *The Politics of Maternity Care*, 107.
8. Vellay to Dick-Read, Sept. 28, 1951; Dick-Read to Vellay, Oct. 29, 1951; both in PP/GDR/D.221, WL; Dick-Read, *L'accouchement sans douleur*.
9. Lamaze and Vellay, "L'accouchement sans douleur," 302–03, 304; see also H. Zaidman, "L'analgésie obstétricale par la méthode psycho-prophylactique," *Santé publique*, Oct. 1, 1953, 1. For an extensive discussion of the common pain medications for use during labor in France and their potential dangers, see Jeanson, *Principes et pratique de l'accouchement sans douleur*, 14–21.
10. Chertok, "L''accouchement naturel' et l''accouchement psychoprophylactique,'" 5106.
11. Lamaze and Vellay, "L'accouchement sans douleur par la méthode psychophy-sique," 3, 4; L. M., "Une nouvelle méthode d'accouchement," *Revue de l'économe* 19 (Oct. 1953): 1194.

12. Leon Chertok, "Reply to the Foregoing: Editor," *American Journal of Psychiatry* 120 (Dec. 1963): 606. On these tensions, see Donald Caton, "Who Said Childbirth Is Natural? The Medical Mission of Grantly Dick-Read," *Anesthesiology* 84 (Apr. 1996): 961–62.

13. Renée Sarfaty, "L'accouchement sans douleur," *Mode du jour*, Sept. 11, 1952, 1, 22; Dick-Read, *L'accouchement sans douleur*.

14. Grantly Dick-Read, "L'accouchement sans douleur," *Votre santé*, Apr. 15, 1954, May 15, 1954, June 1, 1954, press clippings, box E, UFM. The Read method was also associated in France with a variety of phrases, including "accouchement sans crainte" and "accouchement peu douloureux." A. Economides, "État actuel de la pratique de l'accouchement sans douleur en France," *Revue de la nouvelle médecine* 2 (Jan. 1956): 72. The team at Les Bluets saw Dick-Read's rising profile as a testament to the growing recognition of their own method. Lamaze, Vellay, and Hersilie, "Essai d'interprétations des causes d'échec," 129.

15. Other books and articles soon followed from Dick-Read's supporters in France and elsewhere on the Continent, adding to the sudden and confusing barrage of childbirth preparation information to which expectant mothers in France were exposed in the popular press. For example, Renée Girod and Monica Jaquet, *Je vais être maman: Grossesse, accouchement, gymnastique prénatale* (Zurich: Édition Pro Juventute, 1954); "La nouvelle méthode d'accouchement sans douleur," *Bonnes soirées*, Jan. 30, 1955, 63; F. Lepage and G. Langevin-Droguet, *La prépa-ration à l'accouchement sans crainte*, 2nd rev., exp. ed. (Paris: Masson et Cie, 1965). Chertok captures well the terminological confusion, stating that "doc-trinal arguments reign in lieu of [a solid theoretical foundation], which explains the diversity of names given to [non-pharmacological methods of obstetric pain relief]: psychoprophylactic, psycho-physical, neuro-physical, childbirth without anxiety, without fear, without suffering, without agony, without apprehension, eased pain, etc." L. Chertok, "Étude de la psycho-prophylaxie des douleurs de l'accouchement," *La Semaine des hôpitaux* 32 (Aug. 1956): 2619.

16. E.g., "L'accouchement sans crainte," *Le Monde*, Jan. 28, 1954. Dr. Armand Notter of Lyon produced the 1954 educational film "L'accouchement sans appréhen-sion," based on Dick-Read's work, for use in childbirth education classes. Notter chose to avoid confusion with Lamaze's approach by giving it a title that dis-tinguished it from the method of Soviet origin, yet UFF activists in Lyon still struggled with the general public to maintain clarity concerning this distinction. Paule Roussat to UFF Social Commission, Paris, Jan. 6, 1955, box M, UFM.

17. Rivière and Chastrusse, "La douleur en obstétrique," 260–61; [H.] Vermelin, "L'accouchement sans douleur," *La Sage-Femme française*, Jan. 1955, 3; Jeanson, *Principes et pratique de l'accouchement sans douleur*, 195–96; Vincent, "Catherine est née 'sans douleur' grâce à l'accouchement naturel," 28; Joffroy, "Nathalie née sans douleur," 80; "Sept futures mamans sur dix sont encore contre l'accouchement sans douleur," *France soir*, Jan. 11, 1956.

18. Roger Hersilie, "Voici ce que les femmes ont gagné," *Heures claires*, Oct. 1956, 4. Similar frustration seeps into A. Economides, "État actuel de la pratique de l'accouchement sans douleur en France," 73; " 'L'accouchement sans crainte' du Docteur Read diffère-t-il de la méthode psychoprophylactique? En quoi?" *Regards* [1955], 20, press clipping, box I, UFM.

19. Similarly, see F. Lamaze, "Les maternités soviétiques et l'accouchement sans douleur," *Revue de la nouvelle médecine* 2 (May 1955): 63; Lamaze, *Qu'est-ce que l'accouchement sans douleur*, 32–33, 84–88.

20. Pierre Theil, "Préface," in Dick-Read, *L'accouchement sans douleur*, iv–v.
21. Dick-Read to Herbert Thoms, May 2, 1950, PP/GDR/D.196, WL.
22. Dick-Read to Thoms, Feb. 29, 1952, PP/GDR/D.196, WL.
23. Dick-Read to Prof. [A. Iu.] Lurye [sic], Feb. 26, 1952, PP/GDR/D.218/55, WL; "Russians Taking Credit, says Dr. Grantly Read," *Eastern Evening News*, Jan. 17, 1956, press clipping, PP/GDR/C.138/33, WL. See also A. Noyes Thomas, *Doctor Courageous: The Story of Dr. Grantley Dick-Read* (New York: Harper, 1957), 110–11.
24. Angus McPherson to Frank Bamping, Oct. 9, 1953; Program, "Painless Childbirth in Practice by Pavlovian Methods," public lecture by Lamaze, Nov. 27, 1953; Bamping to Mary Barber, Dec. 6, 1953; all in GC/106, WL; Founded in 1923, the Society for Cultural Relations with the USSR (SCR) was the British partner to the USSR's All-Union Society for Foreign Cultural Relations (VOKS). The SCR formed a Medical Section in 1946 to promote the exchange of information and cultivate ties between medical professionals in the UK and USSR. "Epidemiology Section," *British Medical Journal*, Dec. 7, 1946, 881. On VOKS and the SRC, see Ludmila Stern, *Western Intellectuals and the Soviet Union, 1920–1940: From Red Square to the Left Bank* (New York: Routledge, 2007), 124–27.
25. Organ of the Communist Party of Great Britain, *The Daily Worker* painted a rosy picture of psychoprophylactic practice in the USSR and contrasted it to the "shameful" situation in Great Britain. Understaffed maternity wards were ill-equipped to offer women the kind of support and companionship needed during an unanesthetized birth. An equally important obstacle to the spread of psychoprophylaxis was a narrow-minded medical community that had previously obstructed Dick-Read's effort to promote his "very similar" method. Unlike their Soviet or French sisters, British women allegedly "continue to produce their babies in the bad, old, fear-ridden way—in many parts of the country without even the relief of a gas-and-air machine." Sheila Lynd, "She Smiled as her Baby Was Born," *Daily Worker*, Sept. 26, 1953. Who, exactly, continued to bear children in "the bad, old, fear-ridden way" at this juncture is unclear. Historian A. Susan Williams observes that with the coming of the NHS in 1946 the "marked disparity" in access to pain relief between rich and poor came to an end, calling Lynd's accusation into question. Williams, *Women and Childbirth in the Twentieth Century*, 143.
26. Eileen Travis, "A Thousand Painless Births: British Nurses Learn about New Russian 'Relax' System," *Daily Mail*, June 3, 1954.
27. Dick-Read to Ricardo V. Gavensky, Aug. 13, 1955, PP/GDR/D.217/55, WL.
28. For examples of the conflation of the Read method and psychoprophylaxis, see Ryle, "Wither Natural Childbirth?," 725; L. W. St[atius] Van Eps, "Psychoprophylaxis in Labour," *The Lancet* 266 (July 16, 1955): 112–15.
29. Dick-Read to Kyuya Tamura, Oct. 14, 1955, PP/GDR/D.220/55, WL.
30. Dick-Read to Chertok, Dec. 11, 1956, PP/GDR/D.216/55, WL.
31. Brian Welbeck, "Russians Pirate Painless Birth," *Reynolds News*, Jan. 22, 1956.
32. Seabra-Dinis to Dick-Read, Oct. 28, 1955, PP/GDR/D.220/55, WL.
33. Dick-Read to Seabra-Dinis, Dec. 2, 1955, PP/GDR/D.220/55, WL.
34. Seabra-Dinis to Dick-Read, Dec. 15, 1955; Dick-Read to Seabra-Dinis, Dec. 29, 1955, PP/GDR/D.220/55, WL.
35. Meeting minutes, NCT, May 7, 1959, PP/GDR/D.249/57, WL. Formed in 1947, the Sigerist Society took its name in honor of Henry E. Sigerist, a historian of medicine, Soviet sympathizer, and advocate for universal health insurance in

the United States. See Jeanne Daly, *Evidence-Based Medicine and the Search for a Science of Clinical Care* (Berkeley: University of California Press, 2005), 129. On Sigerist's career and its political dimensions, see Elizabeth Fee and Edward T. Morman, "Doing History, Making Revolution: The Aspirations of Henry E. Sigerist and George Rosen," in *Doctors, Politics and Society: Historical Essays*, ed. Dorothy Porter and Roy Porter (Amsterdam: Editions Rodolpi B. V., 1993), 275–311; Elizabeth Fee and Theodore M. Brown, eds. *Making Medical History: The Life and Times of Henry E. Sigerist* (Baltimore: Johns Hopkins University Press, 1997), esp. 197–314. On his objection to Lamaze breathing as exhausting to the mother and of no real benefit, see Dick-Read, *Childbirth without Fear*, 297. Dick-Read endorsed slow, deep breathing. Psychoprophylaxis utilized a varied repertoire of breathing patterns, but the lighter, more rapid panting style referred to here was considered most helpful during transition.

36. Meeting minutes, NCT, May 7, 1959, PP/GDR/D.249/57, WL.
37. Kitzinger, "Strategies of the Early Childbirth Movement," 94.
38. On the French Catholic pronatalist agenda, see Antoine Prost, "Catholic Conservatives, Population, and the Family in Twentieth Century France," *Population and Development Review* 14 (Mar. 1988): 147–64.
39. Catholic hospitals in Jallieu and Cambrai, to the north of Paris, prepared women for childbirth using psychoprophylaxis. F. Lamaze, "L'accouchement sans douleur par la méthode psycho-prophylaxie," Jan. 1955, typescript, box J-2, UFM. Catholics played an early role promoting psychoprophylaxis in the United States as well. For example, St. Mary's Hospital in St. Louis, Missouri, was among the first institutions to develop psychoprophylaxis courses for expectant mothers outside the northeast. See *ASPO News*, Spring 1965, 1.
40. "L'accouchement sans douleur: Discours du Souverain pontife Pie XII (8 janvier 1956)," Jan. 8, 1956, http://frblin.perso.neuf.fr/ccmf/05textesstsiege/pie12/pie12sante1956a.pdf.
41. Vellay and Vellay-Dalsace, *Témoignages sur l'accouchement sans douleur*, 157.
42. F. Lamaze, typescript, Jan. 16, 1956, box H, UFM.
43. See press clippings from, among other places, Belgium, Switzerland, Algeria, Congo, Morocco, Tunisia, and, of course, France, box D, UFM. The leftist press in France prominently featured news of the pope's decree. See, for example, "Le pape Pie XII approuve l'accouchement sans douleur," *Femmes françaises*, Jan. 21, 1956, 8.
44. "L'accouchement sans douleur: Discours du Souverain pontife Pie XII."
45. His reaction can only be guessed at, as I found no direct comment on the 1956 papal decree among Dick-Read's published or unpublished writings. For Anglophone press coverage, see, for example, "The Pope Approves an 'Easy' Childbirth Method," *Daily Sketch*, Jan. 9, 1956; "Painless Birth Pope Says: Bible Does Not Ban It," *Daily Mirror*, Jan. 9, 1956; "Pope Pronounces on Painless Childbirth," *Manchester Guardian*, Jan. 9, 1956; Barrett McGurn, "Pope Pius Approves Painless Birth Method," *New York Herald*, Jan. 9, 1956; Arnaldo Cortesi, "Pope Sanctions Painless Births," *New York Times*, Jan. 9, 1956.
46. Vellay and Vellay-Dalsace, *Témoignages sur l'accouchement sans douleur*, 195.
47. Geneviève Grattesat, interview with the author, July 9, 2010. Under a pseudonym, derived from the name of the town where she lived, Grattesat published an article on psychoprophylaxis. Clairbois, "Oui, il est possible d'accoucher sans douleur," 12–14. On Grattesat and the place of *La Quinzaine* in France's progressive Catholic movement, see Thierry Keck, *Jeunesse de l'église,*

1936–1955: Aux sources de la crise progressiste en France (Paris: Éditions Karthala, 2004), 246–51. On the Catholic Left and its relationship to the PCF, see Yvon Tranvouez, *Catholiques et communistes: La crise du progressisme chrétien, 1950–55* (Paris: Cerf, 2000).

48. A letter from Dr. Bricart of Ostend, Belgium, comments on the evaporation of resistance to psychoprophylaxis in Catholic-run maternity wards following the pope's decree. It seems safe to infer that to the extent that the method's supporters met with religious opposition elsewhere, such as in provincial France, the matter was similarly put to rest. Vellay and Vellay-Dalsace, *Témoignages sur l'accouchement sans douleur*, 333.

49. Karmel, *Thank You, Dr. Lamaze*, 4.

50. Stenogramma vsesoiuznogo soveshchaniia po dal'neishemu razvitiiu psikhopro-filakticheskoi podgotovki beremennykh k rodam, Feb. 10–14, 1956, TsDAVO, f. 342, op. 15, spr. 4267, ark. 132; Obezbolivanie v rodil'nykh uchrezhdeniiakh goroda Stalingrada v 1951 godu i v 1-m polugodii 1952 goda, Oct. 17, 1952, GARF, f. r-8009, op. 22, d. 249, l. 52.

51. Spravka o khode vypolneniia prikaza MZ SSSR no. 142 i resheniia Kollegii MZ SSSR no. 33 "O vnedrenii metod psikhoprofilakticheskoi podgotovki zhensh-chin k rodam," 1955, TsDAVO, f. 342, op. 15, spr. 3491, ark. 10.

52. In some areas, overall access to pain relief in childbirth actually declined after the launch of the psychoprophylactic campaign. In the southern Russian city of Saratov, for example, over 80 percent of births in 1951 involved the use of pain relief. As of 1954, only 66.6 percent of Saratov's maternity cases benefited from either pharmacological or psychological methods of pain relief, a drop of 17 percent. Stenogramma vsesoiuznogo soveshchaniia, TsDAVO, f. 342, op. 15, spr. 4267, ark. 131.

53. Two years after Order no. 142, only about 15 percent of midwives in Ukraine's Ternopol' region, for example, had received any instruction in the psycho-prophylaxis. Spravka o sostoianii rodovspomozheniia v Ternopol'skoi oblasti, [1953], TsDAVO, f. 342, op. 15, spr. 1782, ark. 48. On ethno-linguistic obstacles, see unsigned memo from Zakarpatskii oblzdrav [to Shchukin?], [1955], TsDAVO, f. 342, op. 14, spr. 3491, ark. 56.

54. Stenogramma vsesoiuznogo soveshchaniia, TsDAVO, f. 342, op. 15, spr. 4267, ark. 255, 257–58.

55. Ibid., ark. 352.

56. Ibid., ark. 219.

57. Ibid., ark. 36. Confusion arises over how many lessons there were because not only did their number vary over time, but some were conducted one-on-one with the patient and others in a group setting, only the latter of which were what most Western observers would have considered childbirth preparation "classes." British nurse Molly Lobban, who traveled to the USSR in 1965 on a study tour, clarifies that the psychoprophylactic course at that time "comprised six talks, the first and last given individually by doctors. The other four are given by midwives to groups of mothers." Molly Lobban, "N. M. Study Tour of the USSR," ii.

58. Stenogramma vsesoiuznogo soveshchaniia, TsDAVO, f. 342, op. 15, spr. 4267, ark. 231.

59. Approximately one-third of the women prepared in psychoprophylaxis in 1951 at Kharkov's Maternity Ward no. 4 received preparation upon arrival. By early 1954, this figure rose to nearly half. These numbers may have been high, but

they were not exceptional. At another maternity ward in Kharkov, 29 percent of women received only express preparation in the first six months of 1954. Spravka o khode vypolneniia prikaza MZSSSR no. 142, TsDAVO, f. 342, op. 15, spr. 3491, ark. 5. See also Protokol soveshchaniia rasshirennogo soveta rodovspomozheniia Khar'kovskoi oblasti, Aug. 24, 1953, DAKhO, R-5125, op. 2, spr. 311, ark. 2; Stenogramma vsesoiuznogo soveshchaniia, TsDAVO, f. 342, op. 15, spr. 4267, ark. 37–42, 45. For criticism of express preparation, see Stenogramma vsesoiuznogo soveshchaniia, TsDAVO, f. 342, op. 15, spr. 4267, ark. 208, 228, 231, 249–50, 351.

60. Protokol soveshchaniia rasshirennogo soveta rodovspomozheniia, DAKhO, R-5225, op. 2, spr. 311, ark. 2; Stenogramma konferentsii akusherok Khar'kovskoi oblasti, Jan. 17, 1955, DAKhO, R-5125, op. 2, spr. 546, ark. 71–76.

61. Stenogramma vsesoiuznogo soveshchaniia, spr. 4267, ark. 143, 144. See also spr. 4267, ark. 187, 189; both in TsDAVO, f. 342, op. 15.

62. Stenogramma vsesoiuznogo soveshchaniia, TsDAVO, f. 342, op. 15, spr. 4267, ark. 452.

63. Figurnov, *Painless Childbirth*, 14.

64. P. A. Beloshapko and A. M. Foi, *Obezbolivanie i uskorenie rodov* (Moscow: Medgiz, 1954). See also F. E. Varshavskaia, *Klinicheskie ispytaniia deistviia naibolee dostupnykh v shirokoi praktike metodov i sredstv obezbolivaniia rodov. Aftoreferat dissertatsii na soiskanie uchenoi stepeni kandidata meditsinskikh nauk* (Leningrad: 1-i Leningradskii meditsinskii institut im. akad. I. P. Pavlova, 1954), 4; Stenogramma konferentsii akusherok, DAKhO, R-5125, op. 2, spr. 546, ark. 21–22.

65. A. P. Nikolaev, *Ocherki teorii i praktiki obezbolivaniia rodov* (Leningrad: Medgiz, 1953), 100, 125.

66. Prikaz no. 219-m, MZ SSSR "O provedenii vsesoiuznogo soveshchaniia po dal'neishemu vnedreniiu psikhoprofilaktiki i podgotovki beremennykh k rodam," Oct. 3, 1955, TsDAVO f. 342, op. 15, spr. 4267, ark. 1–4.

67. Stenogramma vsesoiuznogo soveshchaniia, TsDAVO, f. 342, op. 15, spr. 4267, ark. 239. Select papers from the 1956 all-union conference on psychoprophylaxis are published in *Akusherstvo i ginekologiia* 32 (May–June 1956), summarized in Chertok, "Étude de la psycho-prophylaxie," 2619–26.

68. Stenogramma vsesoiuznogo soveshchaniia, TsDAVO, f. 342, op. 15, spr. 4267, ark. 55–56, 130. One male obstetrician observed the peculiarity of men propounding the theory that childbirth was naturally painless. He was greeted with applause when he noted that "men speak very authoritatively that there should be no pain, that these are all remnants that should be struggled against. It is necessary to draw the attention of our women doctors to this matter, which I am deeply convinced cannot be decided only by men." Stenogramma vsesoiuznogo soveshchaniia, TsDAVO, f. 342, op. 15, spr. 4267, ark. 485–86. Nikolaev claimed that, without any psychological or pharmacological intervention, between 7 and 14 percent of all labors were painless. A. P. Nikolaev, "Osnovnye printsipy i puty obezbolivaniia v rodakh," in *Obezbolivanie v rodakh: Trudy konferentsii v g. Leningrade, 29–31 ianvaria 1951 g.*, ed. A. P. Nikolaev (Moscow: Izdatel'stvo akademii meditsinskikh nauk SSSR, 1952), 29.

69. Stenogramma vsesoiuznogo soveshchaniia, TsDAVO, f. 342, op. 15, spr. 4267, ark. 416.

70. Ibid., ark. 158. V. F. Matveeva, chair of the Department of Obstetrics and Gynecology at the Kharkov Medical Institute, pointed out that the objective was for childbirth to be painless, and if psychoprophylaxis was not working, then

pharmacological means were simply indispensable. Stenogramma konferentsii akusherok, DAKhO, R-5125, op. 2, spr. 546, ark. 21.

71. Stenogramma vsesoiuznogo soveshchaniia, TsDAVO, f. 342, op. 15, spr. 4267, ark. 251–52, 380, 420, 534. Obstetricians endorsed, among other drugs, lidol, promedol (trimeperidine), and tekodin (oxycodone).

72. Stenogramma vsesoiuznogo soveshchaniia, TsDAVO, f. 342, op. 15, spr. 4267, ark. 29–30, 47, 103, 122, 162, 240,315, 358, 398, 430, 411.

73. Ibid., ark. 116.

74. Ibid., ark. 158. The previous year he described it as "the most important issue" in midwifery because it was the foundation for all prenatal preparation and education. Even as it focused on reducing fear and the consequent pain, the lessons provided an opportunity for midwives to keep a watchful eye over their patients and to help them prepare for the postpartum phase. Stenogramma konferentsii akusherok, DAKhO, R-5125, op. 2, spr. 546, ark. 70.

75. Stenogramma vsesoiuznogo soveshchaniia, TsDAVO, f. 342, op. 15, spr. 4267, ark. 426, 520, 532.

76. Ibid., ark. 423.

77. Ibid., ark. 68.

78. For example, ibid., ark. 192. See also Stenogramma oblastnogo soveshchaniia rabotnikov zdravookhraneniia Khar'kovskoi oblasti, July 10, 1952, DAKhO, f. R-5125, op. 2, spr. 182, ark. 5.

79. For example, see Stenogramma vsesoiuznogo soveshchaniia, TsDAVO, f. 342, op. 15, spr. 4267, ark. 26, 129, 158, 172, 181, 222, 248, 286, 375.

80. Order no. 142 was republished in translation in an effort to promote psychoprophylaxis abroad, though it was not taken up with equal enthusiasm everywhere within the Soviet sphere of influence. E. g., *Vremenna instruktsiia za obezbolivane na razhdaneto po psikhoprofilaktichniia metod na Velvovski* (Sofia: Nauka i izkustvo, 1952). On Czechoslovakia, see Ema Hrešanová, *Kultury dvou porodnic: Etnografická studie* (Plzeň: Vydavatelství ZČU v Plzni, 2008), 71–72.

81. Stenogramma vsesoiuznogo soveshchaniia, TsDAVO, f. 342, op. 15, spr. 4267, ark. 31,72; Jeanson, *Principes et pratique de l'accouchement sans douleur*.

82. Stenogramma vsesoiuznogo soveshchaniia, TsDAVO, f. 342, op. 15, spr. 4267, ark. 32.

83. Ibid., ark. 78. Lamaze and his collaborators had done work on the use of psychoprophylaxis in breech deliveries, which may have inspired Vel'vovskii to consider the applicability of psychoprophylaxis in births with complications. Ibid., ark. 109.

84. Ibid., ark. 233–34; I. Z. Vel'vovskii, *Sistema psikhoprophilaktiki bolei v rodakh. Aftoreferat dissertatsii na soiskanie uchenoi stepeni doktora meditsinskikh nauk* (Khar'kov: Khar'kovskii meditsinskii institut, 1957); I. Z. Vel'vovskii, *Sistema psikhoprofilakticheskogo obezbolivaniia rodov* (Moscow: Gosudarstvennoe izdatel'stvo meditsinskoi literatury, 1963).

85. Helen Heardman, *A Way to Natural Childbirth: A Manual for Physiotherapists and Parents-to-Be* (Edinburgh: Livingstone, 1948); Helen Heardman, *Relaxation and Exercise for Natural Childbirth* (Edinburgh: E. & S. Livingston, 1950). Two MCA nurses trained by Heardman were among the earliest US practitioners of the Read methods, which they taught along with Heardman's exercises. Like Dick-Read, Heardman visited the United States to promote Natural Childbirth.

Thoms to Dick-Read, Feb. 10, 1948; Thoms to Dick-Read, Apr. 3, 1950; both in PP/GDR/D.196, WL.

86. Stenogramma vsesoiuznogo soveshchaniia, TsDAVO, f. 342, op. 15, spr. 4267, ark. 88, 108, 169, 289, 412. Dick-Read advocated a series of exercises similar to certain simple, restful yoga poses. While he believed that these exercises enhanced breathing and improved flexibility during labor, he was quick to emphasize that exercise "is beneficial for many women, it is not essential for normal birth." Dick-Read, *Childbirth without Fear*, 320.

87. B. L. Gurtovoi, "Zaochnaia shkola psikhoprofilakticheskoi podgotovki k rodam: Zaniatie pervoe," *Zdorov'e*, Mar. 1969, 24; E. I Safronova, *Vliianie kompleksnoi psikhofizicheskoi podgotovki na techenie beremennosti i iskhody rodov dlia materi i ploda. Aftoreferat dissertatsii na soiskanie uchenoi stepeni kandidata meditsinskikh nauk* (Khar'kov: Khar'kovskii meditsinskii institut, 1966), 14.

88. A. P. Nikolaev, *Obezbolivanie rodov* (Leningrad: Meditsina, 1964), 80–81; A. A. Lebedev, "Fiziopsikhoprofilaktika v akusherstve," *Akusherstvo i ginekologiia* 42 (Jan. 1966): 40. In 1954 the method's precise name had been changed from "psychoprophylaxis of labor pain," which emphasized its anesthetizing properties, to "psychoprophylactic preparation of expectant women for labor," which stressed the method's didactic and behavioral goals. See Stenogramma vsesoiuznogo soveshchaniia, TsDAVO, f. 342, op. 15, spr. 4267, ark. 213.

89. Nikolaev, *Obezbolivanie rodov*, 81, 88; Kon''iukturnyi obzor po razdelu akushersko-ginekologicheskoi pomoshchi v Leningradskoi oblasti, 1969, GARF f. A-482, op. 54, d. 3616, l. 75.

90. S. A. Iagunov, *Fizkul'tura v periode beremennosti* (Leningrad, 1938); S. A. Iagunov, "Fizkul'tura: Znachenie fizicheskoi kul'tury v periode beremennosti," *Fel'dsher i akusherka* (Apr. 1950): 33–38; S. A. Iagunov, *Fizkul'tura vo vremia beremennosti i v poslerodovom periode* (Leningrad: Medgiz, 1959); S. A. Iagunov and L. N. Startseva, "Primenenie sredstv fizicheskoi kul'tury i vrachebnogo kontrolia v rodakh," *Akusherstvo i ginekologiia* 35 (Mar. 1959): 14–19. Vel'vovskii traces the Soviet integration of physical therapy to Iagunov and Startseva in his *Sistema psikhoprofilakitcheskogo obezbolivaniia rodov*, 278. See also Safronova, *Vliianie kompleksnoi psikhofizicheskoi podgotovki*, 4.

91. Gurtovoi, "Zaochnaia shkola psikhoprofilakticheskoi podgotovki," 23–25; N. A. Lebedeva, "Budushchim materiam," *Zdorov'e*, Nov. 1960, 24; M. A. Petrov-Maslakov, *Obezbolivanie rodov* (Moscow: Meditsina, 1967). *Zdorov'e* was a popular magazine, with a circulation of 800,000.

92. A. Kh. Dobbin, "'Estestvennye' rody: Opyt avstraliiskogo vracha," *Akusherstvo i ginekologiia* 33 (Mar.–April 1957), 41–44. The effort to date psychoprophylaxis to a period earlier than the Read method made its way into the American literature, too. Citing Vellay as the source, one article incorrectly claimed that "by 1930" Nikolaev, Vel'vovskii, and Platonov had "abandoned hypnosis in favor of a method that would attack not only the symptoms but the causes of pain." Pricilla Richardson Ulin, "The Exhilarating Moment of Birth," *American Journal of Nursing* 63 (June 1963): 61.

93. Vel'vovskii, *Sistema psikhoprofilaktiki bolei v rodakh*; Vel'vovskii, *Sistema psikhoprofilakticheskogo obezbolivaniia rodov*, 261–87.

94. Iu. F. Zmanovskii, *Dinamika izmenenii vysshei nervnoi deiatel'nosti beremennykh pod vliianiem psikhoprofilakticheskoi podgotovki k rodam. Aftoreferat dissertatsii na soiskanie uchenoi stepeni kandidata meditsinskikh nauk* (Moscow: 1-i Moskovskii Ordena Lenina Meditsinskii Institut im. I. M. Sechenova, 1962), 4.

95. Vel'vovskii, *Sistema psikhoprofilaktiki bolei v rodakh*, 5.

96. F. A. Syrovatko, "Teoriia i praktika psikhoprofilakticheskoi podgotovki bere-mennykh k rodam," *Akusherstvo i ginekologiia* 33 (July–Aug. 1957): 6–7; A. P. Nikolaev, "Osnovnye itogi tvorcheskogo primeneniia fiziologicheskogo ucheniia I. P. Pavlova v akusherstve i ginekologii," *Akusherstvo i ginekologiia* 33 (Sept.–Oct. 1957): 54–56; A. P. Nikolaev, *Obezbolivanie rodov*, 13–14; Vel'vovskii, *Sistema psikhoprofilakticheskogo obezbolivaniia rodov*, 274.

97. Assemblée Nationale, Proposition no. 5868, Loi tendant à l'enseignement et au développement de la méthode d'accouchement sans douleur par psychothéra-pie, Mar. 13, 1953, box L, UFM.

98. Ibid.; "Résolution tendant à l'expérimentation dans quelques maternités de l'Assistance publique des méthodes d'accouchement sans douleur," *Bulletin municipal officiel de la ville de Paris: Débats des assemblées de la ville de Paris et du département de la Seine* 74 (Jan. 26, 1954): 1113–114; "Le Conseil municipal de Paris: 15 millions pour développer l'accouchement sans douleur," *France-URSS*, Mar. 1954, 15; "Le Conseil municipal de Paris et l'accouchement 'sans douleur,'" *Médecine et hygiène*, Apr. 30, 1954, press clipping, box L, UFM; "Accouchement sans douleur: Des hôpitaux parisiens vont être équipés," *L'Humanité*, Feb. 3, 1954; F. Le Guay, "Conditions pratiques de réalisation de l'accouchement sans douleur à la Maternité des Métallurgistes," *Revue de la nouvelle médecine* 1 (May 1954): 145; "Au Conseil municipal de Paris: L'accouchement sans douleur," *L'Humanité*, Nov. 30, 1954.

99. René Angelergues, "'L'opération Read' et la vérité sur l'accouchement sans dou-leur," *L'Humanité*, June 15, 1954.

100. On the RPF, see Jean Charlot, *De Gaulle et le Rassemblement du People Français, 1947–1955* (Paris: Armand Colin, 1998); Richard Vinen, *Bourgeois Politics in France* (New York: Cambridge University Press, 1995), 216–33.

101. Rapport no. 10558, Assemblée Nationale, Mar. 30, 1955, box L, UFM. Emphasis mine.

102. "Une interview du Dr. Lamaze," 12; Proposition de loi no. 884 tendant à l'enseignement et au développement de la méthode d'accouchement sans douleur par psychoprophylaxie, Assemblée Nationale, Feb. 29, 1956, box L, UFM; Rapport No. 2190 au nom de la Commission de la famille, de la population et de la santé publique sur la proposition de loi (no. 884) de Mme Rabaté et plusieurs de ses collègues tendant à l'enseignement et au développement de la méthode d'accouchement sans douleur par psychopro-phylaxie, box L, UFM; Caron-Leulliez and George, *L'accouchement sans dou-leur*, 74, 105; Laurence Lentin, "Vous y croyez vous?" *Heures claires*, Mar. 9, 1957, 26.

103. Fernande Harlin, *Préparez-vous à une heureuse maternité* (Paris: Denoël, 1951), front cover. The book's preface emphasizes both Dick-Read's work and similar, Scandinavian influences (7–8).

104. Ch[arles] Devemy to unspecified recipient, May 20, 1957, box E, UFM. Emphasis added. On Harlin, see Caron-Leulliez and George, *L'accouchement sans douleur*, 31.

105. Chertok, "Étude de la psycho-prophylaxie," 2619–26.

106. Lepage and Langevin-Droguet, *La préparation à l'accouchement sans crainte*.

107. Dick-Read to Lepage, Mar. 6, 1957, PP/GDR/C.25/21, WL.

108. Lepage to Dick-Read, Mar. 14, 1957, PP/GDR/C.25/21, WL.

109. Dick-Read to Luigi Bacialli, Apr. 23, 1959, PP/GDR/D.216/55, WL.

110. Journée d'études sur les méthodes psychologiques en analgésie obstétricale, conference program, Apr. 7, 1957, PP/GDR/C.86/26, WL. Read supporters at the conference included Paris's Maurice Mayer; Dick-Read did not appear on the program, but the text of his address and subsequent correspondence make his attendance and presentation clear. Mayer and Bonhomme, "La méthode de l'accouchement naturel, son utilisation en pratique hospitalière," 751–66.

111. Letter of invitation from La Société de Médecine Psychosomatique to Dick-Read, Mar. 3, 1957, PP/GDR/C.86/26, WL. Lamaze and Vellay appeared on the program, but Lamaze had died the previous month and it is unclear whether or not Vellay canceled due to the upheaval at Les Bluets in the wake of Lamaze's untimely demise. Vel'vovskii had been invited, but could not attend.

112. Dick-Read to Chertok, May 22, 1957, PP/GDR/C.86/26, WL.

113. G. Fuzet, summary of USTM report, [1957]; Propositions relatives au fonctionnement de la maternité et à la poursuite de notre combat pour l'accouchement sans douleur, [1957]; F. Le Guay, Rapport sur la maison de santé maternité, [1957]; Rapport de l'équipe d'A.S.D. sur les propositions de l'USTM, Mar. 29, 1957; all in box A, UFM. USTM leaders may here have been following the lead of Soviet administrators, who, as noted above, had begun to shift prenatal preparation courses to midwives beginning in 1954.

114. Quoted in Gutmann, *The Legacy of Dr. Lamaze*, 183.

115. Jean Dalsace to André Lunet, Mar. 6, 1957, box A, UFM. The letter is reprinted and translated, slightly differently than I have here, in full in Gutmann, *The Legacy of Dr. Lamaze*, 197. For a discussion of Dalsace's life and work, see R. Palmer, "Jean Dalsace, 1893–1970," *Gynécologie et obstétrique* 70 (Jan.–Feb. 1971): 7–14.

116. Pierre Vellay to USTM, Mar. 6, 1957, box A, UFM. The Medical Commission at Les Bluets repeated these accusations in a letter to the polyclinic's administration, Mar. 8, 1957, box A, UFM. Of course, Lunet rejected the accusation that somehow he and other USTM representatives had Lamaze's blood on their hands and they expressed to Lamaze's widow and the Les Bluets community in general their sorrow at Dr. Lamaze's death. For Lunet's defense of his relationship with Lamaze, see his letter to Madame Lamaze, n.d., box A, UFM.

117. "Le docteur Lamaze est mort," *L'Humanité*, Mar. 7, 1957; "Le docteur Lamaze et l'accouchement sans douleur," *L'Humanité*, Mar. 7, 1957; "L'hommage du Comité Central du Parti Communiste Français," *L'Humanité*, Mar. 7, 1957. Letters of condolence arrived the next day from across Europe, including from Moscow's Institute of Obstetrics. "Hommage au docteur Lamaze," *L'Humanité*, Mar. 8, 1957.

118. "Fernand Lamaze," *L'Express*, Mar. 8, 1957, 23.

119. "Indécence communiste," *Le Figaro*, Mar. 11, 1957.

120. "Après la mort du docteur Lamaze," *Le Monde*, Mar. 12, 1957; Francois Le Guay, "Un profond dégoût," *L'Express*, Mar. 22, 1957, 35. See also François Le Guay, "Une lettre de l'union des métallurgistes (C.G.T.)," *Le Figaro*, Mar. 25, 1957; La Commission médicale du Centre de santé Docteur–P.-Rouquès, "Pas de désaccord," *L'Express*, Mar. 22, 1957, 35.

121. Gutmann, *The Legacy of Dr. Lamaze*, 200. While she does not adopt their argument that the union contributed to Lamaze's death, Gutmann rightly points out the hypocrisy of those in the press and other public venues who claimed to take pride in Lamaze's work and to support his campaign for psychoprophylaxis, after having just tried to slash his budget and end his efforts to train doctors and midwives in psychoprophylaxis.

122. As already noted, Le Guay resigned and Fuzet's original plan for budgetary reductions went forward. Albert Carn replaced Le Guay as director of Les Bluets and oversaw the restructuring of the maternity ward. André Bourrel and the three most senior midwives on the psychoprophylactic team all quit with Pierre Vellay. Bourrel and his wife, midwife Micheline Bourrel, eventually found a professional home at the Maternité des Lilas, which in the 1970s gained notoriety for the work of Frederick Leboyer and his practice of "childbirth without violence." Caron-Leulliez and George, *L'accouchement sans douleur*, 123; "Histoire," *Maternité des Lilas*, Dec. 10, 2010, http://www.maternite-des-lilas.com/content/histoire.

123. Madame Rouat to André Lunet, July 10, 1957, box A, UFM.

124. Claude Bazin to Lunet, Aug. 16, 1957, box A, UFM.

125. [René] Angelergues, [Henri] Vermorel and [Pierre] Vellay, "Évolution de la méthode psycho-prophylactique," *Bulletin officiel de la Société internationale de psycho-prophylaxie obstétricale* 2 (Apr.–Dec. 1960), 115–33. On the turn among psychoprophylaxis advocates toward psychoanalysis in France, see L. Chertok, "Theories of Psychoprophylaxis in Obstetrics (Prophylaxis or Therapy)," *American Journal of Psychiatry* 119 (June 1963): 1154–59. Angelergues's move to a more ecumenical approach to psychology followed the course of some of his Soviet colleagues amid and in the wake of de-Stalinization. See Léon Chertok, "Reinstatement of the Concept of the Unconscious in the Soviet Union," *American Journal of Psychiatry* 138 (May 1981): 575–83; *Dialogue franco-soviétique sur la psychanalyse*, compiled by Léon Chertok (Toulouse: Privat, 1984).

126. Marianne Caron-Leulliez, "L'accouchement sans douleur: Un enjeu politique en France pendant la guerre froide," *Canadian Bulletin of Medical History/Bulletin canadien d'histoire de la médecine* 23 (2006): 85; Chertok claims that this figure approached 50 percent by 1963. Chertok, "Reply to Foregoing," 607.

127. "100 médecins de 22 pays confrontent leurs expériences sur l'accouchement sans douleur," *L'Humanité*, July 12, 1962. According to Vellay, about 40 percent of French women received training in psychoprophylaxis as of 1963, suggesting that perhaps figures in *L'Humanité* were inflated. Not only are there questions about quality of preparation and standards of practice, but even as psychoprophylaxis was gaining in popularity and enjoying the central government's financial largesse through a universal health care system that covered the costs of preparatory courses and paid leave from work to attend them, some women refused training. A lack of time, discipline, or faith in the method's efficacy were among reasons women gave for turning down the opportunity to access psychoprophylactic courses. Pierre Vellay, typescript, [1963], accession (hereafter cited as accn.) 2000–M173, box 1, fol. 2, Lamaze International Records (hereafter cited as LI), SL; Claude Revault d'Allonnes, "Une enquête préliminaire sur l'accouchement sans douleur," *Revue française de sociologie* 1 (Apr.–June 1960): 205.

128. Lawrence Z. Freedman, address at the memorial service for Dick-Read, transcript, July 8, 1959, MC515/BACE/1.10, SL.

129. A phrase commonly used in the 1960s to describe the kind of birth experience women sought as an alternative to one under heavy anesthesia, it served as the title to one of the era's most popular books. Irwin Chabon, *Awake and Aware: Participating in Childbirth through Psychoprophylaxis* (New York: Delacorte Press, 1966).

CHAPTER 5

1. Isidore Bonstein, *Psychoprophylactic Preparation for Painless Childbirth* (London: William Heinemann Books, 1958).
2. Kelliher, "Natural Childbirth in Boston."
3. C. D. McGratty to J. E. Maltby, [1956], PP/GDR/C.20/20, WL. For similar remarks, see "Not Really Scientific, Says Scot," *The Bulletin*, Jan. 9, 1957, press clipping, PP/GDR/C.137/33, WL.
4. Karmel, *Thank You, Dr. Lamaze*, 14.
5. Elaine Zwelling, "Looking Back in Time: An Interview with Madame Blanche Cohen," *Journal of Perinatal Education* 8 (Dec. 1999): 4; Karmel, *Thank You, Dr. Lamaze*. The book was quickly published in a French translation done by Vellay and his wife Aline. Marjorie Karmel, *J'ai accouché sans douleur*, trans. A. Dalsace-Vellay and P. Vellay (Paris: A. Fayard, 1960).
6. Dick-Read, notes for NCT board meeting comments, [1959], PP/GDR/D.249/57, WL.
7. For example, over time the number of breathing patterns recommended for different stages of labor became quite complex and cumbersome, though it is the panting breaths that are most widely associated with psychoprophylaxis in popular culture. By the late 1960s, there were about twenty distinct breathing patterns in the Lamaze method as practiced in the United States. See Birth Reports, Nov. 1968–Mar. 1969, MC515/BACE/12.10, SL.
8. Waldo L. Fielding and Lois Benjamin, *The Childbirth Challenge: Commonsense versus "Natural" Methods* (New York: Viking, 1962), 9.
9. Though from a twenty-first century perspective, American birth stories of the 1950s and early 1960s appear circumspect, they were far more direct than before World War II. By the early 1960s, birth stories were widely published in newspapers, magazines, and books, and quite graphic educational films were in use in childbirth education courses, such as those taught by the MCA. "Education for Childbearing and Parenthood," transcript, Mar. 2–3, 1961, box 5, fol. 1, MCA, LHSL.
10. Mary Cantwell, "Hers," *New York Times*, Feb. 14, 1980.
11. Elisabeth Bing, *My Life in Birth* (Washington, DC: Lamaze International, 2000), 83–96. Before Karmel's work appeared, Bing had read Bonstein, *Psychoprophylactic Preparation for Painless Childbirth*.
12. Bing, *My Life in Birth*, 87. See also Elaine Zwelling, "The History of Lamaze Continues: Interview with Elisabeth Bing," *Journal of Perinatal Education* 9 (2000): 15–21; "Interview with Elisabeth Bing," *American Baby CBE Reporter: A Supplement to American Baby Magazine*, Spring 2001, 3.
13. ASPO Organizing Committee Constitution and membership list, n.d., accn. 2000–M58, carton (hereafter cited as car.) 1, LI, SL.
14. ASPO Annual Report, Dec. 1962, accn. 2000–M58, car. 1, LI, SL.
15. Minutes, ASPO Executive Meeting, Nov. 1, 1961, accn. 2003–M153, box 1; ASPO Annual Report, Dec. 1962, accn. 2000–M58, car. 1; both in LI, SL. The manual was published as Elisabeth Bing, Marjorie Karmel, and Alfred Tanz, *A Practical Training Course for the Psychoprophylactic Method of Childbirth* (New York: American Society for Psychoprophylaxis in Obstetrics, 1961). It earned the moniker Red Manual thanks to its red cover. Bing published a similar manual intended for use in childbirth preparation courses. See Elisabeth Bing, *Six Practical Lessons for An Easier Childbirth* (New York: Grosset & Dunlop, 1967).
16. Bing, *My Life in Birth*, 88.

17. Prepared remarks, [Elisabeth Bing], WBAI broadcast, Mar. 1961, typescript, accn. 2004–M29, fol. 2, LI, SL. I infer that the remarks were Bing's because the text was found among her papers and has notations and corrections in her handwriting, though it is possible that Segal, Tanz, or another early ASPO leader delivered them.

18. Muriel A. Golden to Harold Winkler, Mar. 24, 1960 [*sic*?], accn. 2004–M29, fol. 2, LI, SL. Handwritten at the top of her notes for the program, Bing gives the broadcast date as March 1961, but Golden's letter puts it as March 1, 1960. It seems doubtful that Golden's letter refers to a different broadcast. I suspect the year on Golden's letter is just a typographical error.

19. WBAI Program Portfolio, June 9, 1963, 14, WBAI Folio, Pacifica Radio Archives, Internet Archive, http://ia600308.us.archive.org/23/items/wbaifolio411wbairich/wbaifolio411wbairich.pdf; Minutes, ASPO Executive Committee Meeting, Mar. 18, 1963, accn. 2000–M173, car. 2, LI, SL. Les Bluets' Hersilie responded to CBS's request for the use of excerpts from the Vellay film by offering a different film, *Accoucher sans douleur*, made after Vellay's departure from Les Bluets. Records do not make clear which film, if any, was in fact broadcast on CBS. Perry Miller to Roger Hersilie, Feb. 4, 1963; Hersilie to Miller, Feb. 8, 1963; both in box M, UFM. Pierre Vellay made *Naissance* in 1961. ASPO rented copies of it to interested groups around the country. ICEA Film and Record Directory, 1972, MC515/BACE/5.16, SL.

20. E.g., Alan Guttmacher, review of *Childbirth without Fear*, *Parents*, May 1945, 158–59; Nicholson J. Eastman, *Expectant Motherhood*, 3rd ed. (Boston: Little, Brown, 1957), 157; Duncan E. Reid and Mandel E. Cohen, "Evaluation of Present Day Trends in Obstetrics," *Journal of the American Medical Association* 142 (Mar. 4, 1950): 615–23; Carl T. Javert and James D. Hardy, "Measurement of Pain Intensity in Labor and Its Physiologic, Neurologic, and Pharmacologic Implications," *American Journal of Obstetrics and Gynecology* 60 (Sept. 1950): 552–63. Deeply upset about Reid and Cohen's article, Dick-Read fretted over the negative impact of the article that he characterized as "much publicized." Dick-Read to Thoms, Mar. 27, 1950, PP/GDR/D.196, WL.

21. Waldo L. Fielding and Lois Benjamin, "The Medical Case against Natural Childbirth," *McCall's*, June 1962, 106. See also Fielding and Benjamin, *Childbirth Challenge*.

22. Natalie Gittelson, "The Case against Natural Childbirth," *Harper's Bazaar*, Feb. 1961, 137.

23. Ibid., 136.

24. Ibid., 137, 179.

25. Fielding and Benjamin, "Medical Case against Natural Childbirth," 185. See also Fielding and Benjamin, *Childbirth Challenge*, 51–52.

26. Fielding and Benjamin, "Medical Case against Natural Childbirth," 184.

27. Ibid., 183.

28. Mardi J. Horowitz and Nancy F. Horowitz, "Psychologic Effects of Education for Childbirth," *Psychosomatics* 8 (July–Aug. 1967): 197.

29. Fielding and Benjamin, *Childbirth Challenge*, 18. See also Arnold A. Hutschnecker, "Medicine and Psychiatry in the USSR," *Psychosomatics* 1 (Sept.–Oct. 1960): 257–59.

30. Fielding and Benjamin, *Childbirth Challenge*, 35.

31. Bing, *My Life in Birth*, 88. As for American physicians and their understanding of and interest in psychoprophylaxis's Soviet origins, it is evident in, for

example, Thomas L. Ball, "The Psychoprophylactic Preparation of Pregnant Women for Childbirth in the Union of Soviet Socialist Republics," *Transactions of the New York Academy of Sciences*, ser. 2, 22 (June 1960): 578–80.

32. David A. Meyer, "The Physician as Teacher," *ASPO Newsletter* 1 (Winter 1961): 1.
33. Ulin, "Exhilarating Moment of Birth," 62. Other publications simply made no mention whatsoever of the method's Soviet origins. A particularly vivid example of this historical erasure comes from Great Britain, where a psychiatrist drew a seemingly straight line from Grantly Dick-Read to psychoprophylaxis, mentioning Swiss physician Bonstein as the conduit for transfer to the United States and briefly referencing Lamaze, but offering no credit to Soviet pioneers. A. Balfour Sciare, "Psychoprophylaxis in Obstetrics," *Nursing Times*, Oct. 8, 1965, 1373–74.
34. Pierre Vellay, "The Aim of Psychoprophylaxis," typescript, Apr. 17, 1963, accn. 2000–M173, box 1, fol. 2, LI, SL. See also Horowitz and Horowitz, "Psychologic Effects of Education for Childbirth," 197.
35. This change was codified in 1965, when ASPO adopted new bylaws. Accn. 2000–M58, car. 1, LI, SL.
36. Jean Anderson, with Heinz Luschinsky, Benjamin Segal, and Alfred Tanz, "The Medical Case for Natural Childbirth: A Reply to Dr. Waldo Fielding," *ASPO Special Publication* (New York: ASPO, 1962), 1. On ASPO's effort to organize a response from its supporters, see Form letter from Judith Frisch to ASPO members, July 12, 1962, accn. 2000–M112—2000–M192, box 1, fol. 1, LI, SL.
37. Medical interventions that ASPO supported as useful when medically indicated, but not appropriate as routine procedures, included episiotomies, forceps deliveries, and the use of anesthetics and analgesics. See Anderson et al., "Medical Case for Natural Childbirth."
38. *ASPO Newsletter* 1 (Winter 1961): 1.
39. Prepared remarks, [Elisabeth Bing], WBAI broadcast, Mar. 1961, typescript, accn. 2004–M29, fol. 2, LI, SL.
40. Quoted in "Psychoprophylaxis: Program for Painless Parturition," *Ob/Gyn Observer* 1 (July–Aug. 1962): 8.
41. I located ninety-three of these early physician reports, which were recorded from 1961 to 1964. ASPO Outline Form, Obstetrician's Report, accn. 2003–M153, box 1, LI, SL. Bonstein was the first to introduce this assessment form in the United States. Bonstein, *Psychoprophylactic Preparation for Painless Childbirth*.
42. ASPO Outline Form, Obstetrician's Report, Nov. 11, 1961, accn. 2003–M153, box 1, LI, SL.
43. Barbara Katz Rothman, *In Labor: Women and Power in the Birthplace* (New York: Norton, 1982), 90.
44. Though she credits the effectiveness of the Lamaze method to Segal's ability to guide her through its proper application, Mrs. L. also likely had moved past transition into the second stage of labor, which most women experience as far less painful, even completely painless.
45. Mrs. L., interview with the author, Chapel Hill, NC, Oct. 4, 2011.
46. Deborah Ruth Wolf Tanzer, "The Psychology of Pregnancy and Childbirth: An Investigation of Natural Childbirth," Ph.D. diss., Brandeis University, 1967.
47. Abraham Maslow, *Religions, Values, and Peak Experiences* (Columbus: The Ohio State University Press, 1964).
48. Tanzer, "The Psychology of Pregnancy and Childbirth," 294–95.
49. Ibid., 298.
50. Ibid., 308.

51. Ibid., 303.
52. Deborah Tanzer, *Why Natural Childbirth? A Psychologist's Report on the Benefits to Mothers, Fathers, and Babies* (New York: Doubleday, 1972); Deborah Tanzer, "Natural Childbirth: Pain or Peak Experience," *Psychology Today* (October 1968): 18–21, 69. For the ASPO reprint, see accn. 2000-M58, car. 2, LI, SL.
53. *ASPO Newsletter* 1 (Fall 1960), 1. Despite their disinterest in promoting psychoprophylaxis at home, Soviet authorities took offense at the growing understanding of France as the leader in this field. "Paris is a charming city, but why should it become the center for the spread of Soviet psychoprophylaxis which originated in Kharkov?" a Comrade Markov was reported to have complained in the Leningrad Communist Party's weekly organ *Nedelia*. "Paris avant Moscou?" *France-URSS* (Feb. 1966), press clipping, box 145, 88AS Association France-URSS, ANF.
54. Heinz Luschinsky to Vellay, June 15, 1962, accn. 2000–M112—2000–M192 [2000–M173], box 1, fol. 1, LI, SL; Anderson's rebuttal to Waldo Fielding appeared in French translation in that journal. Jean Anderson, "Le cas médical de l'accouchement naturel," *Bulletin officiel de la Société internationale de psycho-prophylaxie obstétricale* 4 (Oct.-Dec. 1962): 195–202. *Bulletin officiel de la Société internationale de psycho-prophylaxie obstétricale* ran from 1959 to 1978, with issues usually appearing two to four times annually.
55. Registration form, First International Congress of Psychosomatic Medicine and Maternity, Paris, July 8 12, 1962, accn. 2003–M153, box 1, LI, SL. See also *Bulletin officiel de la Société internationale de psycho-prophylaxie obstétricale* 4 (Apr.–June 1962), which was devoted entirely to coverage of the conference. Vel'vovskii submitted a paper that was read at the conference, but he was unable to attend. He did meet Vellay, however, when the latter visited him in Kharkov in 1965. Pierre Vellay, "Impressions sur mon voyage en URSS: Hommage au Professeur Velvovski," *Bulletin officiel de la Société internationale de psycho-prophylaxie obstétricale* 8 (Jan.–Mar. 1966), 147–54.
56. *1er Congrès international de médecine psychosomatique et maternité* (Paris: Gauthier-Villars, 1965). In addition to her observations on childbirth practices around the world, Mead had written extensively and negatively about Soviet childrearing, asserting that Russian swaddling practices resulted in a citizenry in "fear of [its] own ungoverned impulses and the corresponding belief in the importance of a strong state authority, reinforced by modern Bolshevik training in the value and importance of control." "Reds' Tyrant Bias Laid to Babyhood," *New York Times*, Sept. 23, 1951. See also Margaret Mead, *Soviet Attitudes toward Authority: An Interdisciplinary Approach* (New York: William Morrow, 1955).
57. Niles Newton, "The International Congress on Psychosomatic Obstetrics: A Personal Account," typescript, 1962, box 72, fol. 14, MCA, LHSL. Elsewhere, the Soviet commitment to and practice of psychoprophylaxis as a stand-alone solution to obstetric pain continued to be overestimated. "Obstetrics and Gynecology in the USSR," *WHO Chronicle*, Feb. 1966, 56–57.
58. Pierre Vellay to Physician Members of the ASPO, confidential memorandum, 1963, 2000–M173, car. 2, LI, SL; Patricia Richardson Ulin, "Pierre Vellay: Exporter of Obstetric Reform," *American Journal of Nursing* 63 (June 1963): 62–63. Launched in 1961, the ICEA serves as an umbrella organization for childbirth education organizations that promoted various strains of natural childbirth.

59. [Pierre Vellay], "The Vellay Tour Is over Now," typescript, [1963], 2000–M173, car. 2, LI, SL.

60. Vellay to Physician Members of the ASPO, confidential memorandum, 1963, 2000–M173, car. 2, LI, SL. Joseph B. De Lee promoted this procedure, which was intended to hasten birth. See Joseph B. De Lee, "The Prophylactic Forceps Operation," *American Journal of Obstetrics and Gynecology* 1 (1920): 34–44; Judith Walzer Leavitt, "Joseph B. De Lee and the Practice of Preventative Obstetrics." *American Journal of Public Health* 78 (Oct. 1988): 1353–59. Flora Hommel was one of the first proponents of psychoprophylaxis in the United States. Unfortunately, I could not draw on her rich archive of personal papers, which only became publically accessible as this book went to press. Flora Hommel Papers, Walter P. Reuther Library, Wayne State University, Detroit, MI.

61. Mrs. L., interview with the author, Oct. 4, 2011, Chapel Hill, NC.

62. Elisabeth Bing, Marjorie Karmel, and Alfred Tanz, *A Practical Training Course for the Psychoprophylactic Method of Childbirth (Lamaze Technique)* (New York: American Society for Psychoprophylaxis in Obstetrics, 1969), 9–10. All subsequent citations refer to this 1969 edition, and not the 1961 edition cited previously.

63. "British Impressions of 'Natural' Americana," *ASPO News* 3 (Winter 1964): 1.

64. See, for example, advice to avoid taking tranquilizers or sedatives during pregnancy in Virginia Apgar, "Advice to the Mother-to-Be," *The American Baby*, Jan. 1963, 25A, reprinted in *International Childbirth Education Association Childbirth Preparation Kit*, 3rd rev. ed. (n.p.: ICEA, 1967).

65. A. Notter "Aspects actuels de la psychoprophylaxie obstétricale en Russie, Ukraine et Pologne: Considérations sur les Instituts de Physiologie et les Maternités," *Lyon médical* 93 (Nov. 5, 1961): 972. For similar observations, see Lobban, "N. M. Study Tour of the USSR," iii. Notter had been practicing the Read method in Lyon since 1952, though over time his work evolved to integrate aspects of psychoprophylaxis. Noirez, "L'accouchement sans douleur," 26. On tensions within the Soviet medical community over psychoprophylaxis, see also Chertok, "Psychoprophylaxie ou psychothérapie obstétricale," 7–8.

66. Andrée Audoin, "Conversation avec le père de l'accouchement sans douleur," *L'Humanité dimanche*, July 15, 1962. Nikolaev advocated the use of Andaxin, a sedative with an active ingredient similar to the one in Demerol.

67. Kon"iunkturnyi obzor Khar'kovskogo oblzdravotdela o sostoianii akushersko-ginekologicheskoi pomoshchi naseleniiu oblasti, 1962, TsDAVO, f. 342, op. 15, d. 8542, l. 13. In Kiev that same year 70 percent of births reportedly utilized some form of pain relief. Of these births, 92 percent involved the use of psychoprophylaxis. Only 0.05 percent of all births in Kiev involved pharmacological pain relief. Despite this extremely low figure, obstetricians at conferences and in professional journals supported the use of drugs to alleviate pain, suggesting that supply was likely the chief obstacle to greater application. Svodnye godovye statisticheskie otchety g. Kieva, TsDAVO, f. 342, op. 15, d. 8896, l. 39ob. There was enormous regional variation, with more remote parts of the Soviet Union reporting considerably lower rates of psychoprophylaxis. In general we can say that training was more widely available in urban areas than in rural areas, and found more in European parts of the USSR than in Asian regions. But it is important to remember that, even in central Russia, preparation could be minimal. In 1964, for example, in rural areas of Leningrad region only 21 percent of

women received psychoprophylactic training and even in urban areas only 62 percent of women were prepared. Rates reportedly inched up over the next few years, but of course these numbers say nothing about clinical application and success during labor; they speak only to advance preparation and they are likely inflated. Kon"iunkturnyi obzor akushersko-ginekologicheskoi pomosh-chi naseleniiu Leningradskoi oblasti, 1966, GARF, f. A-482, op. 54, d. 728, l. 5. By the end of the 1960s, some regions stopped providing the Ministry of Public Health with any statistics about psychoprophylactic preparation or pain relief in childbirth. See, for example, Rodovspomozhenie v Bashkirskoi ASSR, kon"iunkturnyi obzor, 1969, GARF, f. A-482, op. 54, d. 3533, ll. 1–72.

68. Vel'vovskii's continued rejection of the use of pharmacological pain relief in combination with psychoprophylaxis was known to his French colleagues, in addition to Notter's comments, through [I. Z.] Velvovsky, "Extrait du livre: *A.S.D. à travers la psychoprophylaxie*," *Bulletin officiel de la Société internationale de psycho-prophylaxie obstétricale* 3 (July–Sept. 1961): 136.

69. Bernard Muldworf, "À propos de l'accouchement sans douleur: 'Mentalité' et 'psychologie' chez la femme enceinte," *La Pensée*, Oct. 1962, 55.

70. Pierre Vellay, "Psychoprophylaxie et anesthésie," *Bulletin officiel de la Société française de psychoprophylaxie obstétricale*, no. 20 (Dec. 1964): 3; Pierre Vellay, "Travail dirigé et psycho-prophylaxie," *Bulletin officiel de la Société international de psycho-prophylaxie obstétricale* 2 (Jan.–Mar. 1960): 31–45. He later recommended the use of the sedative Gamma OH, also called GHB, and popularly known today as the "date rape" drug, which was widely used in childbirth in Western Europe and the United States in the 1960s. Pierre Vellay, "Position de la psychoprophylaxie par rapport à l'analgésie et à l'anesthésie en obstétrique," *Bulletin officiel de la Société française de psychoprophylaxie obstétricale*, no. 23 (Sept. 1965): 15. See also Pierre Vellay, "The Psychoprophylactic Method: Its Evolution, Present Situation, and Prospects," *Bulletin officiel de la Société internationale de psycho prophylaxie obstétricale* 8 (Jan.–Mar. 1966): 57–58.

71. Albert Ayoub, *L'accouchement sans douleur* (Damascus: n.p., 1962), 96.

72. Growing contact between American and French proponents of psychoprophylaxis may have had some influence. French obstetricians gained exposure to these American predilections when they met American colleagues at conferences, toured US facilities, read American journals, or read American research published in the pages of Francophone journals. For example, see the discussion of the use of Pitocin at Boston Lying-In Hospital in Clement Yahia and Priscilla R. Ulin, "Épreuve préliminaire d'un programme psychosomatique de préparation à l'accouchement," *Bulletin-Programme de la Société internationale de psycho-prophylaxie obstétricale* 7 (July 1965): 122.

73. Marianne R. Michel, "L'accouchement sans douleur à 10 ans," *France observateur*, July 17, 1962, 14.

74. Vellay, "Psychoprophylaxie et anesthésie," 15; Pierre Vellay, "Rapport," *Bulletin officiel de la Société française de psychoprophylaxie obstétricale*, no. 31 (Sept.–Dec. 1967): 53.

75. Roger Hersilie, "La place de la méthode psychoprophylactique dans l'analgésie obstétricale," *Bulletin officiel de la Société française de psychoprophylaxie obstétricale*, no. 21 (Mar. 1965): 24–25.

76. Dr. Nauroy, "L'accouchement sans douleur," *Guérir*, Oct. 1963, 9–12; J. Grasset, "Exposé sur l'accouchement dit 'sans douleur,'" *Médicophone: Magazine sonore d'information médicale*, no. 14 (Sept.–Oct., 1962): track 7.

77. René Angelergues quoted in Chertok, "Psychoprophylaxie ou psychothérapie obstétricale," 9.

78. Ibid., 10, 11; Pierre Vellay, "Aspects psychologiques de la psycho-prophylaxie en obstétrique," *Bulletin officiel de la Société internationale de psycho-prophylaxie obstétricale* 3 (Oct.–Dec. 1961): 178, 179.

79. Vellay, "The Psychoprophylactic Method," 55.

80. Vellay, "Rapport," 51.

81. Muldworf, "À propos de l'accouchement sans douleur," 83.

82. Ibid., 60. The author distinguishes between "psychology," which emerges from private, early experiences in the family of origin and "mentalité," which derives from the broader sociocultural values internalized over time through social engagement (56). Muldworf uses mentalité as it was used by the Annales School of history, most notably by Lucien Febvre (1878–1956), to describe society's "mental universe." François Dosse, *New History in France: The Triumph of the Annales*, trans. Peter V. Conroy, Jr. (Urbana: University of Illinois Press, 1994), 61.

83. Muldworf, "À propos de l'accouchement sans douleur," 62. Simone de Beauvoir, *The Second Sex*, trans. Constance Borde and Sheila Malovany-Chevallier (New York: Knopf, 2010).

84. R. Hersilie, "Sexualité et féminité à la lumière de la psychoprophylaxie: Essai de théorisation," *Bulletin officiel de la Société française de psychoprophylaxie obstétricale* no. 30 (May–Aug. 1967): 12.

85. Ibid., 15.

86. "Psychoprophylaxis: Program for Painless Parturition," 8.

87. Betsy Palmer, "A Story for Melissa," *Mothers to Be and Infant Care*, Fall 1962, 70.

88. Vellay, "Aspects psychologiques de la psycho-prophylaxie en obstétrique," 180.

CHAPTER 6

1. Theodore Sturgeon, "Woman of Earth and Sky and Origins...," *ASPO Newsletter*, April 1970, 1.

2. Pierce Barker, "The Eleventh Hour," *ASPO Newsletter*, [Fall 1974], 1.

3. Sam Binkley, *Getting Loose: Lifestyle Consumption in the 1970s* (Durham, NC: Duke University Press, 2007).

4. Richard Block and Lauren Langman, "Youth and Work: The Diffusion of 'Countercultural' Values," *Youth & Society* 5 (June 1974): 415–16.

5. *The Story of Eric* (dir. David Seltzer, 1971).

6. Jeanne Hirsch, "Watching a Childbirth at Home," in *Proceedings of the First International Childbirth Conference*, ed. Dorothy Tennov and Lolly Hirsch (Stamford, CT: New Moon Communications, 1973), 18.

7. Wertz and Wertz, *Lying-In*, 1.

8. Ina May Gaskin, *Spiritual Midwifery* (Summertown, TN: Book Pub Co., 1978); *Spiritual Midwifery* (Videofarm, 1978); *The Farm Midwives: 1000 Births* (Videofarm, 1979); Ina May Gaskin, "Birth Matters: A Midwife's Manifesta," interview by Susan Page, *The Diane Rehm Show* (July 27, 2011).

9. *The Story of Eric.*

10. Anonymous letter, in *Proceedings of the First International Childbirth Conference*, 33. Emphasis in original.

11. Barbara Ehrenreich and Deirdre English, *Witches, Midwives, and Nurses: A History of Women Healers* (Old Westbury, NY: Feminist Press, 1973); Barbara Ehrenreich

and Deirdre English, *Complaints and Disorders: The Sexual Politics of Sickness* (Old Westbury, NY: Feminist Press, 1973); Betty Friedan, *The Feminine Mystique* (New York: W. W. Norton, 1963). Evidence of women's dissatisfaction had surfaced in the late 1940s and 1950s, but, as historian Ruth Rosen writes, "it took Friedan to put that secret onto the national political agenda." Ruth Rosen, *The World Split Open: How the Modern Women's Movement Changed America* (New York: Viking, 2000), 35. See also Stephanie Coontz, *A Strange Stirring: The* Feminine Mystique *and American Women at the Dawn of the 1960s* (New York: Basic Books, 2011).

12. Sandra Sopko and Nancy Ciocca, "New Childbirth Practices Urged by Return to Old," *Bridgeport Telegram*, June 4, 1973; "International Childbirth Confab Set," *Fair Press*, May 9, 1973.

13. "Open Mike," in *Proceedings of the First International Childbirth Conference*, 29.

14. Kathy Linck, "Legalizing a Woman's Right to Choose," in *Proceedings of the First International Childbirth Conference*, 26. Similarly, Suzanne Arms wrote that "the delivery table is hardly the place for woman to fight for her rights." Suzanne Arms, *Immaculate Deception: A New Look at Women and Childbirth in America* (San Francisco: San Francisco Book Co., 1975), 125.

15. Deirdre English, "Society Makes Us Sick," in *Proceedings of the First International Childbirth Conference*, 5.

16. Barbara Davenport-Slack, "Physiological Correlates of Childbirth Pain," in *Proceedings of the First International Childbirth Conference*, 7.

17. Mary Lou Sapone, "The Psychoprophylactic Method of Childbirth (Lamaze)," in *Proceedings of the First International Childbirth Conference*, 16.

18. Elisabeth Bing, "The Future of Childbirth Education," typescript, June 14, 1976, accn. 2000-M64, box 1, LI, SL.

19. Unpublished letter to the editor, *Ms. Magazine*, Sept. 18, 1978, MC331/ *Ms. Magazine* Letters, 1972–80 (hereafter *Ms.* Letters)/6.175, SL. Quoted with the author's permission.

20. Vivian Mills to Sandra Kelly, Ida Bird, Gary Hickernell, Bob Howard and Sunnye Strickland, Feb. 13, 1974, accn. 2000-M135, car. 1, LI, SL.

21. Mills to Maryann Crouch, Feb. 13, 1974, accn. 2000-M135, car. 1, LI, SL.

22. Ibid.

23. Pat Sparks, memorandum to ASPO Board of Directors, June 1, 1971, accn. 2000-M58, car. 1, LI, SL.

24. Kathryn Rose Gertz, "The Truth about Painless Childbirth," *Harper's Bazaar*, Feb. 1975, 128; Gurney Williams III, "What Natural Childbirth Can Mean to You and Your Family," *Family Health*, Dec. 1973, 28, 38.

25. Murray Enkin, "The January Conference on Psychosomatic Ob-Gyn," *ISPOG Newsletter*, Spring 1973, 4; Dorothy Osborne, "Lamaze Method: Husband, Wife Work Together for A Childbirth 'Experience,'" *Observer* (Charlotte, NC), Mar. 15, 1974; Kitty Hanson, "A Change in the American Way of Having Babies," *Sunday News*, Nov. 21, 1976. Mills to Sunnye Strickland, Feb. 8, 1973; Mary S. Alinder to Jack Stiles, June 24, 1974; Mills to Patrick Krolak, Mar. 5, 1974; all in accn. 2000-M135, car. 1, LI, SL.

26. E.g., Ezzat Abouleish, *Childbirth: A Joy—Not A Suffering* (Philadelphia: Dorrance & Company, 1975), 70.

27. Strickland to ASPO Board of Directors, Sept. 20, 1972, accn. 2000-M58, car. 2, LI, SL. For some, there remained meaningful differences between the Read and Lamaze methods. See, for example, Roberta Manning, "Children of The

Revolution," *All You Can Eat* 3 (Dec. 1972): 17; "Biographical Sketches of Lamaze Instructors: Part I of a Series. Mariel Kinsey," *Lamaze Newsletter* (Cambridge, MA), Jan. 1973, 4; Vicki E. Walton, *Have It Your Way: An Overview of Pregnancy, Labor and Postpartum including Alternatives Available in the Hospital Childbirth Experience* (Seattle: Henry Philips, 1976), 16.

28. Central Jersey Chapter of ASPO to ASPO national office, Feb. 6, 1975, accn. 2000–M135, car. 1, LI, SL.

29. Sheila Kitzinger, *Education and Counselling for Childbirth* (London: Baillière Tindall, 1977), 152.

30. Presentation, Los Angeles ASPO Chapter to the ASPO National Board of Directors, Apr. 23, 1971; Connie Castor to Nicholas Wolf, Mar, 9, 1971; Nancy Whitley to Castor, Apr. 10, 1971; Memorandum, Philip E. Sumner to ASPO Board, Apr. 23, 1971; Castor to ASPO membership, Dec. 14, 1971; Meeting Conclusions, Apr. 23, 1971; Memorandum, Sparks to ASPO Board of Directors and chapters, June 1, 1971; all in accn. 2000–M58, car. 1, LI, SL. "Annual Meeting: The Court Decides," *ASPO Presentations* 1 (Nov. 1972): 4–5; Ferris B. Urbanowski, "Crisis: ASPO vs. ASPO," *ASPO Newsletter*, Apr. 1972, 1–3; Ferris B. Urbanowski, "Crisis: ASPO vs. ASPO Continued," *ASPO Newsletter*, June 1972, 3; "Legal Defense Fund," *ASPO Newsletter*, Oct. 1972, 3; Ferris Buck Urbanowski, interview with the author, Jan. 6, 2012.

31. Castor, Polly DeSanto, Pat Hassid, and Judith Hegarty to ASPO teachers and physicians, June 30, 1972; DeSanto to unspecified recipients, Aug. 12, 1972; Castor, DeSanto, and Hassid to unspecified recipients, Mar. 15, 1973; all in accn. 2000–M135, car. 1, LI, SL. Memorandum, Strickland to ASPO Board of Directors, Sept. 20, 1972, accn. 2000–M58, car. 2, LI, SL; Jeannette L. Samsor, *Childbirth Education: A Nursing Perspective* (New York: John Wiley & Sons, 1979); Patricia Hassid, *Textbook for Childbirth Educators* (Hagerstown, MD: Harper & Row, Medical Department, 1978).

32. Annie Coudray, "L'accouchement sans douleur a 13 ans ce mois-ci," *Le Journal du dimanche*, Mar. 28, 1965. See also P. Vellay, "Facteurs essentiels d'échecs en psychoprophylaxie," in *Medicina psychosomatica in obstetritiis et gynaecologia. Berichte* (Vienna: Verlag der Wiener Medizinischen Akademie, 1965), 167.

33. Lévy, "Le mouvement français pour le planning familial et les jeunes," 75–84; Michelle Zancarini-Fournel, *Histoire des femmes en France, XIXe–XXe siècle* (Rennes: Presses universitaires de Rennes, 2005), 144–46; Duchen, *Feminism in France*, 49–66. On May 1968, see Ingrid Gilcher-Holtey, "France," in *1968 in Europe: A History of Protest and Activism, 1956-1977*, ed. Martin Klimke and Joachim Scharloth (New York: Palgrave Macmillan, 2008), 111–24; Michele Zancarini-Fournel, "Histoire(s) du MLAC (1973-1975)," *CLIO. Histoire, femmes et société* 18 (2003): 241–52; Lisa Greenwald, "The Women's Liberation Movement in France and the Origins of Contemporary French Feminism, 1944–1981," PhD diss., Emory University, 1996, 85–129; Michelle Zancarini-Fournel, "'Notre corps, nous-mêmes'," *Le siècle des féminismes*, ed. Élaine Gubin, Catherine Jacques, Florence Rochefort, Brigitte Studer, Françoise Thébaud, and Michelle Zancarini-Fournel (Paris: Les Éditions de l'Atelier, 2004), 209–19; Sandra Reineke, *Beauvoir and Her Sisters: The Politics of Women's Bodies in France* (Urbana: University of Illinois Press, 2011), 54–70.

34. Depouillement de 100 questionnaires en maternité, Nov. 5, 1979, box X-1, UFM.

35. Giséle Tichané, *Accouche et tais-toi: Des femmes parlent* (Paris: Le Centurion, 1980), 159.
36. Mme A., exit survey, [1979], box X-1, UFM.
37. Mme N. to Pierre Rouquès Metallurgists Polyclinic, Oct. 18, 1976; Mme and M. T. to Director, Pierre Rouquès Metallurgists Polyclinic, Dec. 26, 1976; Mme G. to Pierre Rouquès Metallurgists Polyclinic, [1976]; Exit survey, Oct. 18, 1976; Mme and M. H, [to Pierre Rouquès Metallurgists Polyclinic], Apr. 9, 1977; all in box X-1, UFM.
38. Edmonde Morin, "Accouchement, enfantement," *Alternatives*, June 1977, 81.
39. Zila Rennert, Blanche Cohen, and Christiane Goirand, *L'enseignement de l'accouchement sans douleur* (Paris: Vigot Freres, 1975), 15.
40. Tichané, *Accouche et tais-toi*, 98.
41. Marie-José Jaubert, *Les bateleurs du mal-joli: Le mythe de l'accouchement sans douleur* (Paris: Balland, 1979), 132.
42. Mme F. to Pierre Rouquès Metallurgists Polyclinic, Dec. 15, 1975, box X-1, UFM.
43. Mme P. to Pierre Rouquès Metallurgists Polyclinic, Oct. 17, 1976, box X-1, UFM.
44. Marie-José Jaubert, *Ces hommes qui nous accouchent* (Paris: Stock 2, 1982), 199.
45. Jaubert, *Les bateleurs du mal-joli*, 71.
46. Diane E. Hoffman and Anita J. Tarzian, "The Girl Who Cried Pain: A Bias against Women in the Treatment of Pain," *Journal of Law, Medicine, and Ethics*, 29 (Mar. 2001): 13–27.
47. Tichané, *Accouche et tais-toi*, 172. For a germane Foucauldian analysis of gender and obstetric authority, see William Ray Arney, *Power and the Profession of Obstetrics* (Chicago: University of Chicago Press, 1982).
48. Glenda Adams, "Natural Childbirth: Just Another Shuck," *Village Voice*, Sept. 30, 1971, 18.
49. Ibid.
50. *Proceedings of the First International Childbirth Conference*, 33.
51. Letter to the editor, undated [Fall 1978], MC331/Ms. Letters/6.175, SL.
52. Arms, *Immaculate Deception*, 148.
53. Ibid., 140–42.
54. Ibid., 141–43.
55. K. C. Cole, "Can Natural Childbirth Survive Technology?," *Sunday News Magazine*, Jan. 14, 1979, 6.
56. Paul J. Placek and Selma M. Taffel, "Trends in Cesarean Section Rates for the United States, 1970–78," *Public Health Reports* 95 (Nov–Dec. 1980): 542. See also Deborah Larned, "Cesarean Births: Why They Are up 100 Percent," *Ms. Magazine*, Oct. 1978, 24, 27–28, 30.
57. Cole, "Can Natural Childbirth Survive Technology?," 6.
58. Ibid., 6.
59. Bing, "Future of Childbirth Education," accn. 2000–M64, box 1, LI, SL.
60. "Childbirth Technic Hailed As Painless," *New York Times*, Jan. 21, 1943; "Painless Method Is Devised for Childbirth; California Doctor Blocks Spinal Nerves," *New York Times*, June 3, 1944; Stephen Schwartz, "A Holy War Rages over Natural Childbirth," *The Washington Post/Potomac*, Oct. 18, 1970, 43; Abouleish, *Childbirth*, 54; Wolf, *Deliver Me from Pain*, 172–76.
61. Margery Simchak, "Has Epidural Anesthesia Made Childbirth Education Obsolete?" *Childbirth Instructor*, Summer 1991, 18.
62. BACE Training Exam for Childbirth Instructors, 1972, MC515/BACE/5.1, SL.
63. Ibid.

64. Birth report, June 19, 1972, MC515/BACE/13.6, SL.

65. Kitty Hanson, "That Wonderful Feeling," *Daily News*, Nov. 23, 1976.

66. Ministère des Affaires sociales de la santé et de la ville, Haut Comité de la Santé Publique, *La sécurité et la qualité de la grossesse et de la naissance: Pour un nouveau plan périnatalité* (Rennes: Éditions ENSP, 1994), 74; Wolf, *Deliver Me from Pain*, 175; "Travaux de la première journée du séminaire," *Bulletin officiel de la Société française de psychoprophylaxie obstétricale*, nos. 49–51 (1972–73): 7–56.

67. Muller, "Anesthésie péridurale et psycho-prophylaxie obstétricale," 11.

68. Quoted in Poittevin, "P. P. O.," 9.

69. "Travaux de la première journée du séminaire," 16, 21–22; Compte rendu de la réunion, Commission 'Enfance', Jan. 20, 1978, fol. 177, 2AF, Conseil National des Femmes Françaises (hereafter cited as CNFF), Archives du féminisme, l'Université d'Angers, Angers, France (hereafter cited as AFUA); Morin, "Accouchement, enfantement," 80; Muller, "Anesthésie péridurale et psycho-prophylaxie obstétricale," 6–8; Josine Lannoy, "De l'accouchement naturel à l'accouchement électronique: Lequel choisir?," *Femmes d'aujourd'hui*, Nov. 2–8, 1977, 10; Tichané, *Accouche et tais-toi*, 170–71; Jaubert, *Ces hommes qui nous accouchent*, 203.

70. Tichané, *Accouche et tais-toi*, 124.

71. Jaubert, *Ces hommes qui nous accouchent*, 205.

72. Ibid.

73. Quoted in ibid., 206.

74. Ibid., 213.

75. Quoted in ibid., 207.

76. Marian MacDorman, T. J. Matthews, and Eugene Declerq, "Home Births in the United States, 1990–2009," *NCHS Data Brief*, Jan. 26, 2012, http://www.cdc.gov/nchs/data/databriefs/db84.htm. Between 1954 and 1964, the number of live births in the United States exceeded four million births per annum, but then entered a phase of steady decline. In the mid-1970s, it bottomed out, dipping below 3.2 million. Only in 1989 did the number of live births again surpass four million. Maternity wards that had expanded during the baby boom faced a shortfall of patients as American births declined, no doubt a consideration for administrators concerned with the bottom line. "Live Births and Birth Rates by Year," *Infoplease*, accessed May 15, 2012, http://www.infoplease.com/ipa/A0005067.html.

77. "Hospitals Meet Homebirth Halfway," *Medical Tribune*, Jan. 10, 1979, 1.

78. Cole, "Can Natural Childbirth Survive Technology?," 18.

79. Judith Randal, "Childbirth at Home," *Daily News*, Jan. 11, 1979. See also Ruth Watson Lubic, "The Impact of Technology on Health Care—The Childbearing Center: A Case for Technology's Appropriate Use," *Journal of Nurse-Midwifery* 24 (Jan.–Feb. 1979): 6–10; Raymond G. DeVries, "The Alternative Birth Center: Option or Cooptation?," *Women and Health* 5 (Fall 1980): 55; Wendy Kline, *Bodies of Knowledge: Sexuality, Reproduction, and Women's Health in the Second Wave* (Chicago: University of Chicago Press, 2010), 145–49.

80. Hanson, "A Change in the American Way of Having Babies."

81. Frédérick Leboyer, *Pour une naissance sans violence* (Paris: Éditions du Seuil, 1974); Frédérick Leboyer, *Birth without Violence* (New York: Knopf, 1975). I draw the characterization of Leboyer's approach as a philosophy rather than a method of childbirth from Jaubert, *Les bateleurs du mal-joli*, 172.

82. Compte rendu de la reunion, Commission 'Enfance,' Feb. 24, 1978, fol. 177, 2AF, CNFF, AFUA. See also P. A. Chadeyron, "Comment accoucher dans le plaisir," *La Généraliste*, Nov. 21, 1979, 24.

83. Lannoy, "De l'accouchement naturel à l'accouchement électronique," 11.

84. Jean-Marie Cheynier, "La violence de naitre et le besoin de tendresse du nouveau-né (à propos de Frédérick Leboyer)," typescript, n.d. [1977?], box O, UFM.

85. Jaubert, *Ces homes qui nous accouchent*, 24.

86. Jaubert, *Les bateleurs du mal-joli*, 173.

87. Sandy Strickland, "Prepared Childbirth Expert: Pregnancy's Not a Disease," *Jacksonville Journal*, June 26, 1975. On interest in Leboyer among ASPO's rank-and-file members, see, for example, "Has Leboyer Come to Your Town?," *International Childbirth Education Association Actionletter*, Jan. 1976, 3; review of *Gentle Birth, International Childbirth Education Association Actionletter*, Oct. 1978, 7; Hanson, "A Change in the American Way of Having Babies;" Hanson, "That Wonderful Feeling."

88. Strickland, "Prepared Childbirth Expert."

89. Michel Odent, *Bien naître* (Paris: Éditions du Seuil, 1976); Jaubert, *Ces hommes qui nous accouchent*, 28–29; Pascal Grebel, "Accouchement sous l'eau: Révolution ou pétard mouillé?" *Le Quotidien du médecin*, Dec. 14, 1979, 7. On Soviet water birth, see Ekaterina Belooussova, "The 'Natural Childbirth' Movement in Russia: Self-Representation Strategies," *Anthropology of East Europe Review* 20 (2002): 11–18; Karil Daniels, "Water Birth: The Newest Form of Safe, Gentle, Joyous Birth," *Journal of Nurse-Midwifery* 34 (July–Aug. 1989): 198–205; M. Dmitrouk, "Ils sont nés dans l'eau," *Union soviétique*, Feb. 1985, 50; Geneviève Doucet, "La vie comme elle est...," *Elle*, Jan. 28, 1980, 66–67.

90. Michel Odent, *Entering the World: The De-Medicalization of Childbirth*, Christine Hauch, trans. (New York: M. Boyars, 1984); Jaubert, *Les bateleurs du mal-joli*, 177–78. See also *40 Minutes: Birth Reborn* (BBC TV, 1982); Michel Odent, *Birth Reborn* (New York: Pantheon, 1984).

91. Flora Hommel, "Nurses in Private Practice as Monitrices," *American Journal of Nursing* 69 (July 1969): 1447–50; "CWPEA Becoming A National Organization," *Childbirth Without Pain Education Association Newsletter* 11 (Sept. 1970), [4]; Carole Kramer, "In Retrospect—1973," *ASPO Newsletter*, Jan. 1974, 1; *The Birth of a Monitrice: A Comprehensive Guide for Establishing a Lamaze Monitrice Program* (Manchester, CT: Manchester Monitrice Associates, 1977); "What's Going on in ASPO-LA: Monitrice Program," *ASPO Newsletter*, Aug. 1974, 5. According to Marilène Vuille, monitrice practice in France was limited to private hospitals, where babies were delivered by obstetricians. The monitrice supported the woman throughout her labor and the physician stepped in at the time of delivery. In public hospitals, midwives oversaw labor and birth and offered women steady support throughout labor and birth. Marilène Vuille, e-mail to author, Aug. 1, 2012.

92. Carole Kelly, "Lamaze In-Service Programs," *Lamaze Newsletter*, July 1972, 1.

93. Leavitt, *Make Room for Daddy*. For the argument against the father's presence, see Fielding and Benjamin, *The Childbirth Challenge*, 60–62.

94. Robert P. Goldman, "Where Should Dad Be When the Baby Is Born?" *Modesto Bee Parade*, Apr. 30, 1961.

95. Fay Stender, ed., "Husbands in the Delivery Room: Recommendations to Hospital Administrators and Physicians on the Desirability and Safety of the Practice," Apr. 1965, MC515/BACE/16.10, SL.

96. "Father-Attended Deliveries: Pros, Cons on the New Trend," *Medical Tribune*, Mar. 12–13, 1966, 12.

97. Eric Fodor, "Husband's Remarks," *Childbirth without Pain Education Association Newsletter* 11 (Sept. 1970): 8.

98. Elisabeth D. Bing, "Psychoprophylaxis and Family-Centered Maternity: A Historical Development in the USA," *Psychosomatic Medicine in Obstetrics and Gynaecology* (Basel: Karger, 1972), 71.

99. Michael Kimmel, *Manhood in America: A Cultural History*, 3rd ed. (New York: Oxford University Press, 2012), esp. 189–210.

100. "Bradley Speaks for Dads," *ASPO News*, Spring 1965, 5.

101. Robert A. Bradley, "Husband Participation in Childbirth," *The International Childbirth Education Association Report of the 1965 Regional Conferences* (n.p.: International Childbirth Education Association, 1965), 45.

102. Birth report, July 1, 1972, MC515/BACE/13.6, SL. See also, for example, Tom Martin and Shirley Martin, "Lamaze Is for Lovers," *ASPO Newsletter* 10 (Spring 1976): 7; Birth report, May 9, 1972, MC515/BACE/13.6, SL.

103. Sally Olds and Linda Witt, "New Man in the Delivery Room—the Father," *Today's Health*, Oct. 1970, 54.

104. Letter [to Bing?], undated, [1970s?], accn. 2003–M153, box 1, LI, SL. See also Linda R. Cronenwett and Lucy L. Newmark, "Fathers' Responses to Childbirth." *Nursing Research* 23 (May–June 1974): 210–17.

105. John S. Miller, "Parents and Professionals: Partners in Childbearing," *ICEA News*, Sept.–Oct. 1970, 7. On couples' shared prenatal preparation class, see Leavitt, *Make Room for Daddy*, 120–55.

106. *ASPO Focus* 2 (Spring 1975): 1.

107. Doris Haire and John Haire, *Implementing Family-Centered Maternity Care with a Central Nursery* (Hillside, NJ: Childbirth Education Association of New Jersey, 1971), II–16.

108. Benjamin Segal, "A Visit to Maternity House No. 20, Moscow, USSR," typescript, 1970, accn. 2003–M153, box 1, LI, SL.

109. Ibid.

110. shisho4ka comment on germanych, "Vopros k zhenskoi auditorii," *1965* (blog), May 29, 2009, http://germanych.livejournal.com/138984.html.

111. Kurskii oblastnoi otdel zdravookhraneniia. Kon"iunkturnyi obzor po akushersko-ginekologicheskoi sluzhbe v oblasti, 1974, GARF, f. A-482, op. 56, d. 472, l. 33. The birth film likely used in this era in Soviet childbirth preparation classes, including Husband Seminars, was *Materiam i detiam* (Kievskaia kinostudiia nauchno-populiarnykh filmov, 1970).

112. S. N. Akhmadeeva, "Sostoianie gemodinamiki beremennykh zhenshchin pri fiziopsikhoprofilakticheskoi podgotovke k rodam," *Akusherstvo i ginekologiia* 49 (Sept. 1974): 7–11. Efforts continued to be made to apply psychoprophylaxis in other contexts, such as treatment for alcoholism, e.g., L. N. Lezhepekova and B. A. Iakubov, *Voprosy psikhogigieny i psikhoprofilaktiki v rabote prakticheskogo vracha* (Leningrad: Meditsina, 1977), 27–33.

113. O. K. Nikonchik, "K 60-letiiu Velikogo Oktiabria," *Akusherstvo i ginekologiia* 53 (Sept. 1977): 1–6.

114. V. I. Bodiazhina and K. N. Zhmakin, *Akusherstvo* (Moscow: Meditsina, 1970), 185–87; S.-M. A. Omarov, O. M.-G. Aliev, M. I. Chavtaraev, "Obezbolivanie rodov dlitel'noi peridural'noi blokadoi," *Akusherstvo i ginekologiia* 53 (Jan. 1977): 27–29; G. G. Zhdanov, V. K. Rymashevskii, G. M. Ponomarev, "Sovremennye metody

medikamentoznogo obezbolivaniia rodov," *Akusherstvo i ginekologiia* 56 (Feb. 1980): 55–57.

115. Schwartz, "A Holy War Rages over Natural Childbirth," 39.

116. Kon"iunkturnye obzory sostoianii akushersko-ginekologicheskoi pomoshchi naseleniiu Leningradskoi, Lipetskoi, Magadanskoi, Moskovskoi, Novgorodskoi i Novosibirskoi oblasti, 1963, GARF, f. A-482, op. 50, d. 8546; Tekstovoi otchet roddoma no. 1 Dzerzhinskogo raiona g. Khar'kova, 1971, DAKhO, f. R-5125, op. 4, d. 744, l. 15; Ol'ga Valentinovna Grishchenko, interview with author, Apr. 3, 2006.

117. Peter Osnos, "Childbirth, Soviet Style: Labor in Keeping with the Party Line," *Washington Post*, Nov. 28, 1976.

118. Grishchenko, interview with author, Apr. 3, 2006; Jean Ispa, "Soviet and American Childbearing Experiences and Attitudes: A Comparison," *Slavic Review* 42 (Spring 1983): 1–13; klepak, comment on germanych, "Vopros k zhenskoi auditorii"; Nataliia Vorontsova-Iurieva, "Rody v SSSR," *Predmety sovetskoi zhizni* (blog), June 19, 2007, http://community.livejournal.com/soviet_life/53730.html#cutid1.

119. I have slightly revised the translation of this quote as it originally appeared. Belooussouva, "The 'Natural Childbirth' Movement in Russia," 12.

120. madlesha, comment on germanych, "Vopros k zhenskoi auditorii."

121. greenbat, ibid.

122. bormental r, ibid.

CHAPTER 7

1. Margaret V. Wideman and Jerome E. Singer, "The Role of Psychological Mechanisms in Preparation for Childbirth," *American Psychologist* 39 (Dec. 1984): 1367.

2. Boston Women's Health Book Collective, *Our Bodies, Ourselves*, 2nd ed. (New York: Simon and Schuster, 1973), 269–70. On the history of the feminist health care movement, see Sandra Morgen, *Into Our Own Hands: The Women's Health Movement in the United States, 1969–1990* (New Brunswick, NJ: Rutgers University Press, 2002).

3. Wendy Kline, *Bodies of Knowledge*, 127–54; Rochelle Green, "Birthing Alternatives: A Matter of Choice and Turf," *Medical World News*, May 28, 1984, 50; "Frequently Asked Questions about Midwives and Midwifery," *Citizens for Midwifery*. n.d., accessed on Jan. 5, 2012, http://cfmidwifery.org/midwifery/faq.aspx#8.

4. Nearly one in five American women in the early twenty-first century have their labor induced pharmacologically. Jane E. Brody, "As Cases of Induced Labor Rise, So Do Experts' Concerns," *New York Times*, Jan. 14, 2003; "Why Is the National US Cesarean Section Rate So High?" *Childbirth Connection*, last modified June 24, 2013. http://www.childbirthconnection.org/article.asp?ck=10456; Jeremy A. Lauer, Ana P. Betrán, Mario Merialdi, and Daniel Wojdyla, "Determinants of Cesarean Section Rates in Developed Countries: Supply, Demand, and Opportunities for Control," *World Health Report Background Paper* 29 (2010): 1–22; Luz Gibbons, José M. Belizán, Jeremy A. Lauer, Ana P. Betrán, Mario Merialdi, and Fernando Althabe, "The Global Numbers and Costs of Additionally Needed and Unnecessary Cesarean Sections Performed per Year: Overuse as a Barrier to Universal Coverage," *World Health Report Background Paper* 30 (2010): 1–32.

5. Some sources claim that rates are as low as 50 percent. Advocates of natural childbirth put the figure of epidural anesthesia rates at the high end, while those in the obstetrics and anesthesiology communities tend to offer considerably lower figures. Judith P. Rooks, "Epidural Anesthesia as Used during Childbirth in the United States." *Japanese Journal for Midwives* 54 (2000): 9–14; Wilhelm Ruppen, Sheena Derry, Henry McQuay, and R. Andrew Moore, "Incidence of Epidural Hematoma, Infection, and Neurologic Injury in Obstetric Patients with Epidural Analgesia/Anesthesia." *Anesthesiology* 105 (2006): 394.
6. Ministère des Affaires sociales, *La sécurité et la qualité de la grossesse et de la naissance*, 74; Martine Wcislo and Béatrice Blondel, "La naissance en France en 1995: Enquête nationale périnatale," *SESI InfoRapides*, Oct. 1996, http://www.gyneweb.fr/sources/gdpublic/enquete.html; Ruppen et al., "Incidence of Epidural Hematoma, Infection, and Neurologic Injury in Obstetric Patients with Epidural Analgesia/Anesthesia," 394.
7. Ministère des Affaires sociales, *La sécurité et la qualité de la grossesse et de la naissance*, 53. See also "Périnatalité: Le plan du gouvernement, 1995–2000," *Soins: Gynécologie, obstétrique, puériculture, pédiatrie*, no. 156 (May 1994): 43.
8. B. Blondel, G. Bréart, Ch. du Mazaubrun, G. Badeyan, M. Wcislo, A. Lordier, and N. Matet, "La situation périnatale en France: Evolution entre 1981 et 1995," *Journal de gynécologie, obstétrique et biologie de la reproduction* 26 (1997): 770–80; Jennifer Harkins, Brendan Carvalho, Amy Evers, Sachin Mehta, and Edward T. Riley, "Survey of the Factors Associated with a Woman's Choice to Have Epidural Anesthesia," *Anesthesiology Research and Practice* (2010): 1–8. I thank Marilène Vuille for her guidance on the topic of epidural rates and state reimbursement policies in France.
9. "Interview with Elisabeth Bing," 3.
10. Elaine Zwelling, "The History of Lamaze Continues," 20.
11. Judith Rooks, "Nitrous Oxide for Pain in Labor—Why Not in the United States?" *Birth* 34 (Mar. 2007): 4.
12. Ronald Melzack, "The Myth of Painless Childbirth (The John J. Bonica Lecture)," *Pain* 19 (1984): 321.
13. Niels C. Beck and David Hall, "Natural Childbirth: Review and Analysis," *Obstetrics and Gynecology* 52 (Sept. 1978): 371–79; Niels C. Beck, Elizabeth A. Geden, and Gerald T. Brouder, "Preparation for Labor: Historical Perspective," *Psychosomatic Medicine* 41(May 1979): 243–58; Niels C. Beck and Lawrence J. Siegel, "Preparation for Childbirth and Contemporary Research on Pain, Anxiety, and Stress Reduction: A Review and Critique," *Psychosomatic Medicine* 42 (July 1980): 429–47; Niels C. Beck, Lawrence. J. Siegel, Nancy. P. Davidson, Sandra Kormeier, Annette Breitenstein, and David G. Hall, "The Prediction of Pregnancy Outcome: Maternal Preparation, Anxiety, and Attitudinal Sets," *Journal of Psychosomatic Research* 24 (1980): 343–51; Elizabeth Geden, Niels C. Beck, Gerald Brouder, Judy Glaister, and Susan Pohlman, "Self-Report and Psychophysiological Effects of Lamaze Preparation: An Analogue of Labor Pain," *Research in Nursing and Health* 8 (1985): 155–65.
14. Ronald Melzack, Paul Taenzer, Perle Feldman, and Robert A. Kinch, "Labour Is Still Painful after Prepared Childbirth Training," *Canadian Medical Association Journal* 125 (Aug. 15, 1981): 363.
15. Geden, et al., "Self-Report and Psychophysiological Effects of Lamaze Preparation," 155; Ann Japenga, "Tug of War between Two Natural Childbirth Methods: Dr. Robert Bradley Defends His Technique and Criticizes the Widely

Used Lamaze Training as Unnatural," *Los Angeles Times*, Mar. 24, 1987; Smith, Bucklin, and Associates, Organizational Audit prepared for the American Society for Psychoprophylaxis in Obstetrics, Inc., July 11, 1989, accn. 2000–M64, box 1, LI, SL.

16. "Today's Lamaze! (Not Your Ma's Lamaze!!)," *Passion for Birth*. 2012. http://passionforbirth.com/lamaze.html.

17. Judith Lothian and Charlotte DeVries, *The Official Lamaze Guide: Giving Birth with Confidence* (New York: Meadowbrook Press, 2005), 259.

18. Judith A. Lothian and Charlotte DeVries, "Lamaze Breathing: What You Need to Know," *Lamaze International*, April 24, 2012. http://www.lamaze.org/LamazeBreathing.

19. Only about 12 percent of the 117 survey respondents stated that they were currently selling products to parents in their childbirth education classes. "Listed Comments from *Genesis* Member Survey, 1986," accn. 2000–M34, box 1, LI, SL.

20. R. T. to Rob Moran, July 6, 1986, accn. 2002–M34, box 1, LI, SL.

21. Confidential Business Plan, [1986], accn. 2002–M34, box 1, LI, SL.

22. "Blueprint, 1987–89," accn. 2002–M34, box 1, LI, SL.

23. Judith A. Lothian, Debby Amis, and Jeannette Crenshaw, "Care Practice #4: No Routine Interventions," *Journal of Perinatal Education* 16 (Summer 2007): 32.

24. Ibid., 29–34.

25. Contemporary debates in Russia on this issue hew closely to those in the United States in the 1960s and 1970s, with physician opposition playing a key role. "Men's Presence in Maternity Wards during Childbirth Considered Shameful in Russia," *Pravda.ru*, October 18, 2005, http://english.pravda.ru/society/family/18-10-2005/9083-childbirth-0/.

26. Wolf writes that "the meaning of control in the context of birth had changed [in the 1980s]...: natural childbirth conferred control by allowing women to take charge of their labors and deliveries and be the central character. Epidural anesthesia, in contrast, conferred control by allowing laboring women to maintain their composure and socialize normally. These different definitions of the same highly valued cultural concept reflected divergent identities and values of two generations of American women." Wolf is correct, but the contrast is not as black-and-white as she suggests. As earlier chapters have demonstrated, natural childbirth advocates in the 1950s and 1960s saw dignity in self-control and even-keeled comportment. When viewed in this deeper historical perspective, the motives of women in the late 1960s and 1970s seem an aberration to a longer pattern of values and priorities. Wolf, *Deliver Me from Pain*, 177.

27. For examples of this turn toward the rhetoric of choice in the French context, see I. Maury and A.-M. Morice, "Accouchement: Toutes les solutions pour souffrir moins," *Marie Claire*, June 1980, 69–75; Yves Margueritte, "Accouchement: Quelle méthode préférer," *Parent*, Feb. 1980, 58–63.

28. David Edward O'Connor, *The Basics of Economics* (Westport, CT: Greenwood Press, 2004), 60–61.

29. Frederic Jameson, *Postmodernism, or the Cultural Logic of Late Capitalism* (Durham, NC: Duke University Press, 1991), 266.

30. Rick Blizzard, "Revisiting the Diagnosis for Patient Satisfaction," *Gallup*, June 29, 2004, http://www.gallup.com/poll/12181/Revisiting-Diagnosis-Patient-Satisfaction.aspx.

31. See Wolf, *Deliver Me from Pain*, 176–78.

32. Annemarie Mol, *The Logic of Care: Health and the Problem of Patient Choice* (London: Routledge, 2008), 18.

33. Penny P. Simkin and MaryAnn O'Hara, "Nonpharmacologic Relief of Pain during Labor: Systematic Reviews of Five Methods," *American Journal of Obstetrics and Gynecology* 186 (May 2002): S131–59.

34. Lothian and DeVries, *The Official Lamaze Guide*, 261.

35. Tandy Parks, interview with the author, Jan. 9, 2012.

GLOSSARY

Analgesia substance that produces relief from pain

Anesthesia substance that produces a partial or total loss of sensation

Belladonna a drug prepared from a member of the nightshade family by the same name

Codeine analgesic drug derived from morphine

Demerol trademark name of meperidine, a narcotic analgesic; marketed in Western Europe and the Middle East as Dolosol, as Lidol in the USSR

Epidural anesthesia regional anesthetic administered by injection into the epidural space of the spinal cord, creating a loss of sensation below the waist

Gamma-OH also known as gamma hydroxybutyrate, a drug that depresses central nervous system function

Glucose a simple sugar derived from plants and readily absorbed into the bloodstream

Lidol see Demerol

Meperidine see Demerol

Narcotics a class of potentially addictive drugs that numb sensation and induce drowsiness

Nembutol trademark name of the sedative pentobarbital sodium

Nitrous oxide mild anesthetic administered by inhalation, often in combination with oxygen. Also known simply as "gas"

Novocain local anesthetic administered by injection

Opiate sedative narcotic derived from opium or its natural or synthetic derivatives, e.g. morphine, pantapon, Demerol, Promedol

Oxycodone semi-synthetic opiate analgesic. Used with scopolamine as an alternative to morphine-based twilight sleep

Oxytocin hormone used to stimulate uterine contractions

Pantopon see opiate

Parturient a woman in labor

Phenegran see Promethezine

Pitocin see Oxytocin

Promethezine Obstetric use discontinued in 1980s amid concerns over depressed neonatal respiration; this antihistamine alleviates nausea and vomiting.

Promedol Soviet-developed narcotic analgesic and antispasmodic, similar to Demerol.

Sedative a calming and sleep-inducing drug

Sparteine drug used in obstetrics to strengthen and regularize contractions

Tekodin see Oxycodone

Trilene obstetric analgesic administered by inhalation. Seen initially as an alternative to chloroform and ether, it has been abandoned for obstetric use due to fears of toxicity.

Trimeperidine see Promedol

BIBLIOGRAPHY

ARCHIVES

Archives nationales de France (ANF), Paris
    88A5 Association France-URSS
Archives du féminisme, l'Université d'Angers, Angers (AFUA)
    2AF Conseil National des Femmes Françaises (CNFF)
Augustus C. Long Health Sciences Library Archives and Special Collections, Columbia
    University (LHSL), New York
    Maternity Center Association Records (MCA)
Archives de l'Union fraternelle de la métallurgie, L'Institut d'Histoire Sociale CGT de la
    Métallurgie (UFM), Paris
    Collection l'Accouchement sans Douleur
Derzhavnyi arkhiv Kharkivs'koi oblasti (State Archive of Kharkiv Oblast, DAKhO),
    Kharkiv
    f. R-5125 Otdel zdravookhraneniia ispolnitel'nogo komiteta khar'kovskogo
    oblastnogo soveta deputatov trudiashchikhsia (Department of Public Health,
    Kharkov oblast Executive Committee, Council of Worker's Deputies)
        op. 1 1940–50
        op. 2 1944–59
        op. 4 1960–84
    f. R-5833 Lichnyi arkhiv Platonova, K. I. (Personal archive of K. I. Platonov)
        op. 1 1902–1964
Gosudarstvennyi arkhiv Rossiiskoi Federatsii (State Archive of the Russian Federation,
    GARF), Moscow
    fond r-8009 Ministerstvo zdravookhraneniia SSSR (USSR Ministry of Public
    Health, MZ SSSR)
        op. 1 Kantseliariia (Chancellery)
        op. 2 Uchenyi meditsinskii sovet (Academic Medical Council)
        op. 22 Upravlenie rodovspomozheniia (Obstetrics Department)
    fond A-482 Ministerstvo zdravookhranenia RSFSR (MZ RSFSR)
        op. 50 1955–65
        op. 54 1966–73
        op. 56 1974–86
Schlesinger Library, Radcliffe Institute for Advanced Study, Harvard University (SL),
    Cambridge, MA
    MC331 *Ms. Magazine* Letters, 1972–80 (*Ms.* Letters)
    MC515 Boston Association for Childbirth Education Records (BACE)
    accn. 2000-M29, M58, M173 Lamaze International Records (LI)

Tsentral'nyi derzhavnyi arkhiv vyshchykh organiv vlady ta upravlinnia Ukrainy
  (Central State Archive of Higher Agencies of Authority and Administration of
  Ukraine, TsDAVO), Kyiv
    f. 342 Ministerstvo zdravookhraneniia Ukrainskoi SSR (Ministry of Public
    Health of the Ukrainian SSR, MZ USSR)
        op. 14 1943–50
        op. 15 1951–63
Walter P. Reuther Library, Wayne State University, Detroit, MI
    Flora Hommel Papers
Wellcome Library (WL), London
    PP/GDR Personal Papers of Grantly Dick-Read
    GC General Collection
        106 Lamaze Method

INTERVIEWS CONDUCTED BY THE AUTHOR

Buck, Ferris Urbanowski, childbirth educator, Jan. 6, 2012.
Grattesat, Geneviève, former editor of *La Quinzaine*, July 9, 2010.
Grishchenko, Ol'ga Valentinovna, obstetrician, Apr. 3, 2006.
L., Mrs., Lamaze-trained mother, Chapel Hill, NC, Oct. 4, 2011.
Mikhailov, Boris Volodimirovich, chair, Department of Psychotherapy, Kharkiv Medical
    Academy of Postgraduate Education, Apr. 4, 2006.
Park, Tandy, childbirth educator, Jan. 9, 2012.

PERIODICALS

Akusherstvo i ginekologiia
American Journal of Nursing
American Journal of Obstetrics and Gynecology
American Journal of Psychiatry
Anesthesiology
ASPO Focus (n.p.)
ASPO News (New York)
ASPO Presentations (New York)
ASPO Newsletter (Los Angeles)
British Medical Journal
Bulletin officiel de la Société française de psychoprophylaxie obstétricale
Bulletin officiel de la Société international de psycho-prophylaxie obstétricale
Childbirth without Pain Education Association Newsletter
Daily News (New York)
Elle (Paris)
L'Express
Femmes françaises
Le Figaro
France dimanche
France-URSS
Gynécologie et obstétrique
Harper's Bazaar
Heures claires
L'Humanité
L'Humanité dimanche
International Childbirth Education Association Actionletter

Journal of the American Medical Association
Journal of Nurse-Midwifery
Journal of Perinatal Education
Ladies' Home Journal
Lamaze Newsletter (Cambridge, MA)
Medical Tribune
Le Monde
New York Times
Obstetrics and Gynecology
Pravda Ukrainy
Psychosomatic Medicine
Psychosomatics
La Quinzaine
Radar
Regards
Revue de l'économe
Revue française de gynécologie et d'obstétrique
Revue de la nouvelle médecine
La Revue des travailleuses
Slavic Review
Sovetskaia zhenshchina
Union soviétique
Zdorov'e

AUDIOVISUAL SOURCES

40 Minutes: Birth Reborn. Produced by BBC TV. 1982.
L'accouchement sans douleur: Reportage de Francis Crémieux. [Paris]: Voix de son maître, 1955.
Le cas du docteur Laurent. Directed by Jean-Paul Chanois. Produced by Ignace Morgenstern. 1957.
Childbirth without Fear. Directed by Grantly Dick-Read. Produced by Encyclopedia Britannica Educational Corporation. 1956.
Dick-Read, Grantly. *Natural Childbirth: A Documentary Record of the Birth of a Baby Supervised by Dr. Grantly Dick-Read*. 1957.
The Farm Midwives: 1000 Births. Produced by Videofarm. 1979.
Gaskin, Ina May, interview by Susan Page, *The Diane Rehm Show*, WAMU, July 25, 2011.
Grasset, J. "Exposé sur l'accouchement dit 'sans douleur.'" *Médicophone: Magazine sonore d'informations médicales* 14 (Sept.–Oct. 1961): track 7.
Materiam i detiam. Produced by Kievskaia kinostudiia nauchno-populiarnykh fil'mov. 1970.
Spiritual Midwifery. Produced by Videofarm. 1978.
The Story of Eric. Directed by David Seltzer. 1971.

PUBLISHED PRIMARY SOURCES

1er Congrès international de médecine psychosomatique et maternité. Paris: Gauthier-Villars, 1965.
Abouleish, Ezzat. *Childbirth: A Joy—Not A Suffering*. Philadelphia: Dorrance & Company, 1975.
Adams, Glenda. "Natural Childbirth: Just Another Shuck." *Village Voice*, Sept. 30, 1971: 18, 56.

American College of Obstetricians and Gynecologists. *Manual of Standards*. Chicago: ACOG, 1959.

Anderson, Jean with Heinz Luschinsky, Benjamin Segal, and Alfred Tanz. "The Medical Case for Natural Childbirth: A Reply to Dr. Waldo Fielding." *ASPO Special Publication*, July 1962: 1–7.

Apgar, Virginia. "Advice to the Mother-to-Be." *The American Baby*, Jan. 1963: 25A.

Arms, Suzanne. *Immaculate Deception: A New Look at Women and Childbirth in America*. San Francisco: San Francisco Book Co., 1975.

[Arnold], Jill. "Call It a Comeback? The Many Faces of Nitrous Oxide for Labor Pain Relief." *RH Reality Check*. Dec. 16, 2010. http://www.rhrealitycheck.org/blog/2010/12/14/callcomeback-many-faces-nitrous-oxide-labor-pain-relief.

Atlee, H. B. *Natural Childbirth*. Springfield, IL: Charles C. Thomas, 1956.

Ayoub, Albert. *L'accouchement sans douleur*. Damascus: n. p., 1962.

Ball, Thomas L. "The Psychoprophylactic Preparation of Pregnant Women for Childbirth in the Union of Soviet Socialist Republics." *Transactions of the New York Academy of Sciences* series 2, 22 (June 1960): 578–80.

Beauvoir, Simone de. *The Second Sex*. Translated by Constance Borde and Sheila Malovany-Chevallier. New York: Knopf, 2010.

Beck, Niels C., Lawrence. J. Siegel, Nancy. P. Davidson, Sandra Kormeier, Annette Breitenstein, and David G. Hall. "The Prediction of Pregnancy Outcome: Maternal Preparation, Anxiety, and Attitudinal Sets." *Journal of Psychosomatic Research* 24 (1980): 343–51.

Bekhterev, V. M. *Collective Reflexology: The Complete Edition*. Edited by Lloyd H. Strickland. Translated by Eugenia Lockwood and Alisa Lockwood. New Brunswick, NJ: Transaction, 2001.

———. *Suggestion: Its Role in Social Life*. Translated by Tzvetanka Dobreva-Martinova. New Brunswick, NJ: Transaction, 1998.

Beloshapko, P. A. and A. M. Foi. *Obezbolivanie i uskorenie rodov*. Moscow: Medgiz, 1954.

Bing, Elisabeth. *My Life in Birth*. Washington, DC: Lamaze International, 2000.

———. *Six Practical Lessons for an Easier Childbirth*. New York: Grosset & Dunlop, 1967.

Bing, Elisabeth D. "Psychoprophylaxis and Family-Centered Maternity: A Historical Development in the USA." In *Psychosomatic Medicine in Obstetrics and Gynaecology*, 71–73. Basel: Karger, 1972.

Bing, Elisabeth, Marjorie Karmel, and Alfred Tanz. *A Practical Training Course for the Psychoprophylactic Method of Childbirth (Lamaze Technique)*. New York: ASPO, 1969.

———. *A Practical Training Course for the Psychoprophylactic Method of Childbirth*. New York: American Society for Psychoprophylaxis in Obstetrics, 1961.

The Birth of a Monitrice: A Comprehensive Guide for Establishing a Lamaze Monitrice Program. Manchester, CT: Manchester Monitrice Associates, 1977.

Blizzard, Rick. "Revisiting the Diagnosis for Patient Satisfaction." *Gallup*. June 29, 2004. http://www.gallup.com/poll/12181/Revisiting-Diagnosis-Patient-Satisfaction.aspx.

Bodiazhina, V. I. and K. N. Zhmakin. *Akusherstvo*. Moscow: Meditsina, 1970.

Bonnes Soirées. "La nouvelle méthode d'accouchement sans douleur." Jan. 30, 1955.

Bonstein, Isidore. *Psychoprophylactic Preparation for Painless Childbirth*. London: William Heinemann Medical Books, 1958.

Boston Women's Health Book Collective. *Our Bodies, Ourselves*. 2nd ed. New York: Simon and Schuster, 1973.

Bradley, Chester D. "The Urge to Interfere in Obstetrics." *North Carolina Medical Journal* 10 (July 1949): 343–49.

Bradley, Robert A. "Husband Participation in Childbirth." *The International Childbirth Education Association Report of the 1965 Regional Conferences.* n.p., International Childbirth Education Association, 1965.

Braid, James. *The Discovery of Hypnosis: The Complete Writings of James Braid, "The Father of Hypnotherapy."* Edited by Donald Robertson. London: National Council for Hypnotherapy, 2008.

Bramwell, John Milne. *Hypnotism: Its History, Theory, and Practice.* 2nd ed. London: Alexander Moring, 1906.

Bukoemskii, F. V. *Obezbolivanie normal'nykh rodov vdykhaniiami efira i khloroforma.* St. Petersburg: V. A. Vatslika, 1895.

Chabon, Irwin. *Awake and Aware.* New York: Delacorte Press, 1966.

Chadeyron, P. A. "Comment accoucher dans le plaisir." *La Généraliste,* Nov. 21, 1979: 22–24.

Chappell, Marjorie F. *Childbirth: Theory and Practical Training.* Edinburgh: E. & S. Livingstone, 1954.

Chertok, L. "Étude de la psycho-prophylaxie des douleurs de l'accouchement." *La Semaine des hôpitaux* 32 (Aug. 1956): 2619–26.

———. "L''accouchement naturel' et l''accouchement psychoprophylactique.'" *Concours médical* 79 (Nov. 23, 1957): 5105–08.

———. "Psychoprophylaxie ou psychothérapie obstétricale: Évolution des théories sur l'accouchement sans douleur." *Revue de médecine psychosomatique* 3 (1961): 5–15.

Chertok, Leon and Raymond de Saussure. *The Therapeutic Revolution from Mesmer to Freud.* Translated by R. H. Ahrenfeldt. New York: Brunner/Mazel, 1979.

Chertok, Léon, Isabelle Stengers, and Didier Gille. *Mémoires d'un hérétique.* Paris: La Découverte, 1990.

Churlet, Yvette. "Quatre Lyonnaises ont accouché sans peur, sans douleur." *La République—Le Patriote,* Dec. 22, 1953.

Clark, Dale. "A Man's Crusade for Easy Childbirth." *Esquire,* Oct. 1949: 51, 151 52.

Cole, K. C. "Can Natural Childbirth Survive Technology?" *Sunday News Magazine,* Jan. 14, 1979: 6–7, 18, 21, 30, 32.

Comment nous préparer à accoucher sans douleur par la méthode psycho-prophylactique. Paris: Union des Femmes Françaises, 1955.

Cook, Enid and M. Bevan-Brown. *Psychological Preparation for Childbirth.* Christchurch: Christchurch Psychological Society, 1949.

Corbin, Hazel. "Changing Maternity Service in a Changing World." *Canadian Nurse* 46 (Dec. 1950): 949–56.

Coudray, Annie. "L'accouchement sans douleur a 13 ans ce mois-ci." *Le Journal du dimanche,* Mar. 28, 1965.

Coué, Emile. *Self Mastery through Conscious Autosuggestion.* New York: Malkan, 1922.

Cronenwett, Linda R. and Lucy L. Newmark. "Fathers' Responses to Childbirth." *Nursing Research* 23 (May–June 1974): 210–17.

Daily Mirror. "Painless Birth Pope Says: Bible Does Not Ban It." Jan. 9, 1956.

Daily Sketch. "The Pope Approves an 'Easy' Childbirth Method." Jan. 9, 1956.

Demeusy, R. "L'accouchement psycho-prophylactique." *Formulaire dimanche,* July 24, 1955.

Deutsch, Helene. *The Psychology of Women.* Vol. 2. New York: Grune and Stratton, 1945.

DeVries, Raymond G. "The Alternative Birth Center: Option or Cooptation?" *Women and Health* 5 (Fall 1980): 47–60.

Dialogue franco-soviétique sur la psychanalyse. Compiled by Léon Chertok. Toulouse: Privat, 1984.

Dick-Read, Grantly. *Childbirth without Fear.* New York: Harper & Brothers, 1944.

———. *Childbirth without Fear: The Principles and Practices of Natural Childbirth.* 2nd rev. ed. New York: Harper & Row, 1959.

———. *Introduction to Motherhood.* London: William Heinemann Medical Books, 1950.

———. *L'accouchement sans douleur: Les principes et la pratique de l'accouchement naturel.* Translated by Jean-Marc Vaillant. Paris: Éditions Colbert, 1953.

———. *Motherhood in the Post-War World.* London: Wm. Heinemann Medical Books, 1944.

———. *Natural Childbirth.* London: William Heinemann, 1933.

———. *Revelation of Childbirth: The Principles and Practice of Natural Childbirth.* London: Heinemann, 1942.

Dmitrouk, M. "Ils sont nés dans l'eau." *Union soviétique,* Feb. 1985: 50.

Donigevich, M. I. *Metod psikhoprofilaktiki bolei v rodakh.* Kiev: Gosudarstvennoe meditsinskoe izdatel'stvo, 1955.

Dye, John H. *Painless Childbirth, or Healthy Mothers and Healthy Children: A Book for All Women.* Buffalo, NY: Baker, Jones, 1889.

Eastman, Nicholson J. *Expectant Motherhood.* 3rd ed. Boston: Little, Brown, 1957.

"Editorial." *Cahiers de médecine soviétique* 2 (Nov. 1955): 227–28.

Ehrenreich, Barbara and Deirdre English. *Complaints and Disorders: The Sexual Politics of Sickness.* Old Westbury, NY: Feminist Press, 1973.

———. *Witches, Midwives, and Nurses: A History of Women Healers.* Old Westbury, NY: Feminist Press, 1973.

Enkin, Murray. "The January Conference on Psychosomatic Ob-Gyn." *ISPOG Newsletter,* Spring 1973: 4–6.

Fair Press. "International Childbirth Confab Set." May 9, 1973.

Fielding, Waldo L. and Lois Benjamin. "The Medical Case against Natural Childbirth." *McCall's,* June 1962: 106, 183–86.

———. *The Childbirth Challenge: Commonsense versus "Natural" Methods.* New York: Viking Press, 1962.

Figurnov, K. M. *Painless Childbirth: Latest Achievements of Soviet Medicine in Obstetric Analgesia and Anaesthesia.* Moscow: Foreign Languages Publishing House, [1953].

France Soir. "Sept futures mamans sur dix sont encore contre l'accouchement sans douleur." Jan. 11, 1956.

Freud, Sigmund. *On the History of the Psycho-Analytic Movement.* Volume 14 of *The Standard Edition of the Complete Psychological Works of Sigmund Freud.* Edited by James Strachey and Anna Freud, 7–66. London: Hogarth Press, 1975.

Friedan, Betty. *The Feminine Mystique.* New York: Norton, 1963.

Gaskin, Ina May. *Spiritual Midwifery.* Summertown, TN: Book Pub Co., 1978.

Geden, Elizabeth, Niels C. Beck, Gerald Brouder, Judy Glaister, and Susan Pohlman. "Self-Report and Psychophysiological Effects of Lamaze Preparation: An Analogue of Labor Pain." *Research in Nursing and Health 8* (1985): 155–65.

Gelb, Barbara. *The ABC of Natural Childbirth.* New York: Norton, 1954.

germanych. "Vopros k zhenskoi auditorii." *1965* (blog). May 29, 2009. http://germanych.livejournal.com/138984.html.

Girod, Renée and Monica Jaquet. *Je vais être maman: Grossesse, accouchement, gymnastique prénatale.* Zurich: Édition Pro Juventute, 1954.

Goldman, Robert P. "Where Should Dad Be When the Baby Is Born?" *Modesto Bee Parade,* Apr. 30, 1961.

Goodrich, Jr., Frederick W. *Natural Childbirth: A Manual for Expectant Parents.* New York: Prentice Hall, 1950.

Grebel, Pascal. "Accouchement sous l'eau: Révolution ou pétard mouillé?" *Le Quotidien du médecin,* Dec. 14, 1979: 7.

Green, Rochelle. "Birthing Alternatives: A Matter of Choice and Turf." *Medical World News,* May 28, 1984: 42–58.

Guttmacher, Alan. Review of *Childbirth without Fear, Parents,* May 1945, 158–59.

Haire, Doris and John Haire. *Implementing Family-Centered Maternity Care with a Central Nursery.* Hillside, NJ: Childbirth Education Association of New Jersey, 1971.

Hanson, Kitty. "A Change in the American Way of Having Babies," *Sunday News* (New York, NY), Nov. 21, 1976.

Harlin, Fernande. *Préparez-vous à une heureuse maternité.* Paris: Éditions Denoël, 1951.

Hassid, Patricia. *Textbook for Childbirth Educators.* Hagerstown, MD: Harper & Row, Medical Department, 1978.

Heardman, Helen. *A Way to Natural Childbirth: A Manual for Physiotherapists and Parents-to-Be.* Edinburgh: Livingstone, 1948.

———. *Relaxation and Exercise for Natural Childbirth.* Edinburgh: E. & S. Livingstone, 1950.

Iagunov, S. A. *Fizkul'tura v periode beremennosti.* Leningrad: n.p., 1938.

———. "Fizkul'tura: Znachenie fizicheskoi kul'tury v periode beremennosti," *Fel'dsher i akusherka* (Apr. 1950): 33–38.

———. *Fizkul'tura vo vremia beremennosti i v poslerodovom periode.* Leningrad: Medgiz, 1959.

International Childbirth Education Association Childbirth Preparation Class Kit. 3rd ed. n.p.: ICEA, 1967.

"Interview with Elisabeth Bing." *American Baby CBE Reporter: A Supplement to American Baby Magazine,* Spring 2001: 3.

Japenga, Ann. "Tug of War between Two Natural Childbirth Methods: Dr. Robert Bradley Defends His Technique and Criticizes the Widely Used Lamaze Training as Unnatural." *Los Angeles Times,* Mar. 24, 1987.

Jaubert, Marie-José. *Ces hommes qui nous accouchent.* Paris: Stock 2, 1982.

———. *Les bateleurs du mal-joli: Le mythe de l'accouchement sans douleur.* Paris: Éditions du Balland, 1979.

Jeanson, Colette. *Principes et pratique de l'accouchement sans douleur.* Paris: Éditions du Seuil, 1954.

Jottroy, Pierre. "Nathalie née sans douleur." *Paris Match,* Apr. 2, 1955: 75, 80, 82.

Jordan, Edwin P. "Maternal Death Rate Lowered." *Evening Independent,* Sept. 28, 1950.

Kaplan, A. L. *Uchebnik akusherstva i zhenskikh boleznei: Dlia shkol medsester.* 3rd ed. Moscow-Leningrad: Medgiz, 1948.

———. *Uchebnik akusherstva i zhenskikh boleznei: Dlia shkol medsester.* Moscow-Leningrad: Medgiz, 1939.

Karmel, Marjorie. *J'ai accouché sans douleur.* Translated by Aline Dalsace-Vellay and Pierre Vellay. Paris: A. Fayard, 1960.

———. *Thank You, Dr. Lamaze.* 1959. Reprint. London: Pinter & Martin Ltd., 2005.

Kitzinger, Sheila. *Education and Counselling for Childbirth.* London: Baillière Tindall, 1977.

Kopil'-Levina, Z. A. "Metodika obezbolivaniia rodov slovesnym vnusheniem." In *Voprosy psikhoterapii v akusherstve: Rodoobezbolivanie i neukrotimaia rvota beremennykh,* edited by K. I. Platonov, 34–66. Khar'kov: IKPS dorsanotdel IuZhD psikhonevrologicheskii institut, 1940.

"L'accouchement sans douleur: Discours du Souverain pontife Pie XII (8 janvier 1956)." Jan. 8, 1956. ttp://frblin.perso.neuf.fr/ccmf/05textesstsiege/pie12/pie12sante1956a.pdf.

Lamaze, F., P. Vellay, J. Hersilie, R. Angelergues, [A.] Bourrel, and les Sages-Femmes. "Expérience pratiquée à la maternité du Centre 'Pierre-Rouquès' sur la méthode d'accouchement sans douleur par psycho-prophylaxie." *Bulletin de l'Académie nationale de médecin* 138 (Jan. 26–Feb. 2, 1954): 52–58.

Lamaze, Fernand. *La suppression de la douleur liée à la contraction de l'utérus en travail: Méthode psycho-prophylactique.* n. p., [1955].

———. *Qu'est-ce que l'accouchement sans douleur.* Paris: La Farandole, 1956.

Lamaze, Fernand and Pierre Vellay. "L'accouchement sans douleur." *La Semaine médicale* 28 (Jan. 1952): 301–05.

———. "L'accouchement sans douleur par la méthode psychophysique," *Gazette médicale de France* 59 (Dec. 1952): 1445–60.

Lannoy, Josine. "De l'accouchement naturel à l'accouchement électronique: Lequel choisir?" *Femmes d'aujourd'hui*, Nov. 2–8, 1977: 8–13.

Larned, Deborah. "Cesarean Births: Why They Are up 100 Percent." *Ms. Magazine*, Oct. 1978: 24, 27–28, 30.

Lepage, F. and G. Langevin-Droguet. *La préparation à l'accouchement sans crainte.* 2nd rev. and expanded ed. Paris: Masson et Cie, 1965.

Leboyer, Frédérick. *Birth without Violence.* New York: Knopf, 1975.

———. *Pour une naissance sans violence.* Paris: Éditions du Seuil, 1974.

Levi, M. F. *Istoriia rodovspomozheniia v SSSR.* Moscow: Izdatel'stvo akademii meditsinskikh nauk SSSR, 1950.

Lezhepekova, L. N. and B. A. Iakubov. *Voprosy psikhogigieny i psikhoprofilaktiki v rabote prakticheskogo vracha.* Leningrad: Meditsina, 1977.

Lobban, Molly. "N. M. Study Tour of the USSR." *Nursing Mirror*, Aug. 27, 1965: i–v, xvi.

Lothian, Judith and Charlotte DeVries. "Lamaze Breathing: What You Need to Know." *Lamaze International*, April 24, 2012. http://www.lamaze.org/LamazeBreathing.

———. *The Official Lamaze Guide: Giving Birth with Confidence.* New York: Meadowbrook Press, 2005.

Lull, Clifford B. and Robert A. Hingson. *Control of Pain in Childbirth: Anesthesia, Analgesia, Amnesia.* Philadelphia: J. B. Lippincott, 1944.

Lynd, Sheila. "She Smiled As Her Baby Was Born." *Daily Worker* (London), Sept. 26, 1953.

Manchester Guardian. "Pope Pronounces on Painless Childbirth." Jan. 9, 1956.

Manning, Roberta. "Children of the Revolution." *All You Can Eat* 3 (Dec. 1972): 16–17.

Margueritte, Yves. "Accouchement: Quelle méthode préférer." *Parent*, Feb. 1980: 58–63.

Maslow, Abraham. *Religions, Values, and Peak Experiences.* Columbus: Ohio State University Press, 1964.

Maternity Center Association, 1918–1943. New York: [The Maternity Center Association], 1943.

Maury, I. and A.-M. Morice. "Accouchement: Toutes les solutions pour souffrir moins." *Marie Claire*, June 1980: 69–75.

Mayer, Maurice and Jacques Bonhomme. "La méthode de l'accouchement naturel, son utilisation en pratique hospitalière." *La vie médicale*, Dec. 1953: 751–66.

McGurn, Barrett. "Pope Pius Approves Painless Birth Method." *New York Herald*, Jan. 9, 1956.

Mead, Margaret. *Soviet Attitudes toward Authority: An Interdisciplinary Approach.* New York: William Morrow, 1955.

"Medicine: Should It Hurt?" *Time*. July 22, 1946. http://www.time.com/time/magazine/article/0,9171,888278,00.html.

"Men's Presence in Maternity Wards during Childbirth Considered Shameful in Russia." *Pravda.ru*. October 18, 2005. http://english.pravda.ru/society/family/18-10-2005/9083-childbirth-0/.

Melzack, Ronald. "The Myth of Painless Childbirth (The John J. Bonica Lecture)." *Pain* 19 (1984): 321–37.

Melzack, Ronald, Paul Taenzer, Perle Feldman, and Robert A. Kinch. "Labour Is Still Painful after Prepared Childbirth Training." *Canadian Medical Association Journal* 125 (Aug. 1981): 357–63.

Michel, Marianne R. "L'accouchement sans douleur à 10 ans." *France Observateur*, July 17, 1962: 14–15.

Miller, John S. "Parents and Professionals: Partners in Childbearing." *ICEA News*, Sept.–Oct. 1970: 4–7.

Ministère des Affaires sociales, de la Santé et de la Ville, Haut Comité de la Santé Publique. *La sécurité et la qualité de la grossesse et de la naissance: Pour un nouveau plan périnatalité*. Rennes: ENSP, 1994.

Morin, Edmonde. "Accouchement, enfantemant." *Alternatives*, June 1977: 80–82.

Muldworf, Bernard. "À propos de l'accouchement sans douleur: 'Mentalité' et 'psychologie' chez la femme enceinte." *La Pensée*, no. 105 (Oct. 1962): 55–84.

———. *Le divan et le prolétaire*. Paris: Messidor/Éditions sociales, 1986.

Nauroy, Dr. "L'accouchement sans douleur." *Guérir*, Oct. 1963: 9–12.

Nikolaev, A. P. *Obezbolivanie rodov*. Leningrad: Meditsina. 1964.

———., ed. *Obezbolivanie v rodakh: Trudy konferentsii v g. Leningrade, 29–31 ianvaria 1951 g.* Moscow: Izdatel'stvo akademii meditsinskikh nauk SSSR, 1952.

———. *Ocherki teorii i praktiki obezbolivaniia rodov*. Leningrad: Medgiz, 1953.

———. "Teoreticheskie osnovy i sovremennye metody obezbolivaniia rodov." *Vestnik akademii meditsinskikh nauk SSSR* 6 (July–Aug. 1951): 13–23.

Notter, A. "Aspects actuels de la psychoprophylaxie obstétrical en Russie, Ukraine et Pologne: Considérations sur les instituts de physiologie et les maternités." *Lyon médical* 93 (Nov. 1961): 958–98.

Odent, Michel. *Bien naître*. Paris: Éditions du Seuil, 1976.

———. *Birth Reborn*. New York: Pantheon, 1984.

———. *Entering the World: The De-Medicalization of Childbirth*. Translated by Christine Hauch. New York: M. Boyars, 1984.

Olds, Sally and Linda Witt. "New Man in the Delivery Room—the Father." *Today's Health*, Oct. 1970: 52–56.

Osborne, Dorothy. "Lamaze Method: Husband, Wife Work Together for a Childbirth 'Experience.'" *The Observer* (Charlotte, NC), Mar. 15, 1974.

Osnos, Peter. "Childbirth, Soviet Style: Labor in Keeping with the Party Line." *Washington Post*, Nov. 28, 1976.

Palmer, Betsy. "A Story for Melissa." *Mothers to Be and Infant Care*, Fall 1962: 70–71.

Palmer, Greta. "Having Your Baby the New Way." *Collier's*, Nov. 1948: 26–27, 61.

"Périnatalité: Le plan du gouvernement, 1995–2000." *Soins: Gynécologie, obstétrique, puériculture, pédiatrie*, no. 156 (May 1994): 43–45.

Pétain, H. P. "Appel du 20 juin (1940)." In *Le Maréchal vous parle . . . : Recueil des discours et allocations prononcés par le Maréchal Pétain, chef de l'état du 16 juin au 31 décembre 1940*, unpaginated. Le Mans: CEP, 1941.

Petrov-Maslakov, M. A. *Obezbolivanie rodov*. Moscow: Meditsina, 1967.

Petrushevskaia, Liudmila. *Taina doma*. Moscow: Kvadrat, 1995.

Placek, Paul J. and Selma M. Taffel. "Trends in Cesarean Section Rates for the United States, 1970–78." *Public Health Reports*, Nov.–Dec. 1980: 540–48.

Platonoff, C. and G. Z. Velvosky. "Sur l'application de l'hypnose en chirurgie, accouchement et gynécologie." *Revue franco-russe de médecine et de biologie* 1 (June–Sept. 1925): 54–62.

Platonov, K. I. *The Word as a Physiological and Therapeutic Factor: The Theory and Practice of Psychotherapy according to I. P. Pavlov*. 2nd ed. Moscow: Foreign Languages Publishing House, 1959.

Platonov, K. K. *Moi lichnye vstrechi na velikoi doroge zhizni: Vospominaniia starogo psikhologa*. Moscow: Izdatel'svto "Institut psikhologii RAN," 2005.

"Psychoprophylaxis: Program for Painless Parturition." *Ob-Gyn Observer* 1 (July–Aug. 1962): 8.

Rabinovich-Brodskaia, F. I. *Obezbolivanie normal'nykh rodov*. Ivanogo: Gosudarstvennoe izdatel'stvo Ivanovskoi oblasti, 1936.

Regnault, Jules. *Maternité sans douleur: Comment accoucher normalement sans douleur*. Paris: Médicis, 1945.

Rennert, Zila, Blanche Cohen, and Christiane Goirand. *L'enseignement de l'accouchement sans douleur*. Paris: Vigot Freres, 1975.

Rieger, Hans. "Gefahrlose Geburtserleichterung durch Belladonna-Exclud-Zäpfchen." *Die Medizinische Zeitschrift*, Aug. 20, 1955: 1145–47.

"Résolution tendant à l'expérimentation dans quelques maternités de l'Assistance publique des méthodes d'accouchement sans douleur." *Bulletin municipal officiel de la Ville de Paris: Débats des assemblées de la Ville de Paris et du département de la Seine* 74 (Jan. 1954): 1113–14.

Revault d'Allonnes, Claude. "Une enquête préliminaire sur l'accouchement sans douleur." *Revue française de sociologie* 1 (Apr.–June 1960): 202–12.

Rion, Hanna. *The Truth about Twilight Sleep*. New York: McBride, Nast, 1915.

———. [Raion, Ganna]. *Obezboleznennye rody v "sumerechnom sne": Skopolamin-morfinovyi metod po dokladam vrachei i lichnym perezhivaniiam materei*. Translated by M. Bedelar. Moscow: Moskovskoe izdatel'stvo, 1917.

Safronova, E. I. *Vliianie kompleksnoi psikhofizicheskoi podgotovki na techenie beremennosti i iskhody rodov dlia materi i ploda. Aftoreferat dissertatsii na soiskanie uchenoi stepeni kandidata meditsinskikh nauk*. Khar'kov: Khar'kovskii meditsinskii institut, 1966.

Samsor, Jeannette L. *Childbirth Education: A Nursing Perspective*. New York: John Wiley & Sons, 1979.

Sarfaty, Reneé. "L'accouchement sans douleur." *Mode du jour*, Sept. 11, 1952: 1, 22.

Schultze-Rhonhof, F. "Der hypnotische Geburtsdämmerschlaf." *Zentralblatt für Gynäkologie* 46 (1922): 247.

Schurr, Cathleen. *Naturally Yours: A Personal Experience with Natural Childbirth*. New York: Rinehart & Company, 1953.

Schwartz, Stephen. "A Holy War Rages over Natural Childbirth." *Washington Post/ Potomac*, Oct. 18, 1970: 12, 37–39, 41–43, 46, 48, 50–53.

Sciare, A. Balfour. "Psychoprophylaxis in Obstetrics." *Nursing Times*, Oct. 8, 1965, 1373–74.

Shaffer, B. H. "Cultural Exchanges with Soviet Russia." *Editorial Research Reports*. 1959. http://library.cqpress.com/cqresearcher/document.php?id= cqresrre 1959070300#.UmNC_VBkN8E.

Shishkova, V. N. *Obezbolivanie rodov*. Moscow: Medgiz, 1959.

Shishkova, V. N., R. M. Bronshtein, E. I. Ivanova, and P. P. Nikulin. "Psikhoprofilakticheskoe obezbolivanie v rodakh." In *Obezbolivanie v rodakh: Trudy konferentsii v g. Leningrade, 29–31 ianvaria 1951 g.*, edited by A. P. Nikolaev, 54–59. Moscow: Izdatel'stvo akademii meditsinskikh nauk, 1952.

Shub, R. L. *Primenenie vitamina V¹ v akusherstve i ginekologii: Sposob fiziologicheskogo obezbolivaniia i uskoreniia rodov.* Leningrad: Tsentral'nyi institut akusherstva i ginekologii ministerstva zdravookhraneniia SSSR, 1946.

Simchak, Margery. "Has Epidural Anesthesia Made Childbirth Education Obsolete?" *Childbirth Instructor*, Summer 1991: 15–18.

Skrobanskii, K. *Kratkoe rukovodstvo po obezbolivaniiu normal'nykh rodov.* Moscow-Leningrad: Gosudarstvennoe izdatel'stvo biologicheskoi i meditsinskoi literatury, 1936.

Sopko, Sandra and Nancy Ciocca. "New Childbirth Practices Urged by Return to Old." *Bridgeport Telegram*, June 4, 1973.

St[atius] Van Eps, L. W. "Psychoprophylaxis in Labour." *The Lancet* 266 (July 16, 1955): 112–15.

Strickland, Sandy. "Prepared Childbirth Expert: Pregnancy's Not a Disease." *Jacksonville Journal*, June 26, 1975.

Sukhanova, Natalia. *Zal ozhidaniia.* Moscow: Sovremennik, 1990.

Sylvan, Filip. *Natural Painless Childbirth and the Determination of Sex.* London: Kigan Paul, Trench, Trubner, 1916.

Tanzer, Deborah. "Natural Childbirth: Pain or Peak Experience." *Psychology Today*, Oct. 1968: 18–21, 69.

———. "The Psychology of Pregnancy and Childbirth: An Investigation of Natural Childbirth." Ph.D. diss., Brandeis University, 1967.

———. *Why Natural Childbirth? A Psychologist's Report on the Benefits to Mothers, Fathers, and Babies.* Garden City, NY: Doubleday, 1972.

Tennov, Dorothy and Lolly Hirsch, eds. *Proceedings of the First International Childbirth Conference.* Stamford, CT: New Moon Communication, 1973.

"Terapevtychnyi fakul'tet." In *Kharkivs'kyi instytut udoskonalennia likariv: Iuvileine vydannia, 1923–1998.* Kharkiv: Kharkivs'kyi instytut udoskonalennia likariv, 1998.

Thoms, Herbert. *Understanding Natural Childbirth: A Book for the Expectant Mother.* New York: McGraw Hill, 1950.

Tichané, Giséle. *Accouche et tais-toi: Des femmes parlent.* Paris: Le Centurion, 1980.

"Today's Lamaze! (Not Your Ma's Lamaze!!)." *Passion for Birth*, 2012. http://passionfor-birth.com/lamaze.html.

Towler, Jean and Joan Bramall. *Midwives in History and Society.* London: Croom Helm, 1986.

Tracy, Marguerite and Mary Boyd. *Painless Childbirth: A General Survey of All Painless Methods with Special Stress on "Twilight Sleep" and Its Extension to America.* New York: Frederick A. Stokes, 1915.

Travis, Eileen. "A Thousand Painless Births: British Nurses Learn about New Russian 'Relax' System," *Daily Mail*, June 3, 1954.

Varshavskaia, F. E. *Klinicheskie ispytaniia deistviia naibolee dostupnykh v shirokoi praktike metodov i sredstv obezbolivaniia rodov. Aftoreferat dissertatsii na soiskanie uchenoi stepeni kandidata meditsinskikh nauk.* Leningrad: 1-i Leningradskii meditsinskii institut im. akad. I. P. Pavlova, 1954.

Vellay, P. "Facteurs essentiels d'échecs en psychoprophylaxie." In *Medicina psychoso-matica in obstetritiis et gynaecologia. Berichte.* Second International Congress of

Psychosomatic Medicine in Obstetrics and Gynaecology, 163–67. Vienna: Verlag der Wiener Medizinischen Akademie, 1965.

Vellay, Pierre and Aline Vellay-Dalsace, *Témoignages sur l'accouchement sans douleur par la méthode psycho-prophylactique*. Paris: Éditions du Seuil, 1956.

Vel'vovskii, I. Z. *Sistema psikhoprofilakticheskogo obezbolivaniia rodov*. Moscow: Gosudarstvennoe izdatel'stvo meditsinskoi literatury, 1963.

———. *Sistema psikhoprophilaktiki bolei v rodakh. Aftoreferat dissertatsii na soiskanie uchenoi stepeni doktora meditsinskikh nauk*. Khar'kov: Khar'kovskii meditsinskii institut, 1957.

Vel'vovskii, I. Z., K. I. Platonov, V. A. Ploticher, and E. A. Shugom. *Psikhoprofilaktika bolei v rodakh: Lektsii dlia vrachei-akusherov*. Leningrad: Medgiz, 1954.

Velvovsky [Vel'vovskii], I., K. Platonov, V. Ploticher, and E. Shugom. *Painless Childbirth through Psychoprophylaxis*. 1960. Reprint. Honolulu: University Press of the Pacific, 2003.

Vermelin, [H.]. "L'accouchement sans douleur." *La Sage-Femme française*, Jan. 1955: 3, 5, 7, 9.

Vorontsova-Iurieva, Nataliia. "Rody v SSSR." *Predmety sovetskoi zhizni* (blog). June 19, 2007. http://community.livejournal.com/soviet_life/53730.html#cutid1.

Voznesenskaya, Julia. *The Women's Decameron*, translated by W. B. Linton. London: Quartet Books, 1986.

Vremenna instruktsiia za obezbolivane na razhdaneto po psikhoprofilaktichniia metod na Velvovski. Sofia: Nauka i izkustvo, 1952.

Walton, Vicki E. *Have It Your Way: An Overview of Pregnancy, Labor and Postpartum Including Alternatives Available in the Hospital Childbirth Experience*. Seattle: Henry Philips, 1976.

"WBAI Program Portfolio." *Pacifica Radio Archives*. Internet Archive. June 9, 1963. http://ia600308.us.archive.org/23/items/wbaifolio411wbairich/wbaifolio-411wbairich.pdf.

Wcislo, Martine and Béatrice Blondel. "La naissance en France en 1995: Enquête nationale périnatale." *SESI InfoRapides*. Oct. 1996, http://www.gyneweb.fr/sources/gdpublic/enquete.html.

Welbeck, Brian. "Russians Pirate Painless Birth." *Reynolds News*, Jan. 22, 1956.

WHO Chronicle. "Obstetrics and Gynecology in the USSR." February 1966: 56–60.

Williams, Gurney, III. "What Natural Childbirth Can Mean to You and Your Family." *Family Health*, Dec. 1973, 28, 38.

"Why Is the National US Cesarean Section Rate So High?" *Childbirth Connection*. Last modified June 24, 2013. http://www.childbirthconnection.org/article.asp?ck=10456.

Wideman, Margaret V. and Jerome E. Singer. "The Role of Psychological Mechanisms in Preparation for Childbirth." *American Psychologist* 39 (Dec. 1984): 1357–71.

Yahia, Clement and Priscilla R. Ulin. "Épreuve préliminaire d'un programme psychosomatique de préparation à l'accouchement." *Bulletin-Programme de la Société internationale de psychoprophylaxie obstétricale* 7 (1965): 113–26.

Zaidman, H. "L'analgésie obstétricale par la méthode psycho-prophylactique." *Santé publique*, Oct. 1, 1953: 1, 9.

Zmanovskii, Iu. F. *Dinamika izmenenii vysshei nervnoi deiatel'nosti beremennykh pod vliianiem psikhoprofilakticheskoi podgotovki k rodam. Aftoreferat dissertatsii na soiskanie uchenoi stepeni kandidata meditsinskikh nauk*. Moscow: 1-i Moskovskii Ordena Lenina Meditsinskii Institut im. I. M. Sechenova, 1962.

SECONDARY SOURCES

Allen, Valerie. *The Legacy of Grantly Dick-Read*. London: National Childbirth Trust, 1991.

Arney, William Ray. *Power and the Profession of Obstetrics*. Chicago: University of Chicago Press, 1982.

Beinart, Jennifer. "Obstetric Analgesia and the Control of Childbirth in Twentieth-Century Britain." In Garcia et al., eds. *The Politics of Maternity Care: Services for Childbearing Women in Twentieth-Century Britain*, 116–32.

Bell, Marie. "The Pioneers of Parents' Centre: Movers and Shakers for Change in the Philosophies and Practice of Childbirth and Parent Education in New Zealand." PhD diss., Victoria University of Wellington, 2004.

Belooussova, Ekaterina. "The 'Natural Childbirth' Movement in Russia: Self-Representation Strategies." *Anthropology of East Europe Review* 20 (2002): 11–18.

Bernstein, Francis L., Christopher Burton, and Dan Healey, eds. *Soviet Medicine: Culture, Practice, and Science*. DeKalb: Northern Illinois University Press, 2010.

Bieri, Alexander L. *Traditionally, Ahead of Its Time*. Basel: Roche Historical Archives, 2008.

Binkley, Sam. *Getting Loose: Lifestyle Consumption in the 1970s*. Durham, NC: Duke University Press, 2007.

"Biograficheskaia stat'ia: Vel'vovskii, Il'ia (Gilel') Zakharevich (Zel'manovich)." Typescript, courtesy of KhMAPO, 2006.

Block, Richard and Lauren Langman, "Youth and Work: The Diffusion of 'Countercultural' Values," *Youth & Society* 5 (June 1974): 411–32.

Blondel, B., G. Bréart, Ch. du Mazaubrun, G. Badeyan, M. Wcislo, A. Lordier, and N. Matet, "La situation périnatale en France: Évolution entre 1981 et 1995." *Journal de gynécologie, obstétrique et biologie de la reproduction* 26 (1997): 770–80.

Boschert, Sherry. "Nitrous Oxide Returns for Labor Pain Management." *Ob.Gyn. News*. June 18, 2013. http://www.obgynnews.com/specialty-focus/obstetrics/single-article-page/nitrous-oxide-returns-for-labor-pain-management.html.

Brune, Kay. "The Early History of Non Opioid Anesthetics." *Acute Pain* 1 (Dec. 1997): 33–40.

Burton, Chris. "Medical Welfare during Late Stalinism: A Study of Doctors and the Soviet Health System, 1945–53." PhD diss., University of Chicago, 2000.

Caron-Leulliez, Marianne. "L'accouchement sans douleur: Un enjeu politique en France pendant la guerre froide." *Canadian Bulletin of Medical History/Bulletin canadien d'histoire de la médecine* 23 (2006): 69–88.

Caron-Leulliez, Marianne, and Jocelyne George. *L'accouchement sans douleur: Histoire d'une révolution oubliée*. Paris: Les Éditions de l'Atelier, 2004.

Caton, Donald. *What a Blessing She Had Chloroform: The Medical and Social Response to the Pain of Childbirth from 1800 to the Present*. New Haven, CT: Yale University Press, 1999.

Chamberlain, G. "The History of Pain Relief in Labour." In *Pain and Its Relief in Childbirth: The Results of a National Survey Conducted by the National Birthday Trust*, edited by Geoffrey Chamberlain, Ann Wraight and Philip Steer, 1–9. London: Longman, 1993.

Chaperon, Sylvie. *Les années Beauvoir, 1945–1970*. Paris: Librairie Arthème Fayard, 2000.

Charlot, Jean. *De Gaulle et le Rassemblement du Peuple Français, 1947–1955*. Paris: Armand Colin, 1998.

Cohen, Lizabeth. *A Consumers' Republic: The Politics of Mass Consumption in Postwar America*. New York: Vintage, 2003.

Conroy, Mary Schaeffer. "The Soviet Pharmaceutical Industry and Dispensing, 1945–1953." *Europe-Asia Studies* 56 (Nov. 2004): 963–91.

Coontz, Stephanie. *A Strange Stirring: The Feminine Mystique and American Women at the Dawn of the 1960s*. New York: Basic Books, 2011.

———. *The Way We Never Were: American Families and the Nostalgia Trap*. New York: Basic Books, 1992.

Daly, Jeanne. *Evidence-Based Medicine and the Search for a Science of Clinical Care*. Berkeley: University of California Press, 2005.

Davis, Angela. *Modern Motherhood: Women and Family in England, c.1945–2000*. Manchester and New York: Manchester University Press, 2012.

Davis, Rebecca L. *More Perfect Unions: The American Search for Marital Bliss*. Cambridge, MA: Harvard University Press, 2010.

———. " 'Not Marriage At All, But Simple Harlotry': The Companionate Marriage Controversy." *Journal of American History* 94 (Mar. 2008): 1137–63.

Didi-Huberman, Georges. *Invention of Hysteria: Charcot and the Photographic Iconography of the Salpêtrière*. Translated by Alise Hartz. Cambridge, MA: MIT Press, 2003.

Donnison, Jean. *Midwives and Medical Men: A History of the Struggle for the Control of Childbirth*. 2nd ed. New Barnet, Herts, UK: Historical Publications, 1988.

Dosse, François. *New History in France: The Triumph of the Annales*. Translated by Peter V. Conroy, Jr. Urbana and Chicago: University of Illinois Press, 1994.

Dreyfus, Michel. *Une belle santé: Hôpital des Métallurgistes Pierre Rouquès, 50ème anniversaire de la maternité*. Paris: Hôpital des Métallurgistes Pierre Rouquès, 1997.

Duchen, Claire. *Feminism in France: From May '68 to Mitterrand*. London: Routledge & Kegan Paul, 1986.

———. *Women's Rights and Women's Lives in France, 1944–1968*. London: Routledge, 1994.

Eisenberg, Ziv. "Clear and Pregnant Danger: The Making of Prenatal Psychology in Mid-Twentieth-Century America." *Journal of Women's History* 22 (Fall 2010): 112–35.

Etkind, Alexander. *Eros of the Impossible: History of Psychoanalysis in Russia*. Boulder, CO: Westview Press, 1997.

Evans, Janet. "The Communist Party of the Soviet Union and the Women's Question: The Case of the 1936 Decree 'In Defense of Mother and Child.' " *Journal of Contemporary History* 16 (Oct. 1981): 757–75.

Farr, A. D. "Religious Opposition to Obstetric Analgesia: A Myth?" *Annals of Science* 20 (1983): 159–77.

Fayolle, Sandra. "L'Union des Femmes Françaises: Une organisation féminine de masse du Parti communiste français (1945–1965)." PhD diss., Université Paris-I-Panthéon-Sorbonne, 2005.

Fee, Elizabeth and Edward T. Morman. "Doing History, Making Revolution: The Aspirations of Henry E. Sigerist and George Rosen." In *Doctors, Politics and Society: Historical Essays*, edited by Dorothy Porter and Roy Porter, 275–311. Amsterdam: Editions Rodolpi B.V., 1993.

Fee, Elizabeth and Theodore M. Brown, eds. *Making Medical History: The Life and Times of Henry E. Sigerist*. Baltimore: The Johns Hopkins University Press, 1997.

Feldhusen, Adrian E. "The History of Midwifery and Childbirth in America: A Timeline." *Midwifery Today*. 2000. http://www.midwiferytoday.com/articles/timeline.asp.

Filene, Peter G. *Him/Her/Self: Sex Roles in Modern America.* 2nd ed. Baltimore: Johns Hopkins University Press, 1986.

"Frequently Asked Questions about Midwives and Midwifery." *Citizens for Midwifery.* n.d., accessed Jan. 5, 2010. http://cfmidwifery.org/midwifery/faq.aspx#8.

Garcia, Jo, Robert Kilpatrick, and Martin Richards, eds. *The Politics of Maternity Care: Services for Childbearing Women in Twentieth-Century Britain.* Oxford: Clarendon, 1990.

Gibbons, Luz, José M. Belizán, Jeremy A. Lauer, Ana P. Betrán, Mario Merialdi, and Fernando Althabe. "The Global Numbers and Costs of Additionally Needed and Unnecessary Cesarean Sections Performed per Year: Overuse as a Barrier to Universal Coverage." *World Health Report Background Paper* 30 (2010): 1–32.

Gijswijt-Hofstra, Marijke and Roy Porter, eds. *Cultures of Neurasthenia: From Beard to the First World War.* Amsterdam: Rodopi, 2001.

Gilcher-Holtey, Ingrid. "France." In *1968 in Europe: A History of Protest and Activism, 1956-1977,* edited by Martin Klimke and Joachim Scharloth, 111–24. New York: Palgrave MacMillan, 2008.

Goldman, Wendy Z. *Women, the State and Revolution.* New York: Cambridge University Press, 1993.

Gordon, Colin. *Dead on Arrival: The Politics of Health Care in Twentieth-Century America.* Princeton, NJ: Princeton University Press, 2003.

Greenwald, Lisa. "The Women's Liberation Movement in France and the Origins of Contemporary French Feminism, 1944-1981." PhD diss., Emory University, 1996.

Grinval'd, S. G. "Khar'kovskaia shkola psikhoterapii." *Sergei Gennadievich Grinval'd.* 2010. http://grinvald.com/stati/harkovskaya-shkola-psihoterapii.html.

Gutmann, Caroline. *The Legacy of Doctor Lamaze: The Story of the Man Who Changed Childbirth.* Translated by Bruce Benderson. New York: St. Martin's, 2001.

Harkins, Jennifer, Brendan Carvalho, Amy Evers, Sachin Mehta, and Edward T. Riley. "Survey of the Factors Associated with a Woman's Choice to Have Epidural Anesthesia." *Anesthesiology Research and Practice* (2010): 1–8.

Harrington, Anne. *The Cure Within: A History of Mind-Body Medicine.* New York: Norton, 2008.

Heagerty, Brooke Victoria. "Class, Gender and Professionalization: The Struggle for British Midwifery, 1900-1936." PhD diss., Michigan State University, 1990.

———. "Reassessing the Guilty: The Midwives Act and the Control of English Midwives in the Early 20th Century." In *Supervision of Midwives,* edited by Mavis Kirkham, 13-27. Hale, Cheshire, England: Books for Midwives.

"Histoire." *Maternité des Lilas.* Dec. 10, 2010. http://www.maternite-des-lilas.com/content/histoire.

Hoffman, Diane E. and Anita J. Tarzian. "The Girl Who Cried Pain: A Bias against Women in the Treatment of Pain." *Journal of Law, Medicine, and Ethics* 29 (Mar. 2001): 13–27.

Hrešanová, Ema. *Kultury dvou porodnic: Etnografická studie.* Plzeň: Vydavatelství ZČU v Plzni, 2008.

Infoplease. "Live Births and Birth Rates by Year," n.d., accessed May 15, 2012. http://www.infoplease.com/ipa/A0005067.html.

Jameson, Fredric. *Postmodernism, or the Cultural Logic of Late Capitalism.* Durham, NC: Duke University Press, 1991.

Joravsky, David. *Russian Psychology: A Critical History.* Cambridge, MA: Basil Blackwell, 1989.

Jordan, Brigitte. *Birth in Four Cultures: A Crosscultural Investigation of Childbirth in Yucatan, Holland, Sweden, and the United States.* 4th rev. ed. Long Grove, IL: Waveland, 1992.

————. "Childbirth and Authoritative Knowledge." In *Childbirth and Authoritative Knowledge: Cross-Cultural Perspectives,* edited by Robbie E. Davis-Floyd and Carolyn F. Sargent, 55–79. Berkeley: University of California Press, 1997.

Keck, Thierry. *Jeunesse de l'église, 1936–1955: Aux sources de la crise progressiste en France.* Paris: Karthala, 2004.

Kimmel, Michael. *Manhood in America: A Cultural History.* 3rd ed. New York: Oxford University Press, 2012.

King, Leslie. "'France Needs Children': Pronatalism, Nationalism and Women's Equality." *The Sociological Quarterly* 39 (Jan. 1998): 33–52.

Kirkham, Mavis, ed. *Supervision of Midwives.* Hale, Cheshire, England: Books for Midwives, 1996.

Kitzinger, Jenny. "Strategies of the Early Childbirth Movement: A Case-Study of the National Childbirth Trust." In Garcia et al., eds. *The Politics of Maternity Care: Services for Childbearing Women in Twentieth-Century Britain,* 92–115.

Kline, Wendy. *Bodies of Knowledge: Sexuality, Reproduction, and Women's Health in the Second Wave.* Chicago: University of Chicago Press, 2010.

Knaus, William A. *Inside Russian Medicine: An American Doctor's First-Hand Report.* New York: Everest House, 1981.

Knibiehler, Yvonne. *Accoucher: Femmes, sage-femmes et médecins depuis le milieu du XXᵉ siècle.* Rennes: Éditions de l'École Nationale de la Santé Publique, 2007.

————. *La révolution maternelle depuis 1945: Femmes, maternité, citoyenneté.* Paris: Perrin, 1997.

Koontz, Stephanie. *The Way We Never Were: American Families and the Nostalgia Trap.* New York: Basic Books, 1992.

Koos, Cheryl A. "Gender, Anti-Individualism, and Nationalism: The Alliance Nationale and the Pronatalist Backlash against the Femme Moderne, 1933–1940." *French Historical Studies* 19 (Spring 1996): 699–723.

Kuisel, Richard F. *Seducing the French: The Dilemma of Americanization.* Berkeley: University of California Press, 1993.

Lasch, Christopher. *Haven in a Heartless World: The Family Besieged.* New York: Basic Books, 1977.

Lauer, Jeremy A., Ana P. Betrán, Mario Merialdi, and Daniel Wojdyla. "Determinants of Cesarean Section Rates in Developed Countries: Supply, Demand, and Opportunities for Control." *World Health Report Background Paper* 29 (2010): 1–22.

Leap, Nicky and Billie Hunter. *The Midwife's Tale: An Oral History from Handywoman to Professional Midwife.* London: Scarlet Press, 1993.

Leavitt, Judith Walzer. "Birthing and Anesthesia: The Debate over Twilight Sleep." *Signs* 6 (Autumn 1980): 147–64.

————. *Brought to Bed: Childbearing in America, 1750–1950.* New York: Oxford University Press, 1986.

————. "Joseph B. De Lee and the Practice of Preventative Obstetrics." *American Journal of Public Health* 78 (Oct. 1988): 1353–59.

————. *Make Room for Daddy: The Journey from the Waiting Room to the Birthing Room.* Chapel Hill: University of North Carolina Press, 2009.

Lerner, Vladimir, Jacob Margolin, and Eliezer Witztum. "Vladimir Bekhterev: His Life, His Work, and the Mystery of His Death." *History of Psychiatry* 11 (June 2005): 217–27.

Lévy, Marie-Françoise. "Le mouvement français pour le planning familial et les jeunes." *Vingtième Siècle. Revue d'histoire* 75, no. spécial: Histoire des femmes, histoire des genres (July–Sept. 2002): 75–84.

Lewis, Jane. "Mothers and Maternity Politics in the Twentieth Century." In Garcia et al., eds. *The Politics of Maternity Care: Services for Childbearing Women in Twentieth-Century Britain*, 15–29.

Loudin, Irvine. *Death in Childbirth: An International Study of Maternal Care and Maternal Mortality, 1800–1950*. London: Clarendon Press, 1992.

———. *The Tragedy of Childbed Fever*. New York: Oxford University Press, 2000.

MacDorman, Marian, T. J. Matthews, and Eugene Declerq, "Home Births in the United States, 1990–2009." *NCHS Data Brief*. Jan. 26, 2012. http://www.cdc.gov/nchs/data/databriefs/db84.htm.

Marland, Hilary. "'Uterine Mischief': W. S. Playfair and His Neurasthenic Patients." In Gijswijt-Hofstra and Porter, eds. *Cultures of Neurasthenia: From Beard to the First World War*, 117–40.

May, Elaine Tyler. *Homeward Bound: American Families in the Cold War Era*. Rev. ed. New York: Basic Books, 2008.

McIntosh, Tania. "Profession, Skill, or Domestic Duty? Midwifery in Sheffield, 1881–1936." *Social History of Medicine* 11 (Jan. 1998): 403–20.

McLaren, Angus. *Twentieth-Century Sexuality: A History*. Malden, MA: Blackwell Publishing, 1999.

Meckel, Richard A. *Save the Babies: American Public Health Reform and the Prevention of Infant Mortality, 1850–1929*. Baltimore: Johns Hopkins University Press, 1990.

Micale, Mark S. "On the 'Disappearance' of Hysteria: A Study in the Clinical Deconstruction of a Diagnosis." *Isis* 84 (Sept. 1993): 496–526.

Michaels, Paula A. "Comrades in the Labor Room: The Lamaze Method of Childbirth Preparation and France's Cold War Home Front, 1951–1957." *The American Historical Review* 115 (Oct. 2010): 1031–60.

———. *Curative Powers: Medicine and Empire in Stalin's Central Asia*. Pittsburgh: University of Pittsburgh Press, 2003.

———. "Ethnicity, Patriotism, and Womanhood: Kazakhstan and the 1936 Ban on Abortion." *Feminist Studies* 27 (Feb. 2001): 307–33.

Mijolla, Alain de. *France (1893–1965)*. In *Psychoanalysis International*, edited by Peter Kutter, translated by Ruth Hoffman, 1: 66–113. Stuttgart: Friedrich Frommann Verlag, 1992.

———. *La psychoanalyse en France (1893–1965)*. In *Histoire de la psychoanalyse*, edited by R. Jaccard, 2: 9–105. Paris: Hachette, 1982.

Mikhailov, B. V. "Khar'kovskaia psikhoterapevticheskaia shkola." *Mezhdunarodnyi meditsinskii zhurnal* 10 (2004): 43–46.

Miller, Martin A. *Freud and the Bolsheviks: Psychoanalysis in Imperial Russia and the Soviet Union*. New Haven, CT: Yale University Press, 1998.

Moeller, Robert. *Protecting Motherhood: Women and the Family in the Politics of Postwar West Germany*. Berkeley: University of California Press, 1993.

Mol, Annemarie. *The Logic of Care: Health and the Problem of Patient Choice*. London: Routledge, 2008.

Monroe, John Warne. *Laboratories of Faith: Mesmerism, Spiritualism, and Occultism in Modern France*. Ithaca, NY: Cornell University Press, 2008.

Morgen, Sandra. *Into Our Own Hands: The Women's Health Movement in the United States, 1969–1990*. New Brunswick, NJ: Rutgers University Press, 2002.

Moscucci, O. "Holistic Obstetrics: The Origins of 'Natural Childbirth' in Britain." *Postgraduate Medical Journal* 79 (2003): 168–73.

Muel-Dreyfus, Francine. *Vichy and the Eternal Feminine: A Contribution to a Political Sociology of Gender.* Translated by Kathleen A. Johnson. Durham, NC: Duke University Press, 2001.

Nakachi, Mie. "Replacing the Dead: The Politics of Reproduction in the Postwar Soviet Union, 1945–1955." PhD diss., University of Chicago, 2008.

Nestel, Sheryl. "'Other' Mothers: Race and Representation in Natural Childbirth Discourse." *Resources for Feminist Research* 23 (Winter 1994/1995): 5–19.

Noirez, Alain. "L'accouchement sans douleur: De la présence du conjoint à l'accouchement de son épouse. Le vécu de la paternité, le rôle du mari au cours de la gestation. La crise moderne de la paternité." PhD diss., Université Pierre et Marie Curie, Paris-VI, 1976.

Nuland, Sherwin B. *The Doctor's Plague: Germs, Childbed Fever, and the Strange Story of Ignác Semmelweis.* New York: Norton, 2003.

O'Connor, David Edward. *The Basics of Economics.* Westport, CT: Greenwood Press, 2004.

O'Hara, Glen. "The Complexities of 'Consumerism': Choice, Collectivism and Participation with Britain's National Health Service, c. 1961–c. 1979." *Social History of Medicine* 26 (May 2013): 288–304.

Oakley, Ann. *The Captured Womb: A History of the Medical Care of Pregnant Women.* New York: Basil Blackwell, 1984.

Offen, Karen. "Body Politics: Women, Work and the Politics of Motherhood in France, 1920–1950." In *Maternity and Gender Policies: Women and the Rise of the European Welfare States, 1880s–1950s,* edited by Gisela Bock and Pat Thane, 138–59. London: Routledge, 1991.

———. "Depopulation, Nationalism, and Feminism in Fin-de-Siècle France." *The American Historical Review* 89 (June 1984): 648–76.

Oliner, Marion Michel. *Cultivating Freud's Garden in France.* Northvale, NJ: Jason Aronson, 1988.

Oppenheim, Janet. *"Shattered Nerves": Doctors, Patients, and Depression in Victorian England.* New York: Oxford University Press, 1991.

Pickett, Janet A. "History of Obstetric Analgesia and Anaesthesia." In *Textbook of Obstetric Anaesthesia,* edited by Rachel E. Collis, Felicity Platt and John Urquhart, 1–20. London: Greenwich Medical Media, 2002.

Plant, Rebecca Jo. *Mom: The Transformation of Motherhood in Modern America.* Chicago: University of Chicago Press, 2010.

Pollard, Miranda. *Reign of Virtue: Mobilizing Gender in Vichy France.* Chicago: University of Chicago Press, 1998.

Pollock, Ethan. *Stalin and the Soviet Science Wars.* Princeton, NJ: Princeton University Press, 2006.

Prost, Antoine. "Catholic Conservatives, Population, and the Family in Twentieth Century France." *Population and Development Review* 14 (Mar. 1988): 147–64.

———. "L'évolution de la politique familiale en France de 1938 à 1981." *Le mouvement sociale* 129 (Oct.–Dec. 1984): 7–28.

Reineke, Sandra. *Beauvoir and Her Sisters: The Politics of Women's Bodies in France.* Urbana: University of Illinois Press, 2011.

Richards, W., G. D. Parbrook, and J. Wilson. "Stanislav Klikovich, 1853–1910: Pioneer of Nitrous Oxide and Oxygen Analgesia." *Anesthesia* 31 (Sept. 1976): 933–40.

Richmond, Yale. *Cultural Exchange and the Cold War: Raising the Iron Curtain.* University Park: Pennsylvania State University, 2003.

Roberts, Mary Louise. *Civilization without Sexes: Reconstructing Gender in Postwar France, 1917–1927.* Chicago: University of Chicago Press, 1994.

Robinson, Sarah. "Maintaining the Independence of the Midwifery Profession: A Continuing Struggle." In Garcia et al., eds. *The Politics of Maternity Care: Services for Childbearing Women in Twentieth-Century Britain*, 61–91.

Rooks, Judith. "Epidural Analgesia as Used during Childbirth in the United States." *Japanese Journal for Midwives* 54 (2000): 9–14.

———. *Midwifery and Childbirth in America*. Philadelphia: Temple University Press, 1997.

———. "Nitrous Oxide for Pain in Labor—Why Not in the United States?" *Birth* 34 (Mar. 2007): 3–5.

Rosen, Ruth. *The World Split Open: How the Modern Women's Movement Changed America*. New York: Viking, 2000.

Ross, Ellen. *Love and Toil: Motherhood in Outcast London, 1870–1918*. New York: Oxford University Press, 1993.

Rothman, Barbara Katz. *In Labor: Women and Power in the Birthplace*. New York: Norton, 1982.

Roudinesco, Elisabeth. *Jacques Lacan & Co.: A History of Psychoanalysis in France, 1925–1985*. Translated by Jeffrey Mehlman. Chicago: University of Chicago Press, 1990.

———. "Psychoanalysis." In *The Columbia History of Twentieth-Century French Thought*, edited by Lawrence D. Kritzman, Brian J. Reilly and M. B. DeBevoise, translated by M. B. DeBevoise, 100–01. New York: Columbia University Press, 2006.

Sandelowski, Margarete. *Pain, Pleasure, and American Childbirth: From the Twilight Sleep to the Read Method, 1914–1960*. Westport, CT: Greenwood Press, 1984.

Schneider, William. *Quality and Quantity: The Quest for Biological Regeneration in Twentieth-Century France*. Cambridge: Cambridge University Press, 2002.

Shorter, Edward. *From Paralysis to Fatigue: A History of Psychosomatic Illness in the Modern Era*. New York: Free Press, 1993.

Smith, Timothy B. "The Social Transformation of Hospitals and the Rise of Medical Insurance in France, 1914-1943." *The Historical Journal* 41 (Dec. 1998): 1055–87.

Solomon, Susan Gross, ed. *Doing Medicine Together: Germany and Russia between the Wars*. Toronto: University of Toronto Press, 2006.

Soloway, Richard. *Demography and Degeneration: Eugenics and the Declining Birthrate in Britain*. Chapel Hill: University of North Carolina Press, 1990.

Stern, Ludmila. *Western Intellectuals and the Soviet Union, 1920–1940: From Red Square to the Left Bank*. New York: Routledge, 2007.

Stewart, Mary Lynn. *For Health and Beauty: Physical Culture for Frenchwomen, 1880s–1930s*. Baltimore: Johns Hopkins University Press, 2001.

Thebaud, Françoise. *Quand nos grand-mères donnaient la vie: La maternité en France dans l'entre-deux-guerres*. Lyon: Presses Universitaires de Lyon, 1986.

Thomas, A. Noyes. *Doctor Courageous: The Story of Dr. Grantly Dick-Read*. New York: Harper, 1957.

Thomas, Mary. *Post-War Mothers: Childbirth Letters to Grantly Dick-Read, 1946–1956*. Rochester, NY: University of Rochester Press, 1997.

Thomson, Mathew. "Neurasthenia in Britain: An Overview." In Gijswijt-Hofstra and Porter, eds. *Cultures of Neurasthenia: From Beard to the First World War*, 77–96.

Tranvouez, Yvon. *Catholiques et communistes: La crise de progressisme chrétien, 1950–55*. Paris: Cerf, 2000.

Vinen, Richard. *Bourgeois Politics in France*. New York: Cambridge University Press, 1995.

Vuille, Marilène. *Accouchement et douleur: Une étude sociologique.* Lausanne, Switzerland: Antipodes, 1998.

———. "La naissance de l'"accouchement sans douleur.'" *Revue médicale de la Suisse romande* 120 (2000): 991–98.

———. "Le militantisme en faveur de l'accouchement sans douleur." *Nouvelles questions féministes* 24 (2005): 50–67.

Weiss, Jessica. *To Have and To Hold: Marriage, the Baby Boom, and Social Change.* Chicago: The University of Chicago Press, 2000.

Wertz, Richard W. and Dorothy C. Wertz. *Lying-In: A History of Childbirth in America.* Rev. ed. New Haven, CT: Yale University Press, 1989.

Williams, A. Susan. *Women and Childbirth in the Twentieth Century: A History of the National Birthday Trust Fund, 1928–1993.* Phoenix Mill, Gloucestershire: Sutton Publishing, 1997.

Wolf, Jacqueline H. *Deliver Me from Pain: Anesthesia and Birth in America.* Baltimore: Johns Hopkins University Press, 2009.

Yasnitsky, Anton and Michel Ferrari. "From Vygotsky to Vygotskian Psychology: Introduction to the History of the Kharkov School." *Journal of the History of Behavioral Sciences* 44 (Spring 2008): 119–45.

———. "Rethinking the Early History of Post-Vygotskian Psychology: The Case of the Kharkov School." *History of Psychology* 11 (May 2008): 101–21.

Zajicek, Benjamin. "Scientific Psychiatry in Stalin's Soviet Union: The Politics of Modern Medicine and the Struggle to Define 'Pavlovian' Psychiatry, 1939–1953." PhD diss., University of Chicago, 2009.

Zancarini-Fournel, Michelle. *Histoire des femmes en France, XIXe–XXe siècle.* Rennes: Presses universitaires de Rennes, 2005.

———. "Histoire(s) du MLAC (1973-1975)." *CLIO. Histoire, femmes et société* 18 (2003): 241–52.

———. "'Notre corps, nous-mêmes.'" In *Le siècle des féminismes*, edited by Élaine Gubin, Catherine Jacques, Florence Rochefort, Brigitte Studer, Françoise Thébaud, and Michelle Zancarini-Fournel, 209–20. Paris: Les Éditions de l'Atelier, 2004.

INDEX

Page numbers followed by *n* indicate footnotes.